Modern French visual theory

MANCHESTER
1824

Manchester University Press

Modern French visual theory

A critical reader

Edited by Nigel Saint and Andy Stafford

Manchester University Press
Manchester and New York

distributed in the United States exclusively
by Palgrave Macmillan

Published by Manchester University Press
Oxford Road, Manchester M13 9NR, UK
and Room 400, 175 Fifth Avenue, New York, NY 10010, USA
www.manchesteruniversitypress.co.uk

Distributed in the United States exclusively by
Palgrave Macmillan, 175 Fifth Avenue, New York,
NY 10010, USA

Distributed in Canada exclusively by
UBC Press, University of British Columbia, 2029 West Mall,
Vancouver, BC, Canada V6T 1Z2

British Library Cataloguing-in-Publication Data
A catalogue record for this book is available from the British Library

Library of Congress Cataloging-in-Publication Data applied for

ISBN 978 07190 8129 3 hardback
ISBN 978 07190 8130 9 paperback

First published 2013

Typeset
by Action Publishing Technology Ltd, Gloucester
Printed in Great Britain
by Bell & Bain Ltd, Glasgow

Contents

List of plates and figures

Plates

Figures

Notes on contributors

Nathalie Aubert is Professor of French literature at Oxford Brookes University. She has written a range of chapters and articles on European modernism and avant-garde movements, with a special emphasis on the 'visual'. She has published two monographs on Proust (2001 and 2003) and is currently editing a volume on Proust and the visual. Her latest monograph is dedicated to Belgian poet and painter Christian Dotremont: *Christian Dotremont: La conquête du monde par l'image* (2012).

Arthur Bradley is Senior Lecturer in the Department of English & Creative Writing at Lancaster University. He is the author of: *Negative Theology and Modern French Philosophy* (2004); *Derrida's Of Grammatology: A Philosophical Guide* (2008); *The New Atheist Novel: Fiction, Philosophy and Polemic after 9/11* (2010); *Originary Technicity: The Theory of Technology from Marx to Derrida* (2011). He has also co-edited four collections of essays including most recently *The Politics to Come: Power, Modernity and the Messianic* (2010). He is currently writing a new monograph on political theory, biopolitics and religion which is provisionally entitled *Unbearable Life.*

Ralph Dekoninck is Professor of Early Modern Art History at the Université catholique de Louvain (Belgium). He has written on the Jesuit theology and rhetoric of the image, on Renaissance art theory and historiography, on the early modern confrontation between spirituality and aesthetics. He is the author of *Ad Imaginem: Statuts, fonctions et usages de l'image dans la littérature spirituelle jésuite du XVIIe siècle* (2005). He has co-edited *L'idole dans l'imaginaire occidental* (2005); *Emblemata Sacra: The Rhetoric and Hermeneutics of Illustrated Sacred*

Discourse (2007); *Aux limites de l'imitation: L'ut pictura poesis à l'épreuve de la matière* (2009); *L'art en valeurs* (2011).

Patrick ffrench is Professor of French at King's College London. Patrick has written widely on twentieth-century French literature and thought and in particular on the literary review *Tel Quel* and on Georges Bataille. He is the author of: *The Time of Theory: A History of* Tel Quel *(1960–1982)* (1996); *The Cut: Reading Bataille's* Histoire de l'œil (2000); *After Bataille: Sacrifice, Exposure, Community* (2007). He is currently working on the moving body in French literature and culture from Baudelaire to Beckett.

François-Xavier Gleyzon is Assistant Professor of English at the University of Central Florida. In spring 2009 he was visiting professor at UCLA's Center for Medieval and Renaissance Studies. He is the author of: *Shakespeare's Spiral* (2010) and *David Lynch in Theory* (2011), along with a number of articles on English Renaissance literature and visual arts. His forthcoming publications include an edited book on Shakespeare's imagined Orient and two edited volumes on Shakespeare and theory.

Agnès Guiderdoni is Professor of French literature at the Université catholique de Louvain and a research associate at the FNRS (Belgium). She is the co-director of the Centre for Early Modern Cultural Analysis. After a Ph.D. on emblematics, she has developed her research on the concept of figura and figurative languages in the early modern period. Her book *Emblématique et spiritualité* is forthcoming from Éditions Garnier. Among other publications, she has co-edited *Emblemata Sacra: The Rhetoric and Hermeneutics of Illustrated Sacred Discourse* (2007); *Aux limites de l'imitation: L'ut pictura poesis à l'épreuve de la matière (XVIe–XVIIIe siècles)* (2009); *Ut pictura meditatio: The Meditative Image in Northern Art, 1500–1700* (2012).

Paul Hegarty teaches visual culture and philosophy in the Department of French, University College Cork. He is the author of books on Georges Bataille (2000), Jean Baudrillard (2004), and currently focuses on audio culture/sound studies, with his last book being *Beyond and Before: Progressive Rock since the 1960s* (2011), written with Martin Halliwell. A collection edited with Michael Goddard and Benjamin Halligan, entitled *Reverberations*, is soon to be published. He co-runs the record label dotdotdotmusic and performs and releases in numerous guises, primarily in the noise band Safe.

Ian James completed his doctoral research on the fictional and theoretical writings of Pierre Klossowski at the University of Warwick in 1996. Since then he has been a fellow and lecturer in French at Downing College, University of Cambridge. He is the author of *Pierre Klossowski: The Persistence of a Name* (2000); *The Fragmentary Demand: An Introduction to the Philosophy of Jean-Luc Nancy* (2006); *Paul Virilio* (2007); *The New French Philosophy* (2012).

Martine Joly is Honorary Professor *emerita* at the University of Michel de Montaigne (Bordeaux-3), where, having worked on the semiology of the image and of film (1985–2003), she founded the research institute IMAGINES: Image/Histoire/Sociétés. She has been a visiting professor in many countries in Europe and outside of Europe. Her books have been translated into ten languages, among which: *Introduction à l'analyse de l'image* (1994 and 2009); *L'image et les signes: Approche sémiologique de l'image fixe* (1994 and 2011); *L'image et son interprétation* (2002). She has also contributed to the *Dictionnaire de l'image*, with Anne Goliot-Lete *et al.* (2006 and 2008).

Shirley Jordan is Professor of French Literature and Visual Culture at Queen Mary University of London. She has published on twentieth- and twenty-first century art and art criticism, on new women's writing in French and on experimental self-narrative across media. Publications include: *The Art Criticism of Francis Ponge* (1994); *Contemporary French Women's Writing* (2004); *Private Lives, Public Display: Intimacy and Excess in French Women's Self-Narrative Experiment* (2012). Current projects include: a monograph on inhospitality in Marie NDiaye; and a co-edited volume on city photography.

David Packwood teaches at Warwick University and received his Ph.D. on Poussin from the University of Birmingham in 2005. He has published various reviews and articles on art history for English, American and Canadian journals. Recent publications include: 'Socrates Becomes Narcissus: Moral Mediation and Artistic Representation in Achille Bocchi's *Symbolicarum quaestionum*' (*Kuntstexte*, spring 2011); 'From *Pictor Philosophus* to *Homo Economicus*: Renegotiating Social Space in Poussin's *Self-Portrait* of 1649–50' (in D. Warren Sabean and M.

Stefanovska (eds), *Space and Self in Early Modern European Cultures*, 2012). He has participated in a symposium on Hubert Damisch (University of Amsterdam, in 2009); and in colloquia on the early-modern body (College Art Association, Los Angeles, 2009, and Universities of York and Durham, 2010).

Nigel Saint is Lecturer in French in the School of Modern Languages and Cultures at the University of Leeds. He is the author of: *Marguerite Yourcenar: Reading the Visual* (2000); articles on Georges Perec, Pierre Lecuire, Louis Marin and Pascal Convert and is co-editor of *Robert Desnos: Surrealism in the Twenty-First Century* (2006). He is currently working on Convert and Didi-Huberman.

Andy Stafford is Senior Lecturer in French in the School of Modern Languages and Cultures at the University of Leeds. He is the author of: *Photo-texts. Contemporary French Writing of the Photographic Image* (2010); co-editor, with Claude Coste, of Roland Barthes's seminar notes (1968–69) on Balzac's 'Sarrasine' (2011); and co-editor, with Charles Forsdick, of a forthcoming volume on the twentieth-century French periodical. He is a member of the editorial board of *Francophone Postcolonial Studies.*

Bernard Vouilloux is Professor of Twentieth-Century French Literature at the Université de Paris IV-Sorbonne, specialising in literature and the visual arts. His research is on the links between the verbal and the visual, literature and painting, poetics and aesthetics. As well as numerous articles, he has published seventeen books, including: *La Peinture dans le texte: XVIIIe–XXe siècles* (1994); *Langages de l'art et relations transesthétiques* (1997); *Le Tableau vivant: Phryné, l'orateur et le peintre* (2002); *L'Œuvre en souffrance: Entre poétique et esthétique* (2004); *Le Tournant « artiste » de la littérature française: Écrire avec la peinture au XIXe siècle* (2011).

Acknowledgements

We would like to thank Matthew Frost at Manchester University Press for his patient and enthusiastic support for this project. The same goes for our contributors, who will be as pleased as we are to see this volume assembled at last; we owe a special debt to David Packwood for his advice throughout its planning and execution. Our warmest thanks go to Bernard Vouilloux for agreeing to do the long and rewarding interview with which we close. We would also like to thank the anonymous readers of our original submission made to Manchester University Press, Nigel Armstrong, Marie-Claire Barnet, Ridha Boulaâbi, Alain Cantillon, Pierre-Philippe Fraiture and Sue Lowell Books. Finally, Pascal Convert has very generously provided the reproductions of his work used on our cover and in Chapter 10.

Introduction

Nigel Saint and Andy Stafford

> La plus belle image n'a pas de forme 大象無形
> (Chinese proverb, cited by A. Meddeb, *Phantasia*, 29–30)

> Celui qui peint et dessine serait-il définitivement l'ennemi rancunier ou l'otage consentant de celui qui écrit?
> (G. Titus-Carmel, *Épars*, 223)

Origins of the project

Some of the stories about art and culture in twentieth- and twenty-first century France have become legends: Apollinaire was arrested (wrongly) for stealing the *Mona Lisa*; Malraux looted art treasures in Cambodia and later saved the buildings of Paris; and Lacan once owned Courbet's scandalous *L'Origine du monde* but kept it hidden from view. More recently, the Centre Pompidou transformed modern debates about the architecture of museums; and the Louvre, with a vast display of architecture, art, gardens and commerce that dominates central Paris and is integral to Jean Nouvel's vision for 'le Grand Paris', is extending its reach to the unexpected locations of Lens and Abu Dhabi. This diverse array of individual motivations, cultural policy and historical developments is underpinned by many different theoretical frameworks and histories of art and culture. This volume addresses these theories and histories by considering interactions between French thought and the visual arts primarily from 1945 onwards.

While all modern French writing on the visual arts needs to be situated in a national tradition reaching back to the *Discourses of the French Royal Academy of Painting and Sculpture* (Jouin 2010), which began in the middle of the seventeenth century, and Diderot's *Salons* from the period 1759–81 (Diderot 1975–83), recent theoretical writing about the visual arts can be particularly situated in the context of the French structuralist and poststructuralist intellectual revolutions, with reference as well to transformations in German historiography and art history since Burckhardt's *Civilization of the Renaissance in Italy* ([1860]

1990). This wide-ranging context is one of the topics discussed in Chapter 14 of this volume in the interview with Bernard Vouilloux, the author of some seventeen books mainly on French literature and visual culture in the modern period (e.g. Vouilloux 1998, 2004a, 2004b, 2005, 2010, 2011), who responds to our project and helps us to reach some conclusions about the trajectories of modern French art theory. We think that readers of our selected theorists will be very conscious too of the contexts of phenomenology, psychoanalysis, semiology and deconstruction which this volume acknowledges and discusses in detail. In so doing, it also seeks to focus the debate on questions of spectatorship and subjectivity, writing, the specific power of the visual, hybridity in thought and in commentary on the visual, and the non-fusional interweaving of media.

After setting out the reasons for our selection of theorists, the present introduction then seeks to map some of the background contexts to our contributors' chapters, proposing a working definition of the visual, discussing the context of a changing art history, the role of psychoanalysis and links between philosophy and the visual arts. We then look in more detail at the question of representation and language through brief discussions of three seminal thinkers – Michel Foucault, Roland Barthes and Jacques Derrida – not included in the volume because they are well represented in other critical readers and anthologies, but who form a crucial intellectual context for the work of most of our selected theorists. This contextual survey is followed by an outline of post-colonial visual theory and an overview of studies of visual theory and culture. Lastly we explain the structure of the volume in more detail and provide summaries of each chapter.

This critical reader has emerged from a sense we both have of a wide interest across the disciplines in French theoretical writing on the visual. Much of this interest has involved a focus on the crucial role played by the ideas of the best-known group of philosophers and theorists from this period: Sartre, Lévi-Strauss, Foucault, Derrida, Lacan, Levinas, Serres, Lyotard, Kristeva, Deleuze, Irigaray and Barthes. In our view there is already, to varying degrees, a significant body of critical work devoted to the work of these thinkers relating to aesthetics, visual theory, the visual arts and the visual image. One place to look for such discussion, following on from Norman Bryson's path-breaking anthology *Calligram: Essays in New Art History from France* (1988), is Martin Jay's *Downcast Eyes: The Denigration of Vision in Twentieth-Century French Thought* (1994), despite its apparently negative title.

There are also the many studies devoted to these theorists and there will doubtless be further work done in the future on their philosophies of the visual. At present some have received more attention than others, with most nevertheless already finding their way into anthologies and readers.

A different corpus of thinkers is envisaged here, consisting of figures that can be said to have devoted a large part of their work to the visual. Their work is attracting widespread and increasing attention. Our chosen thinkers have links with traditional methods of interpretation and have interests in a wide range of media. We have in mind the following: Arasse, Baudrillard, Buci-Glucksmann, Damisch, Debray, Didi-Huberman, Heinich, Marin, Merleau-Ponty, Metz, Nancy, Schefer and Stiegler. We do not propose this list as a definitive corpus, but as an important and necessary addition to the thinkers mentioned in the first list; this is another issue explored with Vouilloux in the interview. We recognise that Merleau-Ponty and Baudrillard have received considerable critical attention and therefore can be said to belong to both our 'categories', but their important contributions to art theory and practice make them essential for our survey of visually oriented theorists. A similar argument could be made about Kristeva, and Rancière too, but fortunately there are many studies of the former, and, in Rancière's case, accounts of his recent work on art and representation are growing in number (see Rockhill and Watts 2009; Davis 2010). We also believe that the analysis of the work of Merleau-Ponty and Baudrillard, and indeed Metz, presented here provides fresh insights into their role as visual thinkers.

Each thinker is presented and discussed by a different critic. We want to encourage a multiplicity of topics, approaches and histories, since we believe that a comprehensive synthesis of this field would constitute a different project. However, we do engage, where relevant, with the ways in which our corpus of thinkers has been involved in the diverse and evolving French art world and institutions of art history, thus offering an approach that respects the singularity of the thinkers and also plots connections with a number of contexts (exhibitions, art history, art criticism and differences between French and UK traditions of art theory). We contend that our combination of decontextualised and contextualised perspectives will enhance the cross-disciplinary appeal of our selected theorists.

The visual and the subject

With the work of Walter Benjamin in particular in mind, we subscribe to the view that modernity brings a new significance attached to the phenomenon of the visual. New technologies mean a 'second industrial revolution' in the major cities of Europe, with photography, panoramas, cinema and urban development. There are new types of literature, including visual poetry, stream-of-consciousness novels, gruesome crime fiction, illustrated magazines and newspapers, and fine art books and journals. Meanwhile, explored by psychoanalysis, dreams bring challenges to interpretation and newly released visual power. There is increasing attention to the social and political situation of women, foreigners and the working class; there are new disciplines and modes of enquiry, including the anthropological, historical and scientific. Interest in the images of the past takes the form of an enquiry into personal and collective memory, the temporality of the present and the critical force of images. On account of photography and film, from the Crimean War onwards, there are new debates about the limits to what can and what should be represented, notably in relation to images of genocide and atrocity. In the modern period a multilayered understanding emerges of the idea of the visual, alongside new notions of the material, the mechanical and the verbal. The visual plays an integral part therefore in the modern transformation of the notion of the subject and subjectivity, made hugely complex but also, arguably, liberated. As representation becomes more and more complicated, for some writers and critics impossible, an image, according to Georges Didi-Huberman, can nevertheless still wrestle with the world: 'Tout acte d'image s'arrache à l'impossible description d'un réel' [Every image act saves itself from the impossibility of describing the real] (2003: 156).

This book will show, that as a result of this new attention to the visual, the language used to describe it is modified and updated. New and revised vocabularies of the visual appear and keywords are revisited, such as mimesis, imitation, resemblance, representation, dissemblance, opacity, realism, icon, spectacle, phantasia and the formless. It is a time of new dictionaries (Bataille in *Documents*, 1929–30), new interpretations of culture (Mauss, Huizinga, Warburg) and new ways of writing history (*Annales*). Overall the period is marked by a split between those who move deliberately away from idealism and metaphysics and those who seek to conserve these values and systems. In the modern period, many facets of the image are therefore explored from diverse disciplinary angles – theological, philosophical, historical, political – as a critical reading of images develops and ranges between official art history within discrete national borders to international approaches, semiotic analyses, theories of reception, different models of time and the impact of new technologies (and the reinvestigation of older ones too: Mills and Tresch 2011).

Modern accounts of subjectivity and time reflect the transformations that have occurred in the status of the image. Writing about Cy Twombly, Barthes makes the simple but crucial point that 'the subject' means two things, the idea or topic addressed and the persons involved in the creation and reception of the cultural production (1979b: 175). Louis Marin in particular looked at the relationship between a work of art or literature and the spectator and reader, investigating the enmeshed experience of looking, of responding and of performing an identity, and therefore at the construction of subjectivity (Marin 1994; see Chapter 6 in this volume). Marin built on Lacan's analysis of the mirror stage as the foundation of identity (Lacan 1970, 1973) and on Foucault's work relating to the controls placed on subjects by the discourse prevalent in any society at a given time (Foucault 1971). Drawing on this work, but amplifying the drama of the subject, Griselda Pollock has discussed how images are seen as the mediation of history and subjectivity, 'assembling and encountering what we don't yet know about ourselves through investigation of memory and return, repetition and persistence' (2007: 12). Marin and Nancy are included in this volume, while the chapter on Didi-Huberman engages with the work of Pollock (Chapters 6, 9 and 10 respectively).

The widespread use of the term 'visual' reflects a shift, discussed by Stephen Bann (2002) and many others, away from a positivist and hierarchical view of art and its interpretation towards an interest in the power of the image as it exists in all media. One point of departure for our privileging of the term 'visual' rather than 'art' is Didi-Huberman's *Devant l'Image: Question posée aux fins d'une histoire de l'art* (1990). Didi-Huberman makes an argument that has links with some of the approaches of other thinkers treated in our volume, namely that the concentration on the term 'art' had led historically and institutionally to a dependence on the dichotomy of visibility and legibility, omitting from consideration parts of a visual image that are impossible to read as the signs of some pre-existing text. As Vouilloux reminds us, Didi-Huberman is certainly not the first or only thinker to use the term 'visual' and this volume allows us to show the difference in outlook between Didi-Huberman and Régis Debray, who at the time wrote in much more general terms than Didi-Huberman about the visual and its reception: 'nous étions *devant* l'image, nous sommes *dans* le visuel' [we used to be *in front of* the image, now we are *in* the visual] (Debray 1992: 383).

We are interested in how our thinkers, who mostly work in the period, or in the wake, of structuralism and poststructuralism, have contributed new approaches to understanding images, regarding their impact on audiences, their contexts, the reasons for their beauty, their effects on the category 'art', their presence in other disciplines and their histories, transmission and futures. Keywords that appear in the headings we use for arranging these aspects of the visual image are phenomenology, semiotics, art history, genealogy, representation, mediology, sociology, memory, body, image and digital. As W. J. T. Mitchell and Mark Hansen note in relation to the term media in their introduction to *Critical Terms for Media Studies*, cross-fertilisation between ideas can be encouraged by using coherent categories to divide up a field, so that the field, in our case the visual, can then enable connections to emerge (2010: viii). To enhance this aim, we have asked our contributors to allude to other thinkers in the volume.

We are nevertheless mindful of Bann's warning about the risk of imprecision when the term 'visual' is employed (2002: 217). A further aspect of our approach is that, on the one hand, we wish to link contemporary visual theories to art practice and to art history; on the other, the volume insists upon the French-speaking, if not francophone and/or post-colonial, dimensions of contemporary visual theory. In view of the absence of a chapter on a non-metropolitan, French-speaking visual theorist, we discuss this gap and juxtapose it with an analysis of how the importance of metropolitan French visual theory goes far beyond France's borders.

Art history and semiotics

When French theorists of Marin's generation (b. 1931) such as Derrida, Pierre Bourdieu, Hubert Damisch, Gilles Deleuze and Foucault, engaged with interpretations of visual culture, they sought out perspectives with comparable philosophical backgrounds to theirs (Marin 1995: 109). Hence they were drawn especially to Panofsky on account of his German heritage, through the school of Warburg, and his development of a coherent neo-Kantian view of art and its function provided ideal material for them, resulting in thorough engagements with, and critiques of, his methods, especially the encapsulating sense of the overall meaning of an image (the final 'iconological' stage in an interpretation). Damisch and Marin, along with Jean-Louis Schefer, Julia Kristeva and Jean-Claude Lebensztejn, also pursued a semiotic approach to art, questioning the relationship between painted subjects, symbols, narrative and final significance or meaning. In particular, as Mieke Bal and Norman Bryson point out in 'Semiotics and Art History' (1991), the idea of context is problematised because it can be seen to function as an artificial construction with a relationship to the image that is understood as causal but is in fact circular, whereas a work and its 'context' are open both to the mobility of meaning that operates between signs and to historicity (*ibid.*: 176–80). The art historian Edgar Wind once told Louis Marin that to solve the puzzle of the back of the portrait medal of Leon Battista Alberti, with its enigmatic combination of an eye with wings radiating flames and the inscription 'Quid tum' ('What then?'), Marin just needed to wait until he found the source for the inscription and that that would explain everything. 'Trouver *le* texte, c'est l'idéal de l'iconographie' [The iconographer's ideal is to find the key textual source], Marin notes, whereas in the article he had shown Wind he had been interested in how the dual process of condensation and displacement in 'dream-work', as well as its subsequent interpretation by an analyst, as proposed in Freud's *Interpretation of Dreams*, could be a model for the study of the circulation of enigmatic messages in the medal (Marin 1971: 109–23; 1994: 64–5; Freud 1999: 211–36). Finding the precise source for 'Quid tum' would not, in Marin's view, put an end to the flow of meanings.

Where Panofsky had argued that thought should take precedence over sensation when analysing images, semioticians in the 1960s and 1970s considered that the language of images should be treated more 'neutrally' (as Foucault put it in his essay on Velázquez's *Las Meninas*, see below), that interpretation could be more firmly anchored in the works under discussion. A Poussin landscape, for example, would be discussed in terms of the spatial arrangement of figures and their interaction through gesture or looking, through the representation of any narrative and the position of the spectator (Marin 1971). Another way of understanding the approach is to think of it as an alternative to the academic hierarchies associated with *ut pictura poesis*, the Latin tag from Horace used by critics to discuss the rules regarding subject matter, treatment and style that a painter should adhere to if he/she wished to achieve the poetic and rhetorical standards envisaged by the Royal Academy (Lee 1967; Duro 1997). These rules or methods of categorisation therefore involved the production of and investment in degrees of cultural capital and familiarity with erudite contextual knowledge. By contrast therefore, a certain democratisation is encouraged by the semiotic method in the engagement with the visual. At the same time, the most influential semiotic work also engaged with the terms of the Academy, on the one hand in terms of the period in which the work was created and its reception, and on the other hand expanding the appreciation of the spatial arrangement of a painting. What emerged from the encounter between semiotics and art history was a greater attention to representation as a system and to the role of the artist, model, artwork, society and critic in any commentary on the visual. On the other hand, the work of Schefer, Damisch and Marin, for example, became less 'neutral' from the 1980s onwards and far more interested in the strategies of writing and new approaches to theory required to convey the 'enigmatic body' projected by the image, the 'dream perspectives' in Renaissance art and the 'figurability' of representation in Philippe de Champaigne (see Chapters 4, 6 and 11 in this volume).

Psychoanalysis

In his study of Pascal Quignard and the image, Bernard Vouilloux draws on Lacan to argue that the *ut pictura poesis* tradition seeks to pacify the image, offering it to the eye but not to the gaze; Barthes makes a similar point at the end of *La Chambre claire* about the reception of disturbing photographs from the past (Vouilloux 2010: 45–6; Barthes 1980: 180–4). In the aftermath of Sartre's *L'Imaginaire* (1940) and Merleau-Ponty's *Phénoménologie de la perception* (1945), there was a psychoanalytical turn in art history, visual culture and theory, notably with, as we have already mentioned, Lacan's *Écrits* ([1966] 1970) and *Quatre Concepts fondamentaux de la psychoanalyse* (1973), Lyotard's *Discours, figure* (1971), the *Vocabulaire de la psychanalyse* (1967) by Laplanche and Pontalis (as well as the journals *Nouvelle Revue de la psychanalyse* and *Macula*), and the work of Julia Kristeva and other *Tel Quel* writers, succeeded by Rosalind Krauss and Yve-Alain Bois in the USA and Laura Mulvey, Pollock and Bal in Europe. As can be seen in this volume, Lacan's thought was fundamental to the development of our corpus of thinkers. As Maria Scott has argued, the discussion of anamorphosis in the *Quatre Concepts* proposed a model of reading images and a theorisation of the relationship between desire and death that is illustrated and dramatised in the scene of a narrative painting (Lacan 1973; Scott 2008; Bowie 1991). In this volume David Packwood explains how Damisch decided between Freudian and Lacanian models of reading when constructing his analytical iconology (see Chapter 4).

The critical material available on Kristeva is extensive. Her idea of abjection, expounded in the widely read *Pouvoirs de l'horreur: Essais sur l'abjection* (1980), is useful in reading various kinds of art, from Surrealism and the *informe*, to Bacon and Giacometti, as Timothy Mathews has argued (2001, 2007). Kristeva's work also had an impact on exhibitions, notably Tate's 'Paris Post-War' exhibition (1993), followed in 1998 by her own exhibition in the Louvre's 'Parti Pris' series, 'Visions capitales'. The challenge to readers of Kristeva's powerful essays on Giotto and Bellini (1977), as well as *Pouvoirs de l'horreur*, was to find ways of avoiding the absorption of transgressive melancholy and abjection into the mainstream. In a different mode of response, Rancière's work engages with the political status of transgression, arguing for the demise of the separation between the political and aesthetic spheres and for the creation of artworks where both artist and audience have no prior knowledge of the ideas and reactions that the work will induce (2008). Didi-Huberman's dialectical aesthetics of dissemblance has points of intersection with both Kristeva and Rancière but crucially provides a reflection on the complex temporality (like the unconscious) and singularity of images. Didi-Huberman applies an achronological framework to the abject and the transgressive, as we see in Chapter 10, which is devoted to him.

Art and philosophy: third and other meanings

As well as the question of the time of the image, Didi-Huberman emphasises the experience of loss involved in the gaze (1992: 14). In his work on Giacometti, Mathews offers a distinctive and original inflection to this recognition of loss and desire. Situating his enquiry in the space of the art gallery or museum, Mathews considers the vulnerability of seeing and writes about the notion of loss as a shared state to be rethought in terms of mediation and relation (2009: 164–70). His reading stands in relation to both Sartre's essay on Giacometti, 'La recherche de l'absolu' ([1948] 1949), and Genet's *L'Atelier d'Alberto Giacometti* ([1963] 1998), two foundational studies of how to write about Giacometti's aesthetics of space; Genet's essay was Picasso's favourite on an artist (Lord 1986: 350). Mathews takes an approach closer to Genet's interest in the common solitude and singularity of Giacometti's sculptures and his audience.

As well as the terms mediation and relation, we have in mind Barthes's forty-year-old article on the 'third' meaning. Barthes analysed Eisenstein film stills (1970b) in order to talk about another, third aspect of the image that seemed to him to escape the established categories of communication and signification. Barthes sought 'le purement image', which he would later discuss as the punctum in *La Chambre claire* (1980). In between these texts he produced the essay on Cy Twombly, elaborated in two versions, where he considered how Twombly's work gestures towards us. The language of semiotics has not gone entirely, but there is a desire to speak about Twombly's erudite and enigmatic dramas of colour and occasional text in terms of gesture and memory, to consider new categories, to see Twombly's style as beyond intention and authority, consisting instead of irreducible sensations and 'rare' visual achievement, rare because informed by a long tradition, that is nevertheless presented negatively, lightly, with dandyesque panache (1979a: 1028–32; 1979b: 1043–7).

Many essayists on the visual see contemporary artists escaping rules, codes, theory and predictable meanings, as in the texts written about Valerio Adami by Marc Le Bot (1975), Damisch (1974), Jean-François Lyotard (1983b and 2008) and Derrida (1978) or about Gérard Titus-Carmel by Jean-Louis Schefer (1982), Derrida (1978) and indeed Titus-Carmel himself (2003). Patrick ffrench's chapter in this volume considers the way in which, in Schefer's writing, the viewing subject is reconstituted through the experience of the visual (see Chapter 11). In a study of encounters between artists and philosophers in France in the 1970s, concentrating on the 'Figurations' group, Sarah Wilson asks us to consider whether theorists and essayists engage with contemporary art or whether they focus on respectable Old Masters, exploiting the artists' authority to justify their critical choices and manoeuvres (Wilson 2010: 22). A remark by Gérard Genette in his revealing compendium of personal essays, *Bardadrac* (2006), makes a similar point when he notes the tendency among critics to reduce art first to the plastic arts, then to painting, and lastly to the Italian Renaissance, 'quand ce n'est pas cette dernière à la question, pour moi vraiment flagellante, de la perspective' [they even reduce it right down to the question of perspective, in my view truly punishing] (Genette 2006: 139). In this book we discuss new interpretations of the respectable (Arasse on Vermeer, Damisch on

Bellini, Marin on Poussin, Schefer on Uccello) and interpretations of the modern and contemporary or less 'respectable/safe' (Didi-Huberman on Pascal Convert, Heinich on Buren, Schefer on Oshima, Baudrillard on Bauhaus, Warhol, the Pompidou Centre and TV Reality), as well as Merleau-Ponty on Cézanne, Heinich on Van Gogh, Debray on mediology, and Stiegler on technology, time and subjectivity.

The cross-reference between philosophy and the fine arts, prevalent in France from Paul Valéry onwards, is particularly a feature and legacy of the Sartre and Merleau-Ponty generation and their successors. The philosophical enquiry into the meaning and value of art, when it takes Kant's categories as its subject, by way of a key example, focuses on the idea of origins, ends, perfection and failings. The reopening of the question of the Kantian sublime in the 1980s followed the work of Barnett Newman and the critique of Kant's aesthetics set out by Derrida in *La Vérité en peinture* (1978). Lyotard discussed the overwhelming challenge to the concept of representation posed by the sublime, which he sees as explosively impacting on existing categories of experience and impossible to re-present and arrange into a synthesis of aesthetic experience (Lyotard 1983a: 238–40). Nancy contributed to a collective volume on the sublime, along with Lyotard, Marin, Michel Deguy, Philippe Lacoue-Labarthe and others, concentrating on how the sublime is the ultimate question in aesthetics, on the way it refers to the limits of art's self-definition and purpose (Nancy 1988: 57). At the same time, the evidence regarding artists' interest in philosophy suggests a preference for the works of philosophy that are not directly related to art but are instead more generally about time, space, perception and psychology. Examples of influential philosophers include Merleau-Ponty and Deleuze (Mœglin-Delcroix 2003). Critique remains crucial to the spirit of enquiry – artists critique their own work and their writing, writers since Genet have wondered if they are writing nonsense (Genet 1998). In all cases looked at in this volume, and as Vouilloux points out in the interview, self-reflection and auto-critique are a constant feature of writing and theorising about the visual from Merleau-Ponty to Schefer.

Foucault, Barthes and Derrida

There are three theorists we have decided not to focus on in this volume, for the reasons set out above, though we offer below some help to explain their influence on developments in the thinking about the image and art history in the post-1960 period. The figures we want to summarise here with this context in mind are Foucault, Barthes and Derrida.

Two aspects of Foucault's thought have helped to shape his principal impact on visual theory: first, the analysis of representation in chapter one of *Les Mots et les Choses* (1966), which is devoted to Velázquez's *Las Meninas*, with its development in *Ceci n'est pas une pipe* (1968–73) through the distinction between representation and the simulacrum in Magritte's paintings; and, second, his critique of systems of incarceration and surveillance in *Surveiller et punir: Naissance de la prison* (1975). Foucault saw *Las Meninas* (Plate 1) in Madrid in November 1963, an experience that helped him plan his 'livre sur les signes' [book on signs] (Foucault 1994a: 25). His analysis paid close attention to all the areas of the painting (except perhaps the representation of the ceiling) and investigated the way the painting depicted three elements in modern (seventeenth-century) society: the real and symbolic holders of power, namely King, Queen, family and entourage; the artist and his accoutrements; and the spectators. This 'triangle' of representation underlined how complete a system painting had become in Velázquez's hands, with the artist himself prominently positioned in relation both to the worldview that the monarchs represented and to the painting that he is depicted in the act of creating. The idea of an intermediary position between political and pictorial orders of representation was part of what Svetlana Alpers would identify as the crucial contribution of his approach, in which Foucault investigated the relationship between symbolic meaning and its complex representation (Alpers 1983: 31–42). Foucault goes on to discuss the areas of the painting that we cannot make out, so that the painting acknowledges that there are invisible elements in what we see, but he also notes that this lack can be seen as an indication of a self-reflexive awareness of fallibility, that seems in turn overcome by the inclusion in the same painting of both the artist and his models (in the mirror at the back of the room – with some disagreement among critics about whether the figures reflected there are the King and Queen as Velázquez sees them before him and reproduces them (Arasse 2000) or the hidden figures painted on the canvas (Snyder and Cohen 1980; Snyder 1985) or even figures who interrupt the scene of Velázquez painting himself painting *Las Meninas* (Thévoz 1996). Foucault compares Velázquez to a king: 'il règne au seuil de ces deux visibilités incompatibles' [he rules at the threshold of those two incompatible visibilities] (Foucault 1966: 20); more recently Michel

Thévoz has called the Velázquez who masterminds the scene 'un super-Vélasquez qui viendrait mettre en évidence les ficelles de son stratagème' [an Über-Velázquez who finally reveals the workings of his pictorial stratagem] (Thévoz 1996: 46).

Yet Foucault was not content with concluding that this painting challenges the rules of representation by offering 'une métathèse de la visibilité' [a metathesis of visibility] (1966: 24). This would, we may deduce, have ascribed too much authority to the artist. In fact Foucault uses the second half of his essay to emphasise how the painting highlights the relative status of all the figures represented, with all the elements in the triangle absorbed into the world on show. He achieves this by insisting on the need to step back from the process of reflection on representation in order to examine the role of language in the act of scrutiny. He has in mind a way of delaying identification of the figures and their social function, of withholding the interpretation until all the space has been plotted and the lines of sight listed, only then turning to the question of how the figures (mainly the monarchs, princess and artist) are related in this representation. As he does so he retains his analytical mode, using a style of writing that presents itself as neutral: 'Mais si on veut maintenir ouvert le rapport du langage et du visible, si on veut parler non pas à l'encontre mais à partir de leur incompatibilité, de manière à rester au plus proche de l'un et de l'autre, alors il faut effacer les noms propres et se maintenir dans l'infini de la tâche. C'est peut-être par l'intermédiaire de ce langage gris, anonyme, toujours méticuleux et répétitif parce que trop large, que la peinture, petit à petit, allumera ses clartés' [But if one wishes to keep the relation of language to vision open, if one wishes to keep their incompatibility as a starting-point for speech instead of as an obstacle to be avoided, so as to stay as close as possible to both, then one must erase those proper names and preserve the infinity of the task. It is perhaps through the medium of this grey, anonymous language, always over-meticulous and repetitive because too general, that the painting may, little by little, release its illumination] (*ibid.*: 25).

Some grey patches of writing and some repetition are to be found. However, as in his essay on Magritte (1973) which makes a similar point about language and painting but in fact relishes the imaginary skirmishes between the serried ranks of language and the seductive forms of painting, this does not mean that Foucault avoids rhetorical devices in his dramatisation of the power dynamic at play in the painting. Part two of the essay includes the language of the Kantian sublime when referring to the mirror's appearance, 'by means of a violent, instantaneous movement, a movement of pure surprise' (*ibid.*: 10). And the conclusion will emphasise the frailty and ultimate elision of the monarchs by this painting. The concern about language leads him to consider the entire cycle of representation, notably the sources of light and the use of space, organised around an 'X' and a curve which Foucault describes at length, with the mirror as just one of the elements of representation on show. His attention to language forces readers and spectators to consider their status, increasing the sense of ambiguity in the painting and in his final phrase, 'offers itself as representation in its pure form' (*ibid.*: 16). It is clear to us that Foucault's double lesson about pictorial representation and the language of commentary has been heeded in the writing of Arasse, Marin and their contemporaries. Ralph Dekoninck's chapter in this volume (Chapter 3) discusses further Arasse's interest in this 'philosophical' essay by Foucault on *Las Meninas*.

The argument about representation made by Foucault in his essay on *Las Meninas* returns in his essay on Magritte. As Jacques Rancière put it, showing his debt to Foucault, from the nineteenth century onwards resemblance in art was released from the constraints of the regime of representation, namely the requirement to keep what is shown and not shown in balance and to rationalise the depiction of time and space (Rancière 2003: 135–6). In the case of Magritte the prior examples of Klee and Kandinsky are used by Foucault to demonstrate how this regime of mimetic resemblance is no longer required in art, indeed that it has been overcome. Foucault realised that there was a profound difference between the way 'trompe-l'œil' painting had both enhanced and unsettled visual representation and the manner in which Magritte deployed simulacra. 'Trompe-l'œil' and representation had to work together, as Marin also showed (Marin 1988 and 1994: 254), but Magritte realised that simulacra threatened representation completely, reducing its claims to originality and aura, and setting painting free: 'Peinture du "Même", libérée du "comme si". Nous sommes au plus loin du trompe-l'œil' [Painting the same thing, freed from the attempt to imitate. We could not be further from *trompe-l'œil*] (Foucault 1973: 60). Foucault asked us to consider Magritte's *Trahison des images* as a skewed calligram, thereby demonstrating how artificial the claims of language and of painting are when they pretend to represent reality in their respective systems. Representation indeed is seen in his essay as a controlling, stifling and destructive regime that is ridiculed and overturned by Magritte's art. There was an interesting difference in outlook between Foucault and Magritte about the relationship between this approach to painting and thought, with Magritte ascribing creative power and authority to the mind in a way that Foucault's emphasis on self-perpetuating simulacra could not follow (see Foucault 1973: 85–90; Levy 1990).

When writing about the visual beyond art in the modern period Foucault is interested in a new paradigm of productivity and discipline, with human subjects under constant surveillance, visible and made to conform. According to *Surveiller et punir*, we no longer have a staging of an exchange of gazes, but rather an empire of the gaze controlling actions and thoughts. Power saturates society, with a shift from sovereign to social cohesion. In Foucault's study, the gaze is investigated in the hospital, prison, school and army. The Panopticon as conceived by Jeremy Bentham was the figure Foucault used for way the new political anatomy of the nineteenth century oversaw its subjects. Foucault's account of the way this system operated brought together his ideas about power's pervasive presence in society, notably through institutions, and his analysis has enduring power because of the way readers draw parallels with the contemporary era of CCTV, identity surveillance and credit ratings (Welch 2009). The panoptic machine was the focus for Foucault of those forces that impinge on people, channelled through the gaze; and, implicitly for Foucault, the modern world was not the 'spectacle' famously theorised by the Situationist Guy Debord ([1967] 1992), but something far more sinister: 'Notre société n'est pas celle du spectacle, mais de la surveillance; sous la surface des images, on investit les corps en profondeur; derrière la grande abstraction de l'échange, se poursuit le dressage minutieux et concret des forces utiles' [Our society is one not of spectacle, but of surveillance; under the surface of images, one invests bodies in depth; behind the great abstraction of exchange, there continues the meticulous, concrete training of useful forces] (Foucault 1975: 218; 1979: 217). Representation, simulacrum and discipline are all concepts inherited from Foucault by the thinkers in this volume, especially the relationship between the gaze and power in general for the post-1800 period, and representation and illusion for the period after the Renaissance. Our thinkers would also retain in Foucault a distrust of progress in history and histories of art and a sense of the complexities involved in the application of historical context to paintings. As Arasse noted, the chronology employed by Foucault was a powerful and persuasive precedent.

The relationship between language and the visual, and between the image and history, is taken in different directions in the work of Barthes.

'L'Image est ainsi *muette avec force*' [The image is thus *silent with power*], he wrote in his last lectures in 1979 (2003: 97). This negative dialectic sums up well the Barthesian approach to the image, which is often, though not always, considered in relation to language, and especially to written rather than spoken words (to which we will return with Derrida shortly). That said, Barthes famously reduced the commentary possible on the image of the loved one to one single word, 'That' or 'Thus' ('Tel'), as he put it in *Fragments d'un discours amoureux* (1977a). Barthes also spent the final lectures of his life at the Collège de France considering the Japanese Haïku (a seventeen-syllable poem in three lines) as an elliptical, literary form of illumination, which, deeply analogous to the photograph, provoked a 'fascination' with photography, and thereby invited silence as an appropriate speech-act (2003).

However, were we to suggest one key Barthesian approach in this negative dialectic of word and image, it would come in his 1955 critique of a photography exhibition which appeared in *Mythologies* in 1957. Against the sensationalist photographic material dominant in an exhibition, Barthes preferred images that tried to 'nous *désorganiser*' [disorganise us], disturb and disrupt our view; in 'Photo-chocs', following a Brechtian optic, Barthes played on the mismatch between the two media in question, photographic image and written caption (1955b). This mismatch dominates his work on food and especially clothing and fashion across the 1960s: the importance of language to image. The key texts from this period – 'Le Message photographique' (1961), '"La Civilisation de l'image"' (1964a), 'Rhétorique de l'image' (1964b) – raw as they are in bringing semiology, sociology, linguistics and literary theory together, prepare us for the more mature work on the image, especially in relation to Balzac in *S/Z* (1970a), presenting a scenography of writing and reading literature, and in the same year to Eisenstein (1970b), as we have already mentioned, with the idea of obtuse meanings (the 'troisième sens') as a stepping stone to the key notions of *studium* and *punctum* in photography that are brilliantly illustrated in *La Chambre claire* (1980). Having worked extensively in the popular theatre movement in France, Barthes had learned to read, interpret and criticise the visual communication offered by theatre costumes in any one production (1955c), and worked extensively on Roger Pic's pioneering theatre photography of the Berliner Ensemble production of Brecht's *Mutter Courage* in Paris in the mid-1950s (1959, 1960), as well as (we have recently discovered) on images of sport ([1961] 2004).

Visuality, if not considered as a language, is often linked to writing and language in Barthes's work. Margaret Iversen underlines how the Eiffel Tower acts for Barthes as an excellent example of an 'empty visual signifier', whose 'degree zero' meaning contrasts sharply with another monumental structure of the time that is full of meaning and symbolism, the Statue of Liberty in New York (2002: 328–32); whereas the structuralist Barthes of the 1960s has affinities to Merleau-Ponty's work on Saussurean linguistics, the work on artists such as Cy Twombly and André Masson in the 'late' Barthes is shown by Iversen (*ibid.*: 332–5) also to be beholden to Merleau-Ponty's notion of the body within the *langue–parole* distinction established by Saussure. Indeed, Barthes mobilises Saussure's theory of the sign in his essay at the end of *Mythologies*, 'Myth Today' (1957). Here, Barthes famously contemplates a front cover of the tabloid magazine *Paris-Match* from 1955 (that is, at the height of the wars of decolonisation), on which there is a colour photograph of a black boy saluting; using semiology, not only does Barthes impugn the mythical distortion and ideological brainwashing in this (semi-)subliminal message, he also comes to an important understanding of what we do when we look at an image: that is, we name its signified, which is, here, in *Paris-Match*, mythified to become a sign of 'imperiality'. Thus, Barthes coins a neologism that covers this mythical dimension of an image, extending it to 'Basquity' for houses from the Basque region of France, and 'Italianicity' for a poster advertising pasta (1964b). In other words, the visual, the image, for Barthes at least, are but the beginning of, the starting point for, a whole set of internal mumblings by the viewer, in which they persuade themselves of various meanings and ideas in the image. In a similar vein, writing on the Dutch 'masters' of the seventeenth century, he reads signifiers and places signs in their relation to an ascendant bourgeoisie of the time (1953b); similarly, in a piece on the pre-revolutionary French *Encyclopédie* of the eighteenth century, he points to the spatio-ideological nature of the images deployed as illustrations (1964c). Thus the image-text nexus points to a tight tension in Barthes's work between the two media: 'Le texte ne "commente" pas les images. Les images n' "illustrent" pas le texte' [The text does not 'commentate' the images. The images do not 'illustrate' the text], as he wrote in his suggestive (and beautifully illustrated) book on Japan (1970c: 745). As he showed in his review of Jean-Louis Schefer's study on signs in Paris Bordone's *Chess Players*, painting, and visual culture in general by extension, is not necessarily (just?) a 'language' (1969), but both an analysis of codes and a spur to writing (see Chapter 11 on Schefer in this volume).

The 1970s see many essays and writings on the painted image by

Barthes, but interestingly it is the very early Barthes – that from the early to mid-1950s – which returns, in spiral, in his 1970s work on the image. So, early theories on memory, faces and the framing of the image are treated, if not fully, in important precursory fashion in 'Visages et figures' (1953a), on children in advertising (1955a) and on the image of the nineteenth-century historian Jules Michelet (1954). Thus the self as image becomes a key phase in the 1971–75 period – notably in *Roland Barthes par… Roland Barthes* (1975) – morphing into a consideration of the loved one in the *Fragments*, and ending with the search for the lost (and recently deceased) mother in a silent photograph which we (or Barthes?) never get to see, and in a melancholy musing on the person caught and lost in an image (*La Chambre claire*).

If the image is not always fully textualised in Barthes's work, then it certainly is ideologised (though not necessarily a different thing), or (mainly) personalised. Given his (mild) aversion to the cinema, Barthes's work on the image is generally on photography, though not inconsiderably on fine arts – namely, important essays on Twombly, Réquichot, Masson, Steinberg, the last commented upon by Damisch (2002). His work in visual culture involves also an important consideration of the visual nature of the written word (especially in the work of André Masson, and that of Massin). Though no synthesis 'Barthes and the Image' exists there are a number of key secondary texts – Rabaté (1997) generally, and then Shawcross (1997) and Batchen (2009) on photography – which attempt to put some order on the image in Barthesian theory. As for Barthes's influence on theories of visual culture since, these vary enormously. Alloula (1981) is dedicated to Barthes, suggesting the importance of the early Barthes work on stereotyping and myth in photography, and he is clearly an influence on Edward Said and subsequent (visual) theories of orientalism, on body culture and on aspects of film criticism (from Metz onwards).

By contrast, Marriner argues that Derrida's impact on visual studies has been slower than other French theorists (especially Baudrillard during the 1980s), one reason he suggests being Derrida's lack of a 'systematic explanatory vision', in favour of an epistemological critique of the 'logical structures' allowing us to theorise and interpret visual phenomena (Marriner 2002: 349). In other words, Derrida is useful for a consideration of the assumptions, methods and discourses that permeate art history and critical theory. Hence an interest in Derrida for 'frames' and for the interiority–exteriority questions in art, what David Carroll has called 'borderline aesthetics' (1987: 131–54). A good example of Derrida's influence on photography theory is Soulages's notions of photography as art and non-art (1998), as a trace, and as a 'ce qui a été joué' [what has been played (out)], clearly a parody of Barthes's 'ce qui a été' [what has been] which, beholden to André Bazin's seminal essay on the ontology of the photographic image (1945), dominates the ontological notion of photography in *La Chambre claire*. The emphasis on 'jeu' – 'play' in both senses, ludic and mobile within a tight structure – is relevant to Derrida (1967: 409–28), but also to Foucault and to Barthes. Above all, it is our assumptions about representation that Derrida wishes to question. One example of this critique of representation is in his work with photographer Marie-Françoise Plissart, *Droits de regard* (1985), on what is a photo-roman but which becomes an essayistic treatise on the 'gap' in visual representation. Similarly in his opening comments on Cézanne in *La Vérité en peinture*, Derrida is interested in the 'mot' from Cézanne, the 'idiom' of painting (1978: 6–7). Much of Derrida's work on visual culture then is concerned with text–image, or rather with image as text. While much of Barthes's interest in the text–image relationship emerged in the early 1960s, it was heavily inflected after 1967 by the arrival of the work of Derrida, whose promotion of writing over orality certainly led to a cult of *écriture*, against and alongside which the visual and the image had to battle. Indeed both Barthes and Derrida become interested in the written as visual: the letter – alphabets and typography in Barthes (1971), the word and its 'presence' in Derrida (1978).

As with Barthes, the visual in Derrida is largely recondite and dispersed. Unlike Debray (see Chapter 7 in this volume), Derrida is, following Heidegger, highly suspicious of the notions of 'origin' or 'origins'. Furthermore, it is not simply the distant glimmer of a beginning that dismays Derrida, but the (im)possibility of a presence. Both of these critiques of humanism – origins and presence, indeed he sees the (impossible) search for presence as part of lost origins – clearly have an important bearing on the image and on visuality. In particular, 'presence as a supplementary representation does not in fact re-present anything at all, does not substitute itself for something which somehow pre-existed it' (Kearney 1994: 116). Images then, in Derrida's world, are merely signs and we, as viewers of images, merely interpret interpretations. Though influenced by phenomenology (Husserl, Merleau-Ponty), Derrida is also a staunch critic of perception as presence. For him, all is metaphor and every metaphor (even the word itself, meta-phors, carrying beyond) acts so as to make the visible into the invisible. Hence the interest in the trace and, like Barthes, in a critique of 'intentions': for Barthes's 'Death of the Author' we might speak, in relation to Derrida, of the 'Death of the Visual Artist'. Nevertheless, as James shows in this volume (Chapter 9), this question is open to further investigation and Nancy has revisited the question of presence, and examined the way the sense of an image presents itself while withdrawing from what is seen. We also consider this issue in the interview with Vouilloux.

Derrida's critique of representation in *The Truth in Painting* (1978) is certainly related to Foucault, including a distrust of art-historical jargon when applied for the purpose of legislating for the image. As we have noted, Derrida looks at the philosophical foundations of aesthetics, but also at conflicts in interpretation between disciplines. His account of Meyer Schapiro's refutation of Heidegger, in the third section of *The Truth in Painting*, makes many points that might be applied to the reception of Foucault's essay on Velázquez, notably a critique of the assumption that the historical or chronological framework for interpreting images can be defined simply and irrefutably, an awareness of the opacity of the language of interpretation and interest in the notion of the signature of the artist in a contemporary philosophical context. A common way of exploring text–image differences is the use of dialogue and letters as a form of commentary and the use of the dialogic mode within an essay: the discussion passes from one voice to the other/another in Derrida's text, and this duality, or plurality, of voices was influential as a sign of openness and as recognition of the provocations made by the image. This approach to writing and interpretation is taken up in different ways by Marin in *De L'Entretien* (1997), Didi-Huberman in *L'Étoilement: Conversation avec Hantaï* (1998) and Damisch with François Rouan in *Voyage à Laversine* (2004); the attention to writing, in relation to the visual, is therefore a constant preoccupation throughout this volume.

The post-colonial visual

One way of compensating for the striking absence from this volume of a chapter devoted to a non-metropolitan French theorist would be to engage with the huge influence of Derrida on visual theory and on critical practice in francophone culture (in contrast to his slower impact on academic studies of visual culture referred to by Marriner). From 'post-colonial' critics such as Abdelkébir Khatibi, Malek Alloula and Abdelwahab Meddeb (interestingly all North-African francophones:

Moroccan, Algerian and Tunisian respectively; the Congolese V. Y. Mudimbe (1973) providing a rare sub-Saharan example) to the Damisch of *L'Origine de la perspective* (1987) and Duve of *Au nom de l'art: Pour une archéologie de la modernité* (1989) and *Essais datés I* (1987), and then to Lyotard's postmodern work, Derrida's influence can be strongly felt.

In the work of Khatibi for example, we see Derrida's (and Barthes's) conflation of the physical body for the typographical letter, especially in Khatibi's early writing on the tattoo (1971) and in his collaboration with Mohammed Sijelmassi on calligraphy ([1976] 1994), not to mention Khatibi's influential deconstruction of sociology (1985, first published in French in Khatibi 1983) whose 'double criticism' implicitly gestures towards Foucault's 'double lesson' discussed above. Indeed, there is much more work to be carried out on the visual culture dimension of a number of important francophone writers: Tahar Ben Jelloun, Leïla Sebbar, Assia Djebar. Sub-Saharan figures for further study include Mudimbe in his important interventions ([1991] 1999) on African art, as well as Jean-Godefroid Bidima with his Deleuzian approach to the same topic (1997). Mention should also be made of the important contribution made by the research group ACHAC (Association pour la connaissance de l'histoire de l'Afrique contemporaine), especially Pascal Blanchard (see Blanchard and Chatelier 1993), in introducing visual culture into colonial and post-colonial study in France (see publications listed at www.achac.com); more recent, anglophone post-colonial studies have begun to identify a set of non-metropolitan theorists working in French, though not directly in relation to visual culture: see the chapters in Forsdick and Murphy (2009) on Mudimbe, Khatibi, Achille Mbembe, Albert Memmi (especially in relation to 'portraiture'), Assia Djebar (on aesthetics), even Ho Chi Minh as found in photography; see also the special number of the journal *Modern and Contemporary France* (Welch and McGonagle 2011) called 'France and Algeria in Contemporary Visual Culture'. Without the space to discuss the marginalisation of the visual in the francophone domain, we can tentatively suggest that this is an area affected in part by the differences between French semiotics, on the one hand, and Anglo-American gender and post-colonialist studies, on the other, as well as institutional tensions within France, and on which Vouilloux's interview at the end of this volume briefly touches.

Visual studies

It is worth saying that despite the penury of translation from French into English (mainly affecting the novel), 'le French Theory', discussed by François Cusset (2003), has been a central way for French culture, francophone culture, to be imported across the Channel and the Atlantic into the 'monde anglo-saxon', with all the deformation, defamation and dissemination imaginable. A whole raft of readers and anthologies of texts on visual culture and visual theory has emerged across the 1990s and into the new millennium. *Deconstruction and Visual Arts: Art, Media, Architecture*, edited by Brunette and Wills (1994), was significant, especially in the interview with Derrida and in beginning to show how to use deconstruction in visual analysis, theory and culture. *Visual Sense: A Cultural Reader*, edited by Edwards and Bhaumik (2008), follows the trend towards Merleau-Ponty, with an opening chapter by him '(The Intertwining – The Chiasma') and an encasing of the whole book by another French (but very different) phenomenologist, Gaston Bachelard ('Intimate Immunity'), known for his studies of the poetics of space and dreams. The Edwards–Bhaumik take on French theorists is therefore interesting – featuring chapters on Marc Augé (and 'non-lieux' [non-places]) and on Jean-Luc Godard (in the form of an interview). Other similar volumes, for example *A Companion to Art Theory* (Smith and Wilde 2002) and more recently *An Introduction to Visual Culture* (Mirzoeff, 2009), deploy an eclectic and often surprising set of French theorists (qualities that this volume does not necessarily want to avoid). Though the first of these two volumes includes sections on Barthes on art, followed by similar sections on Foucault and Derrida and by regular references to Deleuze and to Thierry de Duve, there is no mention at all of Debray, Didi-Huberman, Heinich, Arasse, Damisch or Marin. Mirzoeff's 2009 volume offers Barthes's 'Rhétorique de l'image' (1964b) and Foucault's 'Des espaces autres' (1994b) and then an original mix of chapters by Michel de Certeau (on everyday life) and by Malek Alloula from his seminal *Colonial Harem* (1981), as well as a section on the 'gaze' indicative of the psychoanalytical and post-colonial 'turns' in visual studies. There will always be missing sections and sometimes theorists omitted entirely, even in the innovative *Critical Terms for Media Studies* (2010), edited by Mitchell and Hansen, where Debray is overlooked (on the other hand, Stiegler, discussed in Chapter 13 in our volume, is a contributor).

Structure of the volume

Our selection of thinkers enables us to outline the important developments in visual theory from the 1940s to the present day, adopting in part a chronological approach and in part a thematic division. Thus readers can first examine two precursors to the principal generation of visual theorists that we are discussing: the phenomenological approach to art and the artist in Merleau-Ponty and the semiological analysis of film narrative and spectatorship developed by Metz. These background chapters supplement the sections above in this introduction devoted to Foucault, Barthes, Derrida, psychoanalysis and the post-colonial. All this material provides crucial contexts for the visual thinking of our corpus of theorists.

After the chapters on Merleau-Ponty and Metz (Part I), our contributors look at the reconfiguration of French art history undertaken by a number of thinkers from the 1950s onwards, following the interdisciplinary spur received from Panofsky in particular. In Part II, Arasse and Damisch offer cases of this new outlook. In our volume they are followed by a thinker who reflects on questions of history and gender relating to modern representation and aesthetics (Buci-Glucksmann). The recent period has also seen further consideration of the relationship between language and the visual arts, between sign systems, between disciplines and between value systems. Part III, in bringing together chapters on Marin, Debray and Heinich, engages with the fundamental questions they have raised regarding how paintings or films construct their narratives, how these media work as systems of representation and how the relationship with their audiences is negotiated.

In Parts IV and V we consider writers who offer particularly original theories of the visual that are hard to limit to a single category. First, we have a philosophical investigation of the status of the image as presence and figure in Chapter 9 on Nancy. Then in Chapter 10 the case of the many works of Didi-Huberman there is a concern for an adequate bodily, critical and emotive response to the visual image, while Schefer's beguiling writing is seen to attend to the perpetual creation of a body out of the meeting of art and writing (Chapter 11). These thinkers reflect on the limits of 'artwriting' and on the experience of these limits. The final two thinkers discussed (Baudrillard and Stiegler) in Part V both engage with the contemporary world and its media and provide accounts of the world, drawing on wide-ranging trajectories of thought and traditions of philosophy, notably regarding space and time. Part VI concludes the volume with the Vouilloux interview, looking at the new understanding of art and representation advanced by our thinkers, and drawing on Vouilloux's interests in aesthetics, the history of art, artwriting, text–image studies and institutions.

Chapter summaries

Part I Precursors: phenomenology and semiotics

Chapter 1 by Nathalie Aubert explores the way in which – from his *Phenomenology of Perception*, written in 1945 in the wake of Husserl's *Ideas I* and of the clear establishment of 'the primacy of perception' – Merleau-Ponty progressively moved away from Husserl's idealist phenomenology centred on single perceptions, logic, geometry and science, towards one centred on the traditions of painting, gesture and speech. With Merleau-Ponty's last and posthumous work *The Visible and the Invisible* (1964), the intention became manifest to take up again the early analyses of the object and the body, with, this time, an unambiguous emphasis on the visual (especially in respect of Cézanne), via the relation between the seer and the visible, in order to try to dissipate their ambiguity and to show that they acquire their full meaning only outside a psychological interpretation, when they are enveloped in a new ontology: the 'madness of vision' of the interaction of the viewer and the viewed. After his sudden death, however, both Merleau-Ponty's optimistic hermeneutic belief in the saturation of the world with meaning and the power of the visual model were questioned as the foundations of epistemological certainty and visual perception became problematic issues in the search for meaning or truth. It is only recently that his approach has been reappraised, in a new consideration of visual experience where truth and certainty are themselves questioned.

Christian Metz is rightly considered to be the founder, in the 1960s, of the semiology of cinema, which is the subject of Chapter 2, by Martine Joly. Metz approaches film through both linguistics and psychoanalysis, focusing on how units of a film are established and elaborating a theory of how meaning is constructed in cinema. One of his principal contributions lies in his demonstration that while cinema is not a language the question of enunciation needs to be studied in its strict cinematic sense, in order to study the way in which an impersonal style is developed in a film. Metz also argues that the spectator needs to be understood 'metapsychologically'. This chapter demonstrates the continuing relevance of the semiotic Metz in an age of poetic realism and digital creation and aims to convey what Roland Barthes meant when he wrote that 'when reading Metz you understand everything he says as if you have learnt it yourself'.

Part II New art histories and genealogies

Chapter 3 by Ralph Dekoninck focuses on art historian Daniel Arasse, whose work is known today for its ability to engage with both the history and the theory of art (at the risk of upsetting some traditional boundaries) and with both the Renaissance and the contemporary period (at the risk of anachronism). He has become an important model for art historians looking for new approaches to try out while at the same time wishing to maintain a sense of the history of the discipline. Visual experience has always been the starting point for Arasse's investigations, based on the premise that history and theory are inseparable. For Arasse the visual is experienced through close attention to details, to the overlooked, to the unexpected and to the optical unconscious, an approach bound to threaten the hold of orthodox views of works of art. Repression in art history, in its ways of seeing and writing, is unearthed by Arasse's mix of detachment and investment, even intimacy. This chapter establishes the manner in which the Arasse method, always derived as closely as possible from the objects of study, and with its restlessness and unexpected framing of images, forges a 'joyful visual science' that renews or even reinvents an art history aiming to expand our experience of painting.

In his seminal *Origine de la perspective* of 1987, Hubert Damisch situates his investigation of this foundational art historical topic between the iconology of Panofsky and the anamorphic gaze of Lacan. Vision and subjectivity are seen to be caught between dream fantasy and the snares of perspective, an approach that Damisch then broadens by looking at parallels between dreams and mythological paintings. In Chapter 4 David Packwood analyses the links that Damisch explores between the space and dynamic of a dream and a studio, looking at Giovanni Bellini's enigmatic *Sacred Allegory*. When he turns to the even more central topic of beauty, in *Le Jugement de Pâris* of 1992, Damisch reverts to Freud and the 'dream-work' in order to acknowledge the workings of the unconscious in the reproduction and dissemination of meaning in art history. Damisch's foregrounding of Freud, and also Kant, in relation to the genealogies of art history deserves a wider audience since it suggests innovative ways of thinking through problems of aesthetics, representation and artistic practice, from the Renaissance to modern art.

François-Xavier Gleyzon's contribution considers the work of Christine Buci-Glucksmann. To understand the work of Buci-Glucksmann is, first of all, to understand the movement intrinsic to every image in all its temporal fluidity. If image-flux is a theory of the image, it proceeds above all through an apostrophe and a spatial contextualisation: 'you imagine that. . .', 'You are in London', thus offering to the reader's gaze a whole aesthetic itinerary in the course of which is deployed not just another *mundus* [*monde*] but also a particular modus operandi [mode] of seeing. Through these spaces and these points of view that invoke Shakespeare, Mannerism and the Baroque and circulate as far as the era of the virtual and technology, the central question of a 'folie du voir' might then be theorised/conceptualised, the contours of which offer us a veritable 'cartographie de l'art'. This is what is at stake in Christine Buci-Gluckmann's work and, at the same time, the critical stake of this chapter: a journey of the gaze, a journey reminiscent of Icarus in which the eye rises in order to be able to contemplate better and thus direct us to the frontiers, to the very limits of the visual. Beyond this limit, representation can no longer represent itself, as it vacillates and then topples into rhetoric and a distinct topology: 'an archaeology of shadows' ('une archéologie de l'ombre'). Working through examples in Shakespeare's *King Lear* and in Pessoa's poetry, this chapter then looks at the question of gender in relation to the limits of representation when conceived in broad philosophical, aesthetic and cultural frameworks.

Part III Representation, mediology and sociology

Louis Marin worked on the theory and practice of representation in philosophy, literature and the visual arts across the centuries, notably in his studies of the Quattrocento, of Thomas More's *Utopia*, of Pascal, Poussin and modern autobiography. Chapter 6 by Agnès Guiderdoni pays particular attention to this. On the one hand, his thought was often devoted to incisive readings of Renaissance and especially early modern texts and images; on the other hand, by working with ideas developed from semiotics, psychoanalysis and linguistics, Marin's investigations of the theoretical foundations of representation were not restricted to these periods. This chapter pays particular attention to Marin's working methods and examines how his experimental thinking about the limits of representation sends us both back to representation's foundations and forward to think about the nature of the figure, how it is defined and how it is conceived. The chapter also draws out and develops Marin's notion of 'figurability', including the challenge of locating the visual in a system of thinking that is (initially at least) anchored in signs: figurability enables us to discuss the unthinkable or unlikely meeting place between text and image. Readers of all the chapters in this volume will notice that studying the place or site of text–image enquiry with Marin offers startling connections across modern French visual theory.

Andy Stafford in Chapter 7 focuses on Régis Debray. If Régis Debray's mediology can be considered a challenge to semiology, then it also expresses the need to get beyond it and to reunite the science of signs with a religious and materialist reading of the visual image. The 'symbolic' nature of semiological insight can then be used to show how the visual differs radically from the written. What we might call a 'visualist turn' – set in motion in the 1990s – thus allows Debray to reread the history of the image as a vehicle for communication, not communication itself: 'moins l'image est médiumnique', he argues, 'plus elle se fait médiatique' [the less an image is a medium for a message, the greater its media impact]; and, by the same token, 'moins un art transmet, plus il communique' [the less an art-form transmits, the more it communicates] (*Vie et mort de l'image* (1992: 86)). Debray therefore sees the image as a 'complexe médiologique' [mediological complex or superstructure], whose various layers this chapter investigates. By examining Debray's tripartite history of the reception of images, the chapter underlines his aim to align an understanding of the power of images with their participation in the development of progressive democracy.

Since the early 1990s Nathalie Heinich has elaborated methodologies for the analysis of the art world which draw on sociology. Less concerned with developing responses to the plastic qualities of art than with exploring the broader ideological apparatus which attributes meaning to it, she approaches art as a social phenomenon, throwing into sharp relief the values and categories on which Western notions and practices of visual culture in its broadest sense depend. Chapter 8 by Shirley Jordan indicates the scope and impact of Heinich's theory, beginning with an analytical summary of her evolving methods and then engaging critically with three key focal points: conceptualisations of 'the artist'; the attribution of value to contemporary art works; and epistemological dialogue. Heinich's analyses of the status of the artist are assessed, from her 1991 case study of Van Gogh and the hagiographic impulse to her work on the contemporary valorisation of artists as 'elite' (*L'Élite artiste*, 2005). Heinich's observations on aesthetic perception and value regimes are then summarised. Finally, the chapter offers several points of comparison and contrast with Baudrillard's critique of images.

Part IV Memory, body, image

Chapter 9 by Ian James analyses the way in which Jean-Luc Nancy's thinking about the visual and plastic arts (film, painting, sculpture) brings together figures of seeing and touching, and of visual and tactile experience. It suggests that, through an intertwining of these figures, Nancy develops an innovative thinking about the relation of the artistic image to lived, embodied experience. Nancy's thinking about the visual arts and about the tactile dimension of visual images enacts both an appropriation and a deconstruction of key moments of existential phenomenology and ontology (in particular the thought of Heidegger). The intersection of figures of seeing and touch in Nancy therefore provides a theory for understanding the status and nature of the artistic image, but also has wider implications for thinking beyond phenomenological accounts of seeing, perception and world disclosure. An examination of Nancy's thinking about presence in this context of visual thought allows for a constructive engagement with the readings of his work provided by Derrida and Badiou.

Since the early 1980s Didi-Huberman's rebellious art history or 'history of images' has sought to relocate the origins of the modern discipline from Vasari, Kant and Panofsky to Freud and Warburg. This overhaul of interpretative practice is intended to revalorise images through sustained reflection on their temporality and their relationship to memory. We are being asked to recognise both our fallibility and our involvement as spectators, while we are also released from the burden of over-determined content. The relocation of foundations may also be seen as a move away from discipline to sensibility, and the chapter explores this idea in a general analysis of Didi-Huberman's writing and in particular of his book on Hantaï. Chapter 10 by Nigel Saint goes on to consider how Didi-Huberman has developed a dialectics of the image that alternates an exposure to the power of images with an investigation of their unruly temporality, drawing on Warburg and Benjamin. This analysis is pursued through a discussion of Warburg's *Mnemosyne Atlas* (1927–29) in relation to the wax sculptures of Pascal Convert (1999–2003). The question of time has permitted Didi-Huberman to forge a method of art history that is applicable to a wide range of periods and styles, involving attention to the way images operate a montage of different times and also allow for the development of a new model of readability and exploration of historical and cultural contexts.

Jean-Louis Schefer's attention to what one might call the affective and trans-historical dimensions of visual theory has assured him a crucial if hidden place in the legacy that French theory has donated to thinking about the visual arts. Schefer attends to what has been called the 'enigmatic body' projected by the image, whether that image is historically distant from us, as in the case of Uccello (*Le Déluge, la peste, Paolo Uccello*), or part of our contemporaneity, as in the case of Oshima (*Polyxène et la vierge à la robe rouge*). This body which he finds in us, in himself, and in 'the ordinary man of cinema' (to cite the title of one of his most significant works, and celebrated by Deleuze), is monstrous, criminal, freakish; it is the body of our childhood and of our nightmares, a body of *sidération* [overwhelming astonishment], for which a specific psychoanalysis is needed. Schefer provides us with that analysis, which says as much about the image itself as about the state we are in. Chapter 11 by Patrick ffrench also situates Schefer's work within its intellectual contexts, whilst attending in particular to the character of the virtual body which his writing projects.

Part V The digital era

Jean Baudrillard was a highly influential thinker in the realm of visual culture, his theory of simulation (in the mid-1970s) seeming to preempt much new media work, recent art and reality TV. Like McLuhan, Baudrillard argued that media were not just tools, but had the capacity to alter cultural reality. Many criticised his most extreme take on this, which was his claim in 1992 that 'the Gulf War did not happen'. For close readers of Baudrillard, what was going on here was a simple application of the notion that simulation precedes the real such that 'the real' cannot be seen except through simulations – which does not at all imply the absence of actual death nor aggression. Curiously, despite the far reach of his ideas in the 1970s, Baudrillard had little to say about digital media as such, and if anything, he claims that they are largely negative in effect. Chapter 12 by Paul Hegarty outlines Baudrillard's early work on visual phenomena: notably art (for example, Warhol), television, architecture and the total visualisation of the world. From this last point, the analysis moves on to comment on his thoughts on new media, especially IT and/or digital, covering questions of surveillance, 'perfect' reproducibility in digital formats, and interaction, ending with a series of questions: had Baudrillard already answered the questions he seems largely to avoid later on? Is the 'real' world subsumed as he suggests? How can Baudrillard's ideas be applied to production within digital media?

Chapter 13 by Arthur Bradley considers Bernard Stiegler's philosophy of technology with particular reference to his work on the digital image. It falls into three parts. First, it offers a brief survey of the central thesis of Stiegler's ongoing project *La Technique et le temps* (1994–), namely that there is an essential and constitutive relation between technical prostheses and the human capacity to temporalise time. Second, there is a focus on Stiegler's diagnosis of the political implications of this relation between technology and time in the contemporary moment. For Stiegler, contemporary capitalism produces what he calls the 'industrialisation of memory': the human capacity to temporalise is, he argues, now subject to a technical, political and economic appropriation that is without parallel in history. Finally, the chapter centres on a specific example of this industrialisation of time: the digital image. In Stiegler's double-edged account, the digital image arguably represents the paradigmatic site of the capitalist industrialisation of memory but it also contains the possibility of a new critical culture of the image.

Part VI Afterword

Chapter 14 is a wide-ranging interview with the prolific art theorist, critic and academic Bernard Vouilloux (b. 1953) that addresses the contexts and keywords of French visual theory, the historiography of art and text–image relations. The discussion deals with the keywords 'representation', 'image' and 'visual' in detail and also covers artwriting, institutions and post-coloniality. Further perspectives on the thinkers we have selected are offered throughout and the discussion looks beyond them to Vouilloux's own work and to other important figures in the field of visual theory since Merleau-Ponty. We also engage with possible future sources of theoretical reflection on the visual, allowing us to suggest some thoughts for further work on French art criticism and practice in our period.

References

Alloula, M. (1981) *Le Harem colonial: Images d'un sous-érotisme*, Paris: Garance; *The Colonial Harem*, trans. M. and W. Godzich, Minneapolis, MN: Minnesota University Press, 1986.

Alpers, S. (1983) 'Interpretation without Representation, or, the Viewing of *Las Meninas*', *Representations* 1 (Feb.), 31–42.

Arasse, D. (2000) 'L'œil du maître', *On n'y voit rien: Descriptions*, Paris: Denoël.

Bal, M. and Bryson, N. (1991) 'Semiotics and Art History', *Art Bulletin* 73(2) (1991), 174–208.

Bann, S. (2002) 'The History of Art History in Britain: A Critical Context for Recent Developments and Debates', in Peter Burke (ed.), *History and Historians in the Twentieth Century*, Oxford: Oxford University Press, 207–29.

Barthes, R. (1953a) 'Visages et figures', republished in Barthes 1993, 224–32.

—— (1953b) 'Le monde-objet', in *Essais critiques*, Paris: Seuil, 1963; republished in Barthes 1993, 1177–84.

—— (1954) *Michelet*, Paris: Seuil; republished in Barthes 1993, 243–374.

(1955a) 'Enfants-vedettes', republished in Barthes 1993, 460–1.

—— (1955b) 'Photo-chocs', in *Mythologies*, Paris: Seuil, 1957; republished in Barthes 1993, 626–8.

—— (1955c) 'Les maladies du costume de théâtre', in *Essais critiques*; republished in Barthes 1993, 1205–11.

—— (1957) 'Le mythe, aujourd'hui' in *Mythologies*; republished in Barthes 1993, 681–719.

—— (1959) 'Sept photos-modèles de *Mère Courage*', *Théâtre populaire* 35 (3e trimestre), 17–32; 'Seven Photo Models of *Mother Courage*', trans. H. F. Bernays, *Tulane Drama Review* 37 (1967), 44–55.

—— (1960) 'Préface à Bertolt Brecht', *Mère courage et ses enfants*, with photographs by Roger Pic, Paris: L'Arche.

—— (1961b) 'Le Message photographique', republished in Barthes 1993, 944–6. ['The Photographic Message', in Barthes 1977b, 15–31]

—— (1964a) '"La Civilisation de l'image"', republished in Barthes 1993, 1410–11.

—— (1964b) 'Rhétorique de l'image', republished in Barthes 1993, 1417–29. ['Rhetoric of the Image', in Barthes 1977b, 32–51]

—— (1964c) 'Les planches de l' "Encyclopédie"', in *Nouveaux essais critiques*, Paris: Seuil, 1972; republished in Barthes 1994, 1348–58.

—— (1969) 'La peinture est-elle un langage?', republished in Barthes 1994, 539–40.
—— (1970a) *S/Z*, Paris: Seuil; *S/Z*, trans. R. Miller, New York: Hill & Wang, 1974.
—— (1970b) 'Le troisième sens. Notes de recherche sur quelques photogrammes de S. M. Eisenstein', republished in Barthes 1994, 866–84. ['The Third Meaning', in Barthes 1977b, 52–68]
—— (1970c) *L'Empire de signes*, Geneva: Slatkine; *Empire of Signs*, trans. R. Howard, London: Cape, 1983.
—— (1971) 'Erté ou à la lettre', republished in Barthes 1994, 1222–40.
—— (1977a) *Fragments d'un discours amoureux*, republished in Barthes 1995, 457–687; *A Lover's Discourse: Fragments*, trans. R. Howard, London: Jonathan Cape, 1979.
—— (1977b) *Image-Music-Text*, ed. and trans. S. Heath, London: Fontana.
—— (1979a) 'Sagesse de l'art', republished in Barthes 1995, 1021–32.
—— (1979b) 'Cy Twombly, ou *Non multa sed multum*', republished in Barthes 1995, 1033–47.
—— (1980) *La Chambre claire. Note sur la photographie*, Paris: Cahiers du Cinéma/Gallimard; republished in Barthes 1995, 1105–99; *Camera Lucida*, trans. R. Howard, London: Fontana, 1984.
—— (1993, 1994, 1995) *Œuvres complètes*, vols 1–3, ed. Eric Marty, Paris: Seuil.
—— (2003) *La Préparation du Roman I et II: Cours et séminaires au Collège de France*, 1978–79 et 1979–80, suivi de *Proust et la Photographie. Examen d'un fonds d'archives photographiques mal connu* [1979–80], ed. Nathalie Léger, Paris: Seuil/IMEC; *The Preparation of the Novel*, trans. Kate Briggs, New York: Columbia University Press, 2011.
—— ([1961] 2004) *Le Sport et les hommes*, text for documentary by Hubert Juin, Montreal: Les Presses de l'Université de Montréal.
Bataille, G. (ed.) (1991) *Documents*, 2 vols, Paris: Jean-Michel Place.
Batchen, G. (2009) *Photography Degree Zero: Reflections on Roland Barthes's 'Camera Lucida'*, Boston, MA: MIT Press.
Bazin, A. (1945) 'Ontologie de l'image photographique', in Bazin, *Qu'est-ce que le cinéma?*, Paris: Cahiers du cinéma, 1958, 6–15; *What Is Cinema?*, trans. Hugh Gray, Berkeley, LA and London: University of California Press, 2005, 9–16.
Bidima, J.-G. (1997) *L'Art négro-africain*, Paris: Presses Universitaires de France.

Blanchard, P. and Chatelier, A. (eds) (1993) *Images et Colonies*, Paris: Syros–ACHAC.

Bowie, M. (1991) *Lacan*, London: Fontana.

Brunette, P. and Wills, D. (eds) (1994) *Deconstruction and Visual Arts: Art, Media, Architecture*, Cambridge: Cambridge University Press.

Burckhardt, J. ([1860] 1990) *The Civilization of the Renaissance in Italy*, trans. S. G. C. Middlemore, with intro. by P. Burke, notes by P. Murray, London: Penguin.

Bryson, N. (1988) *Calligram: Essays in New Art History from France*, Cambridge: Cambridge University Press.

Carroll, D. (1987) *Paraesthetics: Foucault, Lyotard, Derrida*, London: Methuen.

Cusset, F. (2003) *French Theory: Foucault, Derrida, Deleuze & Cie et les mutations de la vie intellectuelle aux États-Unis*, Paris: La Découverte; *French Theory: How Foucault, Derrida, Deleuze & Co. Transformed the Intellectual Life of the United States*, trans. Jeff Fort, Minneapolis, MN: University of Minnesota Press, 2008.

Damisch, H. (1974) 'S. Freud en voyage vers Londres', in H. Damisch and H. Martin, *Adami*, Paris: Galerie Maeght, 8–43.

—— (1987) *L'origine de la perspective*, Paris: Flammarion.

—— (2002) 'Traits', in Marianne Alphant and Nathalie Léger (eds), *R/B: Roland Barthes*, Paris: Seuil/Centre Pompidou/IMEC, 91–4.

—— (2004) *Voyage à Laversine*, Paris: Seuil.

—— and Martin, H. (1974) *Adami*, Paris: Galerie Maeght.

Davis, O. (2010) *Jacques Rancière*, Cambridge: Polity.

Debord, G. ([1967] 1992) *La Société du spectacle*, Paris: Gallimard.

Debray, R. (1992) *Vie et mort de l'image: Une histoire du regard en Occident*, Paris: Gallimard.

Derrida, J. (1967) *L'écriture et la différence*, Paris: Seuil; *Writing and Difference*, trans. A. Bass, Chicago, IL: Chicago University Press, 1978.

—— (1978) *La Vérité en peinture*, Paris: Flammarion; *The Truth in Painting*, trans. G. Bennington and I. McLeod, Chicago, IL: Chicago University Press, 1987.

—— and Plissart, M. F. (1985) *Droit de regards*, Paris: Minuit; *Right of Inspection*, trans. D. Wills, New York: Monacelli Press, 1998.

Diderot, D. (1975–83) *Salons*, 3 vols, ed. J. Seznec and J. Adhémar, Oxford: Clarendon.

Didi-Huberman, G. (1990) *Devant l'Image: Question posée aux fins d'une histoire de l'art*, Paris: Minuit; *Conflicting Images: Questioning the Ends of a Certain History of Art*, trans. John Goodman, University

Park, PA: Pennsylvania State University Press, 2004.
—— (1992) *Ce que nous voyons, ce qui nous regarde*, Paris: Minuit.
—— (1998) *L'Étoilement: Conversation avec Hantaï*, Paris: Minuit.
—— (2003) *Images malgré tout*, Paris: Minuit.
Duro, P. (1997) *The Academy and the Limits of Painting in Seventeenth-Century France*, Cambridge: Cambridge University Press.
Duve, Thierry de (1989) *Au nom de l'art: Pour une archéologie de la modernité*, Paris: Minuit.
—— (1987) *Essais, datés 1974–1986*, vol 1, Paris: La Différence.
Edwards, E. and Bhaumik, K. (2008) *Visual Sense: A Cultural Reader*, Oxford: Berg.
Forsdick, C. and Murphy, D. (eds) (2009) *Postcolonial Thought in the French-speaking World*, Liverpool: Liverpool University Press.
Foucault, M. (1966) 'Les Suivantes', *Les Mots et les Choses: Une archéologie des sciences humaines*, Paris: Gallimard, 19–31; 'Las Meninas', *The Order of Things: An Archaeology of the Human Sciences*, trans. A. Sheridan, London: Tavistock, 1970, 3–16.
—— (1971) *L'Ordre du discours*, Paris: Gallimard.
—— (1973) *Ceci n'est pas une pipe*, illustrations de René Magritte, Montpellier, fata morgana; *This Is Not a Pipe*, with illustrations and letters by René Magritte, ed. and trans. J. Harkness, Berkeley, CA: University of California Press, 1983.
—— (1975) *Surveiller et punir: Naissance de la prison*, Paris: Gallimard; *Discipline and Punish: The Birth of the Prison*, trans. A. Sheridan, New York: Vintage, 1979.
—— (1994a) *Dits et écrits, I: 1954–1969*, ed. D. Defert and F. Ewald, Paris: Gallimard.
—— (1994b) 'Des espaces autres: Hétérotopies', *Dits et écrits, IV: 1980–1988*, ed. D. Defert and F. Ewald, Paris: Gallimard.
Freud, S. (1999) *The Interpretation of Dreams*, trans. J. Crick, with introd. and notes by R. Robertson, Oxford: Oxford University Press.
Genet, J. ([1963] 1998) *L'Atelier d'Alberto Giacometti*, Paris: L'Arbalète.
Genette, G. (2006) *Bardadrac*, Paris: Seuil.
Iversen, M. (2002) 'Barthes on Art', in Paul Smith and Carolyn Wilde (eds), *A Companion to Art Theory*, Oxford: Blackwell, 327–36.
Jay, M. (1994) *Downcast Eyes: The Denigration of Vision in Twentieth-Century French Thought*, London and Berkeley, CA: University of California Press.
Jouin, H. (ed.) (2010) *Conférences de l'Académie royale de peinture et de sculpture*, Paris: Kessinger.

Kearney, R. (1994) 'Jacques Derrida', *Modern Movements in European Philosophy: Phenomenology, Critical Theory, Structuralism*, Manchester: Manchester University Press, 113–33.
Khatibi, A. (1971) *La mémoire tatouée*, Paris: Denoël.
—— with Mohamed Sijelmassi ([1976] 1994) *L'Art calligraphique de l'Islam*, Paris: Gallimard; *The Splendour of Islamic Calligraphy*, trans. James Hughes, London: Thames & Hudson, 1976.
—— (1983) *Maghreb pluriel*, Paris: Denoël.
—— (1985) 'Double criticism: The Decolonization of Arab Sociology', in Halim Barakat (ed.), *Contemporary North African Issues of Development and Integration*, Sydney: Croom Helm, 9–19. [Originally published in Khatibi 1983]
Kristeva, J. (1977) *Polylogue*, Paris: Seuil.
—— (1980) *Pouvoirs de l'horreur*, Paris: Seuil; *Powers of Horror: An Essay On Abjection*, trans. Leon Roudiez, New York, Columbia University Press, 1982.
—— (1998) *Visions capitales*, Paris: Réunion des Musées Nationaux.
Lacan, J. (1970) 'Le stade du miroir comme formateur de la fonction du Je', *Écrits I*, Paris: Seuil, 89–97 [1st edn, 1966].
—— (1973) *Les Quatre Concepts fondamentaux de la psychanalyse (Séminaire XI)*, Paris: Seuil.
Laplanche, J. and Pontalis, J.-B. (1967) *Vocabulaire de la psychanalyse*, Paris: Seuil.
Le Bot, M. (1975) *Valerio Adami: Essai sur le formalisme critique*, Paris: Galilée.
Lee, R. W. (1967) *Ut Pictura Poesis: The Humanistic Theory of Painting*, New York: W. W. Norton.
Levy, S. (1990) 'Foucault on Magritte on Resemblance', *Modern Language Review* 85(1) (Jan.), 50–6.
Lord, J. (1986) *Giacometti: A Biography*, London: Faber.
Lyotard, J.-F. (1971) *Discours, figure*, Paris: Klincksieck.
—— (1983a) *Le Différend*, Paris: Minuit.
—— (1983b) 'Préface', *Adami: peintures récentes*, Paris: Galerie Maeght.
—— (2008) *Que peindre?*, Paris: Hermann.
Marin, L. (1971) *Études sémiologiques: Écritures, peintures*, Paris: Klincksieck.
—— (1988) 'Le Trompe-l'œil, un comble de la peinture', in R. Court *et al.*, *L'Effet trompe-l'œil dans l'art et la psychanalyse*, Paris: Dunod, 75–92.
—— (1994) *De La Représentation*, Paris: Gallimard/Seuil.

—— (1995) *Sublime Poussin*, Paris: Seuil.
—— (1997) *De l'Entretien*, Paris: Minuit.
Marriner, R. (2002) 'Derrida and the Parergon', in Paul Smith and Carolyn Wilde (eds), *A Companion to Art Theory*, Oxford: Blackwell, 349–59.
Mathews, T. (2001) *Literature, Art and the Pursuit of Decay in Twentieth-Century France*, Cambridge, Cambridge University Press.
—— (2007) 'Touch, Translation, Witness in Alberto Giacometti: *La Main, Le Nez*', *French Studies* 61(4) (Oct.), 447–59.
—— (2009) 'Trauma, Witness, Form: Thinking Walter Benjamin with Alberto Giacometti', in J. Chamarette and J. Higgins (eds), *Guilt and Shame: Essays in French Literature, Thought and Visual Culture*, Bern: Peter Lang, 161–76.
Meddeb, A. (1986) *Phantasia*, Paris: Sindbad.
—— (1995) 'La trace, le signe', in Gilbert Beaugé and Jean-François Clément (eds), *L'Image dans le monde arabe*, Paris: CNRS, 107–23.
—— (1997) 'La double mémoire. Méditation sur des photos postcoloniales prises à l'ère coloniale', *Dédale* 5–6 (spring), special issue 'Postcolonialisme', 268–87.
Merleau-Ponty, M. (1945) *Phénoménologie de la perception*, Paris: Gallimard.
Mills, M. and Tresch, J. (eds) (2011) *Audio-Visual*, special issue of *Grey Room*, 43, Cambridge, MA: MIT Press.
Mirzoeff, N. (2009) *An Introduction to Visual Culture*, London: Routledge.
Mitchell, W. J. T. and Hansen, M. B. N. (eds) (2010) *Critical Terms for Media Studies*, Chicago, IL and London: University of Chicago Press.
Mœglin-Delcroix, A. (2003) 'L'inspiration philosophique de l'art contemporain', *Revue d'esthétique* 44(3), 'Les artistes contemporains et la philosophie', 5–11.
Mudimbe, V. Y. (1973) *L'autre face du royaume: Introduction à des langues en folie*, Paris: L'Age d'Homme.
—— ([1991] 1999) '*Reprendre*: Enunciations and Strategies in Contemporary African Arts', in Olu Oguibe and Okwui Enwezor (eds), *Reading the Contemporary: African Art Theory to the Marketplace*, London: Institute of Visual Arts, 31–47. [French trans. by L. Jacob, in M. Quaghebeur *et al.*, *Papier blanc, encre noire: Cent ans de culture francophone en Afrique centrale*, vol. II, Brussels: Éditions Labor, 1992, 491–517]
Nancy, J.-L. (1988) 'L'Offrande sublime', in J.-F. Courtine *et al.*, *Du*

Sublime, Paris: Belin, 37–75; 'The Sublime Offering', J.-F. Courtine *et al.*, *Of the Sublime: Presence in Question*, trans. and afterword Jeffrey S. Librett, Albany: SUNY Press, 1993.
—— (2001) *Le Regard du portrait*, Paris: Galilée.
Pollock, G. (2007) *Encounters in the Virtual Feminist Museum: Time, Space and the Archive*, London: Routledge.
Rabaté, J.-M. (ed.) (1997) *Writing the Image after Roland Barthes*, Philadelphia, PA: University of Pennsylvania Press.
Rancière, J. (2003) *Le Destin des images*, Paris: La Fabrique.
—— (2008) *Le Spectateur émancipé*, Paris: La Fabrique.
Rockhill, G. and Watts, P. (eds) (2009) *Jacques Rancière: History, Politics, Aesthetics*, Durham, NC: Duke University Press.
Said, E. (1978) *Orientalism*, London: Penguin.
Sartre, J.-P. (1940) *L'Imaginaire*, Paris: Gallimard.
—— ([1948] 1949) 'La recherche de l'absolu', *Situations III*, Paris: Gallimard, 289–305.
Scott, M. (2008) 'Lacan's "Of the Gaze as *Objet Petit a*" as Anamorphic Discourse', *Paragraph* 31(3) (Nov.), 327–43.
Shawcross, N. (1997) *Roland Barthes on Photography: The Critical Tradition in Perspective*, Florida, FL: University of Florida Press.
Smith, P. and Wilde, C. (eds) (2002) *A Companion to Art Theory*, Oxford: Blackwell.
Snyder, J. (1985) '*Las Meninas* and the Mirror of the Prince', *Critical Inquiry* 11 (Jun.), 539–72.
Snyder, J. and Cohen, T. (1980) 'Reflexions on *Las Meninas*: Paradox Lost', *Critical Inquiry* 7 (winter), 429–47.
Soulages, F. (1998) *Esthétique de la Photographie: La perte et le reste*, Paris: Nathan.
Thévoz, M. (1996) 'Le miroir et l'*in-fente*', *Le Miroir infidèle*, Paris: Minuit, 36–54.
Titus-Carmel, G. (2003) *Épars: textes & poèmes 1990–2002*, Cognac: Le Temps qu'il fait.
Vouilloux, B. (1998) *Un art de la figure: Francis Ponge dans l'atelier du peintre*, Villeneuve d'Ascq: Presses universitaires du Septentrion.
—— (2004a) L'Œuvre en souffrance: entre poétique et esthétique, Paris: Belin.
—— (2004b) *Tableaux d'auteurs: après l'*Ut pictura poesis, Saint-Denis: Presses universitaires de Vincennes.
—— (2005) *La Peinture dans le texte, XVIII–XXe siècles*, Paris: CNRS.
—— (2010) *La Nuit et le silence des images: Penser l'image avec Pascal*

Quignard, Paris: Hermann.

—— (2011) *Le Tournant 'artiste' de la littérature française: écrire avec la peinture au XIXe siècle*, Paris: Hermann.

Welch, E. J. (2009) 'Stars of CCTV: Technology, Visibility and Identity in the Work of Sophie Calle and Annie Ernaux', *Nottingham French Studies* 48, 55–67.

—— and McGonagle, J. (2011) (eds), 'Untying the Knot? France and Algeria in Contemporary Visual Culture', *Modern & Contemporary France* 19(2), 123–8.

Wilson, S. (2010) *The Visual World of French Theory: Figurations*, New Haven, CT and London: Yale University Press.

Part I
Precursors: phenomenology and semiotics

1

Merleau-Ponty: the madness of vision

Nathalie Aubert

Il y a une sorte de folie de la vision.
(Merleau-Ponty 1968: 106)

Maurice Merleau-Ponty's *Phenomenology of Perception* was published in 1945, at the same time as Sartre's *Existentialism Is a Humanism*; it was also the year they both created *Les Temps modernes*. In his article 'The War Has Taken Place' that appeared in the first issue of *Les Temps modernes*, Merleau-Ponty noted: 'We have learned history and we claim that it must not be forgotten' ([1945] 1964a: 150). At the heart of *Phenomenology of Perception* is a discussion of consciousness of being in the world, and perhaps, more precisely, of being in *this* world. The kind of concrete philosophy that Merleau-Ponty was intending to establish therefore claimed that we could not escape our coexistence with others and for this reason philosophy could not be severed from language and history. His ambition to find truth in our being-in-the world – and this coexistence with others is also one of the stepping stones towards a philosophy aimed at defining the nature of the look – called first of all for a return to the perceived world as the presupposed foundation of all rationality. The perceived world for Merleau-Ponty is always the presupposed foundation of all rationality, all value and all existence even if there is a whole cultural world which constitutes a second level of perceptual experience.

In this chapter, I will first examine Merleau-Ponty's *Phenomenology of Perception* and its thesis of the 'primacy of perception' and progressively follow the philosopher's emphasis on *visual* perception as the archetypal form of all perception. Looking for truth in perception meant that Merleau-Ponty took an unprecedented level of interest in art: I will then examine the way he articulates his 'topography of a phenomenology of painting' (Johnson 1993: 3) and move on to his unfinished text, *The*

Visible and the Invisible, in which he takes up again a number of his early analyses of the object, the body, and the relation between the seer and the visible, in order to show that they acquire their full meaning only outside of a psychological interpretation and when they are enveloped in a new phenomenological ontology.

Merleau-Ponty opens the *Phenomenology of Perception* with a direct question: 'What is phenomenology?' Anchoring his answer in Husserl's works,[1] he provides a deceptively simple definition:

> Phenomenology is the study of essences; and according to it, all problems amount to finding definitions of essences: the essence of perception, or the essence of consciousness, for example. ([1945] 2001: vii)

Immediately, however, things get more complicated:

> But phenomenology is also a philosophy which puts essences back into existence, and does not expect to arrive at an understanding of man and the world from any starting point other than that of their 'facticity'. (*ibid.*)

At the same time, this facticity serves as a basis for a *transcendental* philosophy, which 'places in abeyance the assertions arising out of the natural attitude, the better to understand them' (*ibid.*). The task of phenomenology is the descriptive analysis of essences as they appear to our intellectual intuition. Its realisation requires the search for a foundation, a sphere in which things give themselves absolutely; that is, with a clarity, distinctness and completeness which renders them apodictic, or demonstrably certain. The originality of Merleau-Ponty's approach is that it is seeking this facticity in a world that is always 'already there'.

To try, as Descartes had attempted before, to establish a philosophy that is both a 'rigorous science' *and* an 'account of space, time and the world as we 'live' them' (*ibid.*) appears, against the background of rationalist philosophy, an impossible, contradictory task. And yet this is the very programme of Merleau-Ponty's *Phenomenology of Perception*, which is supposed to account for the paradox of immanence and transcendence that are both present *in* perception. In this book it was Merleau-Ponty's intention to establish a solid basis for the research which would take him forward from the phenomenology of perception to studies on imagination, language, culture, reason and on aesthetic, ethical, political and even religious experience.[2]

With the thesis of the 'primacy of perception', Merleau-Ponty meant to assert first of all that the perceived life-world is the primary reality. Following Husserl's call for a return to 'things themselves', he intended to regain the experience of the intertwining of the subject and the object that had been lost in dualistic philosophies. So doing, Merleau-Ponty found that the question of perception merged with the ontological question in its simplest form, namely an inquiry into the meaning of the being of what is.

Indeed, Merleau-Ponty argues that it is in and through our experience, primordially perceptual, that we are initiated into the thing itself. It is in the 'immanence' of what we 'live' that we find a path towards transcendence. This explains the purpose of the phenomenological return to the things themselves as a return to perception. In *The Primacy of Perception*, Merleau-Ponty establishes that 'the perceived world is always the presupposed foundation of all rationality, all value and all existence' (1964b: 13) even if 'there is a whole cultural world which constitutes a second level about perceptual experience' (*ibid.*: 33). Prior to this 'second level of perceptual experience', there is perception in itself, 'the fundamental basis which cannot be ignored' (*ibid.*). Instead of approaching perception on the basis of consciousness, he approached consciousness as based on perception. This means not only that consciousness is a moment of perception, but that consciousness of self *is* a perception:

> At the outset of the study of perception, we find in language the notion of sensation, which seems immediate and obvious: I have a sensation of redness, of blueness, of hot or cold. It will, however, be seen that nothing could in fact be more confused, and that because they accepted it readily, traditional analyses missed the phenomenon of perception. ([1945] 2001: 3)

Significantly, the first sentence of the first chapter of his study mentions language and how we wrongly assume that we understand perception because we accept a certain type of formulation without questioning what is at the heart of the sensation (of red, blue, hot or cold) itself. Perception is the sensation *and* its expression and that is where we need to start. Merleau-Ponty is unquestionably the first to have clearly understood this, as *Phenomenology of Perception* confirms (in particular the chapter devoted to the *cogito*). Having mentioned the 'traditional analyses' of perception, Merleau-Ponty, referring to the works of Descartes, Kant, Husserl, Heidegger and Sartre, explains how they failed to fully account for the phenomenon of perception. Moving away from the Cartesian model in which perception is not an event of the world but an act of the subject, Merleau-Ponty tried to explore in

Phenomenology of Perception the pre-reflexive phenomenal field which he called 'being in the world' (*ibid.*: xiii), examining the experience of perception prior to the construction of the body as object and the *cogito* as a rational subject. 'Vision' for him could not be reduced, as in the empiricist tradition, to a mere sensation nor could it be an escape into the purer world of eidetic essences. 'The perceived is not limited to that which strikes my eyes' he contended, 'when I am sitting at my desk, the space is closed behind me not only in idea, but also in reality' (1965: 249).

This 'inherence to the world' explains Merleau-Ponty's emphasis on the body; he goes so far as to claim that vision is linked with the other senses, and that touch for example plays a role in our perception of colours. There is no objectifying gaze in his work,[3] rather an 'inherence' to the textured quality of the world surrounding us. The world is apprehended by him on the level of an interactive presence and the lived body is irreducible to a static image observed from without: 'the lived perspective that which we actually perceive, is not a geometric or photographic one' (Johnson 1993: 64). Equally, because the body is not a static image, Merleau-Ponty echoed Bergson in stressing temporality as one of its constituent elements.[4] This position emerges towards the end of *Phenomenology of Perception*, in particular in the chapter dedicated to temporality.[5] Merleau-Ponty's work thus argues that visual images are not instantaneous snapshots of external reality, that they have a duration. Most importantly, this temporal dimension forms the basis of his definition of the visual as a knot of words and images.

Having criticised classical prejudices relating to perception (and in particular the hegemony of a vision-based, vision-centred episteme found in the division between object and subject as presented in both the empiricist and intellectualist tradition) in *Phenomenology of Perception*, he endeavoured, in an unfinished text (edited by Claude Lefort after the author's untimely death in 1961) known as *The Visible and the Invisible*, to take up again a number of his early analyses by concentrating especially on the thing, the body, the relation between the seer and the visible. *The Visible and the Invisible* is the result of Merleau-Ponty's exploration in his latter years of the relationship between perception and language. In *Phenomenology of Perception*, Merleau-Ponty set out an optimistic hermeneutic belief in the saturation of the world with meaning, but came up against how to extract this meaning without losing altogether the directness of the initial contact with the world, with the things themselves; in other words, how the visible and the invisible can interact in a non-contradictory way is one of his key preoccupations.

Appearing at the end of *The Visible and the Invisible*, his 'working notes' allow us to see Merleau-Ponty's thought on language at work. Under the date 27 October 1959, he wrote:

> I describe perception as diacritical, relative, oppositional system – the primordial space as topological (that is, cut out in a total voluminosity which surrounds me, in which I am, which is behind me as well as before me...)
>
> This is right. But there is all the same this difference between perception and language, that I *see* the perceived things and that the significations on the contrary are invisible. ([1964] 1968: 213–14)

Perception is now almost entirely concentrated in the act of seeing:

> We see the things themselves, the world is what we see: formulae of this kind express a faith common to the natural man and the philosopher – the moment he opens his eyes; they refer to a deep-seated set of mute 'opinions' implicated in our lives. But what is strange about this faith is that if we seek to articulate it into theses or statements, if we ask ourselves what is this *we*, what *seeing* is, and what *thing* or *world* is, we enter into a labyrinth of difficulties and contradictions. (*ibid.*: 3; Merleau-Ponty's emphasis)

As we have seen, the contribution that Merleau-Ponty made to phenomenology, was to show that the fundamental concepts of modern philosophy, such as the distinction between subject and object, essence and fact, being and nothingness, concepts that are in constant use, already implicate a singular interpretation of the world and cannot lay claim to special dignity when our intention is precisely to go back to our experience in order to seek in it *the birth of meaning*. And one of Merleau-Ponty's great intuitions is that the return to the birth of meaning, the description of this perceptual process has to be firmly anchored in an elaborate definition of vision: 'True philosophy consists in re-learning to look at the world' ([1945] 2001: xx).

Since *The Phenomenology of Perception*, and even more so *The Visible and the Invisible*, Merleau-Ponty's insistence on the absence of exteriority between vision and the world led him to emphasise that 'to look at the world' is also an interrogation of the question of 'how to *tell* the world'. The first language he questioned was of course his own: 'Consider language, even philosophical language, not as a sum of statements or of "solutions", but as a veil lifted, a verbal chain woven' ([1964]

1968: 199). The ontological affinity between vision and the visible means that vision cannot pierce the ontological texture out of which it is made. This transcendence is what the philosopher calls *chiasm*; equally, the incarnate condition of vision, the fact that vision occurs in the milieu of the world, 'as an envelopment irreducible in principle to frontal grasp' (Barbaras 2004: 156) is what Merleau-Ponty called, following Husserl, the *flesh*. More precisely, since vision cannot be distinguished from the world, it follows that the world cannot be distinguished from vision either. The duality between subject and object, which *merges* at the level of perception requires a new philosophical language to describe this paradoxical interaction or *intertwining*. Merleau-Ponty therefore reached a point where language, by definition supremely constituted by consciousness as an object, and therefore necessarily a substitute, a secondary means of communication, has to be, somehow, conceived on the model of vision.

After the publication of *Phenomenology of Perception*, Merleau-Ponty, understanding that language could no longer be considered simply as a form of corporeal expressivity, decided to concentrate on expression, of the *event* of expression. *The Phenomenology of Perception* makes frequent references to modern painting, to Cézanne in particular, in relation to philosophical questions of space, depth, lighting, colour and colour perception; and its publication in 1945 coincided with that of his work *Cézanne's Doubt*. Rather tellingly, *Cézanne's Doubt* appeared in *Fontaine*, a monthly review of poetry and French letters.[6] This clearly reflected Merleau-Ponty's belief that in order to form a new idea of reason, the philosopher could not restrict his inquiry to the fields of logic and mathematics, but needed to widen it to comprehend the meanings expressed in novels, poems and paintings. Indeed, defining the task ahead for phenomenology, he had concluded his preface to *Phenomenology of Perception* with this comparison:

> It is as painstaking as the works of Balzac, Proust, Valéry or Cézanne – by reason of the same kind of attentiveness and wonder, the same demand for awareness, the same will to seize the meaning of the world or of history as that meaning comes into being. In this way it merges into the general effort of modern thought. ([1945] 2001: xxi)

A central difficulty of Merleau-Ponty's approach to phenomenology is that although there are 'many ways for consciousness to be conscious', as he says in a famous phrase (*ibid.*: 124), we *never* completely escape from the realm of perceptual reality; even the seemingly independent structures of categorical thought (of 'rationality') are ultimately founded in perception. We are always immersed in the world and perceptually present to it. Equally, because our encounter with the 'something' would become lost in darkness, it has to be underpinned by an activity that constitutes it, that tries to grasp its significance. It is not a dogmatic doctrine but a programme of phenomenological research which he left incomplete at his death.

Although *Cézanne's Doubt* was dedicated to the study of two painters: Leonardo da Vinci and Cézanne, Merleau-Ponty was more interested, more attuned to Cézanne's efforts to 'paint from nature'. For, in the French painter, the philosopher found a modern artist who did not seem to be slave to the Renaissance techniques of linear perspective and outline. This 'instinctive' approach to painting, riddled with anxiety and doubt (the discordance between the posthumous recognition of Cézanne's achievements and the critical reception of his works during his lifetime is well documented)[7] results, in Merleau-Ponty's eyes, in a genuinely originary form of expression: 'the artist launches his work just as a man once launched the first word, not knowing whether it will be anything more than a shout' (Johnson 1993: 69). Cézanne himself reportedly said that he did not want to make a picture, but to attempt 'a piece of nature'. When he quoted Cézanne saying 'The landscape thinks itself in me' (*ibid.*: 67), Merleau-Ponty seemed to see a proof that in this painter's work the visible world is reconstructed in the process of appearing to visual sensation, which, for the philosopher epitomised his phenomenology of painting. The painter does not depict representations in his mind but rather paints with his body, which is mingled with the perceived world. This immersion of the viewer in the world on view is the ultimate rejection of the realist paradigm which turned vision into a view of the world rather than *in it*. The self revealed by painting is thus 'not a self through transparency, like thought, which only thinks its object by assimilating it, by constituting it, by transforming it into thought. It is a self through confusion, narcissism, through inherence of the one who sees in that which he sees' (1964b: 162–3).

And yet, although at one with the world, the painter is also apart from it, which is the paradoxical, enigmatic 'madness' of vision. *Eye and Mind*, which was the last work Merleau-Ponty saw published,[8] was conceived, according to Claude Lefort, as a preliminary statement to the book that the philosopher was writing at the time of his death, which became *The Visible and the Invisible*. Tellingly, Cézanne's painting (alongside that of Matisse, Klee and some Dutch artists) is still at the heart of the reflection on science and painting in *Eye and Mind.* Descartes's *Dioptrique* is criticised for failing to appreciate the ontological importance of painting. One can indeed argue, as Merleau-Ponty does, that Descartes is more concerned with drawing than painting when light, lighting, shadows, reflections and colours are 'all the objects of [the painter's] quest' (*ibid.*: 166). Merleau-Ponty concentrates on the body, going as far as arguing that 'we cannot imagine how a *mind* could paint' (*ibid.*: 162):

> It is by lending his body to the world that the artist changes the world into paintings. To understand these transsubstantiations we must go back to the working, actual body – not the body as a chunk of space or a bundle of functions but that body which is intertwining of vision and movement. (*ibid.*)

According to Merleau-Ponty, this is this link between vision and movement that forbids us to conceive vision as an operation of thought 'that would set up before the mind a picture or a representation of the world, a world of immanence and of ideality' (*ibid.*). For Merleau-Ponty, painting reveals the enigma of the body simultaneously seeing and being seen. This is what Merleau-Ponty attempts to describe in terms of chiasma or intertwining between body and world. The body envelops the world, that is to say makes it appear, only to the degree to which it is enveloped by it. Thus, the manifestation of the world for the body is at the same time a manifestation of the world by itself within the body, so that the body's constituting power coincides with the phenomenalising of the world. This intertwining reveals an ontological continuity between the body and the world, a co-belonging deeper than their opposition. To illustrate this, Merleau-Ponty uses the concept of 'flesh'. Flesh designates the co-appearance of the world and the subject as incarnated. In this theoretical elaboration, painting as an art is an essential stepping stone; its creations, a 'figured philosophy': 'In paintings themselves we could seek a figured philosophy' (*ibid.*: 168). By means of painting, Merleau-Ponty is hoping to be able to open up the originary signifying of language, its inscription in the world before the world transmutes this signifying into ideality.

After having described the mute expression of our contact with the world which he sees painting accomplishing (especially in Cézanne's art), Merleau-Ponty shows that pictorial expression announces that of language. If the world can be painted, it is because a scattered sense that contains already all of what painting and language will unfold on their own account is gathered into it. This is the path he chose to resolve the tension between perception and expression that was still at work in *Phenomenology of Perception* where he concentrated on intellectualism and its unwarranted confidence in language which ignored the fact of the world, reducing it to transparent significations. By contrast, the discovery of expression as absence of closure and infinity of sense that came at the time he was writing *The Prose of the World*, implied the unveiling of the world in its authentic, originary appearance. Merleau-Ponty thus offered an approach to expression in which the world is only given as a withdrawal, as a presence which, through its obscurity, gives birth to expression without ever being absorbed into the expressed.

If a number of the categories at work in *The Visible and the Invisible* are borrowed from the description of pictorial expression, the novel, and in particular, Proust's *In Search of Lost Time*, is also able to provide a model for this conception of expression, as one which is a movement preserving and continuing perceptual life (even while transforming it) and which is simultaneously apprehending ideality.[9] The difference between language and perception which dominated *Phenomenology of Perception*, is conceived, from *The Prose of the World* to *The Visible and the Invisible* as two *moments* of one, more fundamental reality:

> The philosopher knows better than anyone that what is lived is lived-spoken, that, born at this depth, language is not a mask over Being, but – if one knows how to grasp it with all its roots and its foliation – the most valuable witness to Being, that it does not interrupt an immediation that would be perfect without it, that the vision itself, the thought itself, are, as has been said, 'structured as a language', are *articulation* before the letter, apparition of something where there was nothing or something else. ([1964] 1968: 126)

Merleau-Ponty argues this on the basis of a new definition of perception, conceived as 'exegesis'. The lived is already 'spoken lived' before the letter. Paraphrasing Lacan, he explains that vision, placed at the same level as thought is 'structured as a language'.

This 'articulation before the letter' (as well as the very use of a botanical metaphor) is a transposition in philosophical terms of what Proust expressed in literary terms with the episode of the hawthorn bush in *Swann's Way*:

> It was in vain that I lingered beside the hawthorns – breathing in their invisible and unchanging odour, trying to fix it in my mind (which did not know what to do with it), losing it, recapturing it, absorbing myself in the

> rhythm which disposed the flowers here and there with a youthful light-heartedness and at intervals as unexpected as certain intervals in music – they went on offering me the same charm in inexhaustible profusion, but without letting me delve any more deeply, like those melodies which one can play a hundred times in succession without coming any nearer to their secret. I turned away from them for a moment so as to be able to return to them afresh [. . .] And then I returned to hawthorns, and stood before them as one stands before masterpieces which, one imagines, one will be better able to 'take in' when one has looked away for a moment at something else; but in vain did I make a screen with my hands, the better to concentrate upon the flowers, the feeling they aroused in me remained obscure and vague, struggling and failing to free itself, to float across and become one with them. They themselves offered me no enlightenment, and I could not call upon any other flowers to satisfy this mysterious longing. (Proust 1988: 151–2)

In this episode, Proust stages powerfully the idea of a sense that 'precedes' its strictly linguistic expression. Language is here considered as an analogue of perceptual life rather than a transforming of its meaning; Proust indicates here, and in other moments of his long novel (bearing all the marks of a quest for truth), the insertion of expression into the world, the world as veiling of sense. And the reason why the author of *In Search of Lost Time* could provide such a model for Merleau-Ponty's conception of language is that Proust understood, better than anyone else, the movement which, in vision, opens upon a texture of Being of which the sensorial – yet enigmatic – messages are only the punctuations:

> No one has gone further than Proust in fixing the relations between the visible and the invisible, in describing an idea that is not the contrary of the sensible, that is its lining and its depth. ([1964] 1968: 149)

Expression is not a veil draped over the world but 'insofar as it is the very becoming of the world, what can open us to it' (Barbaras 2004: 66); or, in other words: 'The eye lives in this texture as man lives in his house' (1964b: 166).

Merleau-Ponty specifically refers to 'the little phrase' which, in Swann's love story with Odette, is like the 'anthem of their love', and he quotes from Proust: 'the notions of light, sound, of relief, of physical voluptuousness, which are the rich possessions with which our inward domain is diversified and adorned' (Proust 1988: 503). For Merleau-Ponty the arts, but also human passions and generally the experience of the visible world, all contribute (no less than science) to the exploration of an invisible which is, for him, the disclosure of a universe of ideas. The difference with science, and an important one in his view, is that these ideas cannot be detached from 'the sensible appearance and be erected into a second positivity' ([1964] 1968: 149). It is worth quoting Merleau-Ponty's comment on Proust's text at length, since it allows us to see the way perception and expression interconnect, and the way, even when speaking of music, Proust is still, in fact, speaking of the visible:

> Swann can of course close in the 'little phrase' between the marks of musical notation, ascribe the 'withdrawn and chilly tenderness' that makes up its essence or its sense to the narrow range of the five notes that compose it and to the constant recurrence of two of them: while he is thinking of these signs and this sense, he no longer has the 'little phrase' itself, he has only 'bare values substituted for the mysterious entity he had perceived, for the convenience of his understanding'. Thus it is essential to this sort of ideas that they be 'veiled with shadows', appear 'under a disguise'. They give us the assurance that the 'great unpenetrated and discouraging night of our soul' is not empty, is not 'nothingness'; but these entities, these domains, these worlds that line it, people it, and whose presence it feels like the presence of someone in the dark, have been acquired only through its commerce with the visible, to which they remain attached. (*ibid.*: 150)

This example from Proust's novel is in a way more telling than those derived from painting, since, it is, after all, a visual art. There is no doubt that Merleau-Ponty deliberately chose a musical example – in a novel where pictorial descriptions abound – to expand and illustrate what 'visible' means for him. The 'visibility' he has in mind is born out of our immersion in the world and of our ability to express it. Expression is anchored in intentionality, which is part of what the process of perception is. The possibility of expression inscribed in things themselves is the guarantee that 'there is something'. There is a 'lining' in the 'texture' of all things that is potentially the bearer of meaning: the 'absence', which Merleau-Ponty also calls 'a certain hollow, a certain interior' is the 'negativity that is not nothing' (*ibid.*: 151); it is, as he says quoting Valéry, something like the 'secret blackness of milk' (*ibid.*: 150). What Vinteuil's sonata's notes offer is a sort of screened presentation of ideas, entrenched behind these few notes, 'perfectly distinct from one another, unequal among themselves in value and in significance' (Proust 1988: 505). Merleau-Ponty concluded, after a passage entirely dedicated to music:

> With the first vision, the first contact, the first pleasure, there is initiation, that is, not the positing of a content, but the opening of a dimension that

can never again be closed, the establishment of a level in terms of which every other experience will henceforth be situated. The idea is this level, this dimension. ([1964] 1968: 151)

Artistic language contains better than ideas, matrices of ideas; all artistic forms are a language capable of introducing us to unfamiliar perspectives instead of confirming us in our own. Cézanne, Proust, among others, supplied Merleau-Ponty with a conception of artistic language which provides us with symbols that never stop developing; their style is what allows them to make manifest the visible world 'the coherent deformation' by which they concentrate 'the still scattered meaning of [their] perception and make it exist expressly' (1964c: 54–5):

> Precisely because it dwells and makes us dwell in a world we do not have a key to, the work of art teaches us to see and ultimately gives us something to think about as no analytical work can. (*ibid.*: 77)

Following Husserl, Merleau-Ponty came to consider that:

> the whole of philosophy [...] consists in restoring a power to signify, a birth of meaning, or a wild meaning, an expression of experience by experience, which in particular clarifies the special domain of language. And in a sense, as Valéry said, language is everything, since it is the voice of no one, since it is the very voice of the things, the waves and the forests. ([1964] 1968: 155)

In the end however, this reliance on artistic language, literary language in particular and the metaphorical shift in his own language, is certainly one of the reasons why — along with his sudden death — his philosophy was considered an impasse by many of his successors. As Claude Lefort pointed out:

> The key notions introduced in some of the essays which appeared in *Signs*, in *The Prose of the World*, in *Eye and Mind*, and especially in *The Visible and the Invisible* [...] had clearly stopped to operate in the way concepts do in metaphysical discourse. Flesh, chiasmus, reversibility, circularity and dehiscence, or dimensions, hinges and pivots, these words did not lend themselves to a strict definition.[10]

One of the problems that the later generation had with Merleau-Ponty's writings was that, as Martin Jay explained: 'Rather than celebrating the mutual imbrication of the discursive and the figural in the flesh of the world, they would question any positive resolution of the conflict between them' (1993: 325–6). Other critics included practitioners of the visible such as the Belgian painter René Magritte who thought that *Eye and Mind* offered a conception of the visible that was too meaningful, too expressive, robbing this realm of its enigmas.[11] Foucault would include Merleau-Ponty in the category of 'transcendental narcissism' which he condemned in *The Archaeology of Knowledge* ([1969] 1989: 203) and Derrida would condemn phenomenology as imprisoned within the 'closure of representation' as he called it. His own intention was to deliver phenomenology from that which 'still holds it within the confines of a metaphysics, the metaphysics of presence' (1973: 94). Finally, it was especially structuralism which induced a crisis in phenomenology,[12] and 'deconstruction' was used as a method to unmask what was considered naive in Merleau-Ponty's 'phenomenological positivism'. This critical discourse coalesced, not always coherently or self-consciously (Jay 1993: 327), into an attack on visuality *in all its forms* coinciding with the proclamation of the death of the subject which disqualified a philosophy essentially centred on the experience of 'being for myself'.

Today, however, we can say that Merleau-Ponty's enduring legacy, his conception of an incarnated reality of vision in the corporeal and social context have been developed again by a number of philosophers (Nancy, and then Rancière)[13] whose reflection on the visual, like his, is often based on art; painting in particular, not as representation of the empirical world – understood in the platonic, metaphysical way – but as *presentation* of world, of sense, of existence.

References

Aubert, N. (2003), *Proust: La traduction du sensible*, Oxford: Legenda.

Barbaras, R. (2004) *The Being of the Phenomenon: Merleau-Ponty's Ontology*, trans. Ted Toadvine and Leonard Lawlor, Bloomington and Indianapolis, IN: Indiana University Press.

Derrida, J. (1973) *Speech and Phenomenon: And Other Essays on Husserl's Theory of Signs*, trans. D. B. Allison, Evanston, IL: Northwestern University Press.

Descombes, V. (1980) *Modern French Philosophy*, Cambridge: Cambridge University Press.

Foucault, M. ([1969] 1989) *The Archaeology of Knowledge and the Discourse on Language*, trans. A. M. Sheridan Smith, London: Routledge.

Jay, M. (1993) *Downcast Eyes*, Berkeley, CA: University of California Press.

Johnson, G. A. (1993) *The Merleau-Ponty Aesthetics Reader*, Evanston, IL: Northwestern University Press.
Lefort, C. (1982) 'Philosophie et non-philosophie', *Esprit* (Jun.), 101–12.
Merleau-Ponty, M. ([1945] 2001) *Phenomenology of Perception*, trans. C. Smith, London: Routledge.
—— ([1964] 1968) *The Visible and the Invisible*, trans. A. Lingis, Evanston, IL: Northwestern University Press.
—— ([1945] 1964a) 'The War Has Taken Place', trans. Dreyfus and Dreyfus in *Sense and Non-Sense*, Evanston, IL: Northwestern University Press.
—— (1964b) *The Primacy of Perception*, trans. J. M Edie, Evanston, IL: Northwestern University Press.
—— (1964c) *Indirect Language and the Voices of Silence in Signs*, Evanston, IL: Northwestern University Press.
—— (1965) *The Structure of Behaviour*, trans. A. L. Fisher, London: Methuen.
Proust, M. (1988) *Swann's Way*, trans. C. K. Scott Moncrieff, London: Penguin Classics.
Rancière, J. (1998a) *La Chair des mots: Politiques de l'écriture*, Paris: Galilée.
—— (1998b) *La Parole muette: Essai sur les contradictions de la littérature*, Paris: Hachette.
—— (2000) *Le Partage du sensible*, Paris: La Fabrique.
Zola, É. (2008) *The Masterpiece*, ed. R. Pearson, trans. T. Walton, Oxford: Oxford World's Classics.

Notes

1 In *Phenomenology of Perception*, Merleau-Ponty, immediately emphasising the possible 'contradictions' of a 'doctrine which says everything', mentioned both Husserl and Heidegger alongside Descartes. For Merleau-Ponty, Husserl's *Cartesian Meditations* is the primary philosophical reference for anybody trying to establish a philosophy which shall be a 'rigorous science' ([1945] 2001: vii).
2 In *The Primacy of Perception*, where Merleau-Ponty addressed the Société Française de Philosophie in order to defend the central thesis of his recently published *Phenomenology of Perception* shortly after its publication, he acknowledged the programmatic aspect of his *Phenomenology of Perception*: [it is] 'only a preliminary study, since it hardly speaks of culture or history' (1964b: 25).
3 This is where he differs significantly with Sartre's analysis of the gaze. For

Sartre's conception of a 'reifying look' goes as far as 'ocularphobia' (see Jay 1993: 276).

4 Bergson's influence on Merleau-Ponty is significant, and fully acknowledged by the author of *Phenomenology of Perception.* Bergson crucially associated perception not with knowledge but with action. For him, perception amounts to the production of images which are in movement because the perceiving subject is a living subject. It is the singularity of this movement explaining the emergence of specific manifestations that accounts for perception. Perceptual manifestation does indeed proceed in this instance from the strict relation between living movement and phenomenal field. In so far as it stems from movement, perception is satisfied with focusing on the thing itself in order to circumscribe it; it is intentional because of its mobility. This is the reason why the way to access perception in a satisfactory way cannot therefore be either by coincidence or fusion with things: an essential component of the process of understanding perception is an interrogation on language.

5 In his analysis, Merleau-Ponty uses both Heidegger and Bergson, even if he thinks that the latter 'was wrong in explaining the unity of time in terms of its continuity' preferring to follow Heidegger's definition in *Sein* und *Zeit* according to which 'temporality temporalizes itself as future-which-lapses-into-the-past-by-coming-into-the-present' (Merleau-Ponty [1945] 2001: 420).

6 *Fontaine: Revue mensuelle de la poésie et des lettres françaises* 6(47) (Dec. 1945), 80–100. The director of the journal was Max-Pol Fouchet. This issue of the journal included essays by Roger Caillois on Bossuet and Pascal, by Georges Blin on Gabriel Marcel, by Paul Éluard and Paul Claudel. It also contained the announcement of the first number of *Les Temps modernes*, the political and philosophical journal edited by Sartre and Merleau-Ponty (see Johnson 1993: 375).

7 It famously caused his break-up with his childhood friend, Émile Zola, who, in *L'Œuvre* [The Masterpiece] had depicted a failed painter, Claude Lantier, who, Cézanne largely assumed, had been based on his friend's perception of him.

8 Significantly, it was finished in July–August 1960, in Le Tholonet, at the heart of Cézanne's countryside. Indeed, it was a place where the painter particularly enjoyed going because of the views one gets on the Mount Sainte-Victoire from the village. *Eye and Mind* appeared in the inaugural issue of *Art de France* 1(1) (Jan. 1961). After his death, it was reprinted in *Les Temps modernes* no. 184–5, along with seven articles devoted to him. Gallimard published it as a book in 1964.

9 As I have tried to show in Aubert (2003).

10 'Les notions clés introduites dans certains essais de Signes, dans La Prose du Monde, dans *L'Œil et l'esprit*, dans *Le Visible et l'Invisible* surtout [...] n'exerçaient plus manifestement la fonction qu'on prête aux concepts dans le

discours métaphysique. *Chair, chiasme, réversibilité, circularité, déhiscence,* ou *dimensions, charnières, pivots,* ces mots ne semblaient plus passibles d'une stricte définition' (Lefort 1982: 101).

11 In a letter to Alphonse de Waelhens of 1962, he wrote: 'The only kind of painting Merleau-Ponty deals with is a variety of serious but futile divertissement, of interest only to well-intentioned humbugs. The only painting worth looking at has the same *raison d'être* as the *raison d'être* of the world – mystery' (quoted in Jay 1993: 326).

12 Although, as Vincent Descombes points out (1980: 77), structuralism was not a philosophical school in the way that the phenomenological school was. Nonetheless: 'The effect of structuralism upon philosophical discourse is [...] incontestable.'

13 Rancière uses the category of the 'flesh' as defined by Merleau-Ponty in a number of his books such as *La Parole muette, La Chair des mots* and *Le Partage du sensible.*

2

Christian Metz: constructing meaning in film

Martine Joly

Christian Metz (1931–93) is rightly considered as the founder of the semiology of cinema. His semiological thought, part of a wider structuralist movement dominant at the time, brought together cinema and linguistics, cinema and psychoanalysis, and later cinema with utterance theory.[1] Never one to be an intellectual 'maître' [guru], Metz was nevertheless exemplary in his openness and innovation, as well as his rigour. In an interview, Marc Vernet reminded Christian Metz of his 'trois régimes d'écriture différents' [three different writing regimes]: 'celui des *Essais*, celui de *Langage et cinéma* (qu'il a) explicitement voulu "bétonné", technique de A à Z, enfin celui du *Signifiant imaginaire*, avec un style beaucoup plus littéraire, plus fluide, parfois presque transparent' [that of the *Essais*, that of *Language and cinema* which he explicitly wanted to be 'rock solid', and finally that of the *Imaginary Signifier* with a much more literary style that is fluid, sometimes even transparent] (Marie and Vernet 1990: 276).

Film as text

It was the 1950s and 1960s that saw the founding of a semiology of cinema, or rather of 'film'. This was a way of looking at cinema that used a form of theorisation which, up until then and only recently, had been found in very diverse theoretical approaches to literature. There were plenty of historical, economic, sociological, above all critical studies. But in the 1960s there was now the start of a new theoretical grouping in France called filmology, with personalities such as André Bazin, Jean Mitry, Albert Laffay, on whom Christian Metz went on to write various in-depth studies.[2] According to Metz, 'définir actuellement la sémiologie du film ... c'est la volonté de traiter les films comme des *textes*, comme des unités de discours, en s'obligeant par là à rechercher les différents *systèmes* (qu'ils soient ou non des codes) qui viennent informer ces textes et s'impliciter en eux' [a definition today of the semiology of film is the wish to consider films as *texts*, as units of discourse which requires the search for the different *systems* which inform these texts and become part of them, whether based on codes or not] (Metz 1971: 14). From his first article onwards, 'Le cinéma: langue ou langage?' (1964), Metz's work on film as discourse will be based, right up to his final publication, on 'l'énonciation au cinéma' [utterance in cinema]. All his work represents a constant questioning of language and its materials, including the ways they work, the signifying processes, and using theories of utterance. Along the way, as with studies of all discourses, there was also bound to be a fundamental questioning of the links between psychoanalysis and language, and the whys and wherefores of psychoanalysis and cinema. The famous issue 4 of the structuralist journal *Communications* brought together a series of seminal articles, in addition to 'Le cinéma: langue ou langage?': Roland Barthes's 'La rhétorique de l'image', Claude Bremond's 'Le message narratif', Tzvetan Todorov's 'La description de la signification en littérature'. Looking back on his first article, we might be struck by the programmatic nature of the piece, and this may be part of our *a posteriori* synthesis of the work of Christian Metz. Indeed, there are three decades that separate *L'Énonciation impersonnelle ou le site du film* from this early article, but in the latter we can already see Metz's future trajectory, as well as that of many of his successors.

For each new research topic Metz begins with a 'dépouillement théorique des écrits précédents' [theoretically based survey of previous writing] (1964: 66). Hence his reference not only to the writers mentioned but also to the Russian Formalists, Eisenstein, or Bela Balàzs. There is work on Chaplin, on the French 'avant-gardistes' such as Epstein, Delluc and Dulac, and then Bazin and Merleau-Ponty; not to mention on contemporaries such as Souriau, Cohen-Séat, Mitry, Robbe-Grillet and Zazzo. Here the Germanist in Christian Metz (*agrégé*, former teacher at the Institut français in Hamburg and interpreter for Radio Hamburg), allowed him to read works by Rudolph Arnheim, and he even thought about translating *Film als Kunst* (*Film as Art*) in his seminar at the EHESS.[3] Just as he would fleece ['dépouiller'] Freud and Lacan for *Le signifiant imaginaire* (1977b), his translation (also unpublished) of Freud's *Witz und sein Beziehung zum Unbewussten* (*Le mot d'esprit et ses rapports avec l'inconscient* [Jokes and their relation to the unconscious]) came with his comments attached, as recalled by those who attended the seminar. Let us not forget that his seminar was very special in that it was both closed and open to the public; closed in the sense that Christian Metz allowed in (and with great generosity besides) only those people he had already spoken to individually about their motives, thereby avoiding the seminar becoming 'mondain' [fashionable], as was the case with certain other seminars at the EHESS at the time; but open, in the sense that he allowed many French and international researchers to attend and to talk about their own work, in such a way as to nourish theoretical research on cinema from as many different points of view as possible. Metz's weekly seminar allowed for an exploration of major and ancillary themes, both complementary and contradictory. In line with the essentially interdisciplinary nature of semiology, there were French and international theoreticians of sound, of 'énonciation' [utterance], gestalt, didactics, media studies, experimental cinema, narrative theory, generative grammar; not to mention sociologists, historians, experimental directors, French and international critics, and young researchers coming from many horizons. 'La sémiologie ... est "interdisciplinaire" par elle-même [...] elle entretient déjà, et couramment, des rapports avec autre chose: critique des idéologies, psychanalyse, féminisme, analyse textuelle, histoire structurale ... sciences de l'éducation, etc.' [Semiology is 'interdisciplinary' by its nature, it already has regular links with other subjects: forms of ideological critique, psychoanalysis, feminism, textual analysis, structural history, educational theory, etc.], as Christian Metz argued in a 1990 interview (Marie and Vernet 1990: 277).

'Le cinéma: langue ou langage?'

As for the links between cinema and linguistics, it fell to Christian Metz to 'épuiser' (research thoroughly) the expression 'langage cinématographique'. In his book *Langage et cinéma* which is based on the article 'Le cinéma: langue ou langage?', we find from the outset a concern with producing a systematic study of the question in its theoretical domain: here, that of linguistics: 'La sémiologie peut et doit s'appuyer fortement sur la linguistique, mais elle ne se confond pas avec elle' [semiology can and must rely heavily on linguistics, but it is not to be confused with it] (1971: 58 n. 4). Thus we can see the appearance, progressively, that is to say 'programmatiquement', of a definition of a semiology of cinema: 'une théorie du fait filmique est non pas spécialement une approche inspirée de la linguistique, mêmė s'il faut passer par ceci pour atteindre à cela' [a theory of the filmic is not especially an approach inspired by linguistics, even if one has to go through one to reach the other] (*ibid.*: 13). Far from it being about an application of linguistics to cinema, as it has been often suggested and much discussed ('on n'applique jamais rien' [you never apply anything], Metz would say in his seminars), instead it is about a confrontation, of a measure, between language, the language system and cinema. If we can agree with the linguist André Martinet that what characterises a language system is the double articulation phoneme–moneme, which is possible only thanks to the isolation of smallest unities of sound and meaning, then it became clear that this isolation was no longer possible when applied to the cinema any more than to the image in general. Christian Metz insisted then on the heterogeneity of cinematographic language and showed that it was indeed a language but a language in the widest sense of the term, one which operates on five types of signifying material: the moving image, the written text, speech, noise and music.

However, if cinematographic language has no small units of meaning, it nevertheless assembles large syntagmatic units, which can be seen in the way they permutate, and these large units are described by Metz as 'segments autonomes' [free-standing segments] and for which he was to try to write an inventory, a 'Grande syntagmatique'. Thus cinematographic language shares with the language system a certain number of rules of functioning: those of developing along the two axes of the syntagm and the paradigm, or also according to the laws of rhetoric (1977b). These observations by Christian Metz were made following the major theoretical advance made by Roland Barthes in 'Éléments de sémiologie',[4] by making semiology part of linguistics and not the other way round as Ferdinand de Saussure had argued in the introduction to his *Cours de linguistique générale*. The cinema appeared then like a 'language without a language system' and furthermore stuck with narrativity. 'Passer d'une image à deux images, c'est passer de l'image au langage' [to move from one to two images, is to move from image to language], declared Christian Metz (1964: 63). He was showing all the while that as long as we do not forget what will later be called la 'suture' [stitching] operated by 'l'esprit humain, ce diachroniste impénitent' [the human spirit, that impenitent diachronist], this language 'ne fait qu'un avec la narrativité du film' [is but one with the narrativity of film] (*ibid.*: 64). Therefore it was necessary to underline the irresistible need to narrativise the montage between two frames, to fictionalise the stitching, just as Koulechov had once shown. Semiological analysis of film then becomes like an 'étude des discours et des "textes" . . . qui rencontrera inévitablement la sociologie, l'histoire des cultures, l'esthétique, la psychanalyse' [a study of discourses and 'texts' which comes inevitably into contact with sociology, cultural history, aesthetics, psychoanalysis] (*ibid.*).

But still, what precisely does the term 'cinema' cover? How is cinema different from film? Here Metz uses the cinema–film distinction made by Gilbert Cohen-Séat (1958), in order to sharpen this distinction and show the extent to which the filmic includes the cinematographic and vice versa, allowing Metz to describe nevertheless certain specificities of cinematographic language, this 'language without a language system'. As for '"grammaires" cinématographiques', was it an acceptable form of terminology for film? Christian Metz pointed out in the first two chapters of *Langage et cinéma* that cinema was not just a 'language', but a 'fait cinématographique', film constitutes a vast complex 'au sein duquel trois aspects prédominent avec force: aspect technologique, aspect économique, aspect sociologique' [at the heart of which three aspects dominate heavily; the technological, the economic and the sociological]; whereas a 'fait filmique' sees in each film an 'espace délimitable' [a definable space], an 'objet voué de part en part à la signification' [an object wholly given over to creating meaning], a 'discours clos' [a closed discourse], which allows itself to be considered 'comme un langage' [like a language] only 'dans son entier' [as a whole entity]. In other words, 'le cinématographique' would cover anything to do with the phenomenon 'cinema': economics (let us not forget the famous comment by the then culture minister André Malraux, 'cinema is also an industry'); sociology ('going to the cinema'); forms of expression (particular language, screen-play, cameras, microphones, actors, settings, etc.); world cinema (European, Indian, American, etc.); whereas the 'filmic', for its part, would be concerned strictly with the work itself, with the film in as much as it displays its cinematographic potential (1971).

La grande syntagmatique

As for the need to classify the various elements in a 'langage cinématographique', Metz went on to establish the first 'grande syntagmatique' (Metz 1968a). Its principle was to elaborate a typology of cinematographic sequences in films with narratives typical of

Hollywood, putting into play the eight types of syntagms that are needed in order to start analysing at a level that reflected the dominant mode in which films are put together, that is montage. So Metz isolated large units, 'segments autonomes', into which went all distinctive elements of the composition ('plan autonome' [free-standing section]/syntagms), of time (descriptive syntagms, parallel or alternate), of compactness (scene/sequence, with or without temporal ellipsis, of variable length). This was no different from the segments of montage found in the major narrative codes that Todorov was studying at the time in his narrative semiotics, alongside Greimas, Barthes and Bremond.

Many have criticised the fact that this typology did not account for the whole functioning of the 'cinématographique', that certain films may have no segment corresponding to the eight segments set out in 'La grande syntagmatique'. In particular, the typology did not correspond to the practice of the 'nouveau cinéma' (Château and Jost 1979). In this type of cinema, variations (or oppositions) would be no longer syntagmatic but paradigmatic. Furthermore, in as much as the 'grande syntagmatique' was interested above all in the visual aspect, Metz has been accused of ignoring the role of sound in cinema. In reality the question of sound, of speech, of the noises and the music, is very evident in the preoccupations of Metz's thought, which had set out at the earliest stage the notion of a language, be it visual or sound material. As for the first objection raised concerning the relations between the 'grande syntagmatique' and Hollywood film – or those between semiology and fictional film – Metz replied by underlining the fact that, given that fictional film is in the predominant category, semiology cannot but start by studying it. In so doing he went on to measure the extent to which his 'grande syntagmatique' was adapted to fit so-called modern cinema (1968a). He pointed out that 'modern' cinema (the *nouvelle vague*, in particular) was renewing narrative forms without abandoning them: 'Nous pensons ... que le principal apport du cinéma "nouveau" est d'avoir enrichi le récit filmique' [We believe that the main effect of the 'new' cinema is to have enriched the filmic] (*ibid.*). Furthermore, Christian Metz recognised that semiology 'doit s'occuper aussi de tous les films qui sont plus ou moins non-fictionnels' [must also consider all films which are more or less non-fictional], but added, with a nod towards his detractors: 'je ne me sens pas obligé de couvrir personnellement ... tout le champ de la sémiologie du cinéma; et pas obligé non plus de remplir personnellement la totalité du programme que j'ai pu esquisser moi-même dans *Langage et cinéma*, par exemple. Il y a d'autres chercheurs (heureusement pour moi!)' [I do not see myself obliged personally to cover the whole field of semiology of cinema, nor personally to carry out in its entirety what I myself set out in *Language and Cinema*. There are other researchers to do this (luckily for me)].[5] He suggested that we should understand semiology 'dans le sens d'analyse structurale du film et des films' [in the sense of structural analysis of film and films], with the aim of realising 'une théorie du fait filmique', which uses first of all a method inspired by linguistics, and then psychoanalysis, and then by theories of utterance, as 'les morceaux de l'acquis peuvent et doivent circuler' [the collected data can and must move around] (1971: 13).

So 'La grande syntagmatique' must not be considered as a universal typology, but one which reveals a dominant model of 'cinema', and which encourages us to isolate a system of oppositions (in accordance with the first rule of modern linguistics) that is operative in each particular film, so as to understand the particular system of signification in use. Metz went on, with Michèle Lacoste, to establish a list of 'segments autonomes' in the film *Adieu Philippine* by Jacques Rozier (1960), despite his declared aversion to 'exemples'. He preferred to work at a much wider theoretical level, he would say. Nevertheless, identifying the eighty-three 'segments autonomes' that make up Jacques Rozier's film, allowed him to arrive at a certain number of conclusions about the length of segments, about the history of styles in cinematography, about the connection between grammar and stylistics in cinematographics, all of which forms the basis of the particular rhetoric that belongs to each work. As it happens, this type of analysis allows us to show how *Adieu Philippine*, a film about 1960s youth and above all this youth's way of speaking about itself, privileges the 'scène' and the 'plan-séquence' as the 'types syntagmatiques les mieux adaptés à la conversation' [scene and sequence layout are the syntagmatic types the best suited to conversation]. This work allowed Metz also to distinguish between the 'séquence cinématographique', the 'unité filmique' (or 'segment autonome'), on the one hand, and the narrative sequence (normally called 'sequence') on the other which he calls the 'unité scénaristique'.

But other precisions, verifications and proposals were made by Christian Metz in his explorations published in *Essais sur la signification au cinéma*, *Essais sémiotiques* and in the journal *Communications*. Here are a number of examples ['postures'] which seem to us to remain fundamental: the distinction between 'illusion de réalité' and 'impression de réalité' is intensified in the cinema thanks to the 'injection "dans l'irréalité de l'image de la réalité du mouvement" et du son (perçu)' [injection 'into the irreality of the image of the reality of movement' and of (perceived) sound] (1965c: 82); Metz's insistence on the fact that what can define the image cannot be reduced to an analogy, even if this notion obviously needs to be preserved. It was important for the semiologist that the '"au delà"' ['beyond'] and the '"en deçà"' [this side] (of analogy) be considered in all the codes which add to the analogy. Indeed these codes construct the analogy (rhetorical codes, socio-cultural codes, linguistic codes) and allow us to refute, at this stage, the 'mythe de la "pureté visuelle"' [myth of 'visual purity'], which is very much present today and regularly invoked to point to the myth of 'pouvoir' commonly attributed to images (1970a: 9). Hence his work on the notion of the 'vraisemblable cinématographique' which is closer to the 'effet-genre', a relativist criterion if ever there was one, and which is impossible to bring up to date, according to Metz, unless there is some form of a 'possible' proposed; this would not be a conventional 'possible' at all, allowing a new form of 'vraisemblable' [verisimilitude] (1968b). Crucial in all this was the essay on 'Trucage et cinéma' (1972: 173–93) which helps us to understand the reception and the efficiency (or inefficiency) of what is known as 'special effects' which dominate in today's cinema. In particular he insisted upon the distinction between invisible effects and visible ones: invisible but perceptible effects bring a satisfaction to the viewer who appreciates that 'l'on ne voit rien' [we see nothing], it is that well done, but enjoying also the feeling of being complicit in a particular type of cinema (1975c).

Impersonal speech

It is in the area of impersonal speech that Metz's research on enunciation in the cinema appears, even if it is true to say that, in chronological terms, this only comes in the final publications Metz. To study this enormous area Metz uses the same method: exploring existing works on enunciation, understanding them fully and working out if and how they might help to think about enunciation in the cinema. In 1983, a whole number of the journal *Communications* (38) is given over to 'Énonciation et cinéma'. In 1987, 'en marge de travaux récents sur l'énonciation au cinéma', Metz published a first consideration of the question in the first number of the journal *Vertigo* (1988) using the same title as that of his final work, *L'Énonciation impersonnelle ou le site du film* (1991). Metz offers us first a problematisation of the very notion of enunciation (coming originally from linguistics), to admit that, once the arguments over the pseudo-transparency of the filmic have ended, we can counterpose an 'énonciation diégétisée (donc imperceptible) à une énonciation énoncée (donc perceptible), qui se signale d'une façon ou d'une autre' [utterance lost in the diegesis (therefore imperceptible) with an utterance that is uttered (therefore perceptible) which signals itself one way or another]. If 'l'énonciation c'est le fait d'énoncer' [utterance is the act of uttering], then to borrow from linguistics appears founded; but to see how it works in films, then we have to abandon the 'human' terms, according to Metz, such as 'énonciateur' [utterer] and 'énonciataire' [utteree]. Indeed Metz considered that utterance in the cinema is never 'personnifiante' but always impersonal because it is always 'accrochée au texte' [tied to the text], its 'site': 'Tout se passe comme si le film ne pouvait manifester l'instance de profération qu'il porte en lui et qui le porte, qu'en nous parlant de caméra, de spectateur, ou en désignant sa propre filmitude, c'est-à-dire dans tous les cas en se montrant du doigt' [Everything happens as if the film can show the moment of its proferation that it carries in it and which carries it only by speaking to us about the camera, the spectator or by pointing to its own filmic status, that is only by pointing to itself] (1991: 214). This proposal, qualified by an 'envolée théorique' written by Metz (*ibid.*: 173), is carried out after close examination of the main forms of address in the cinema: the look towards the camera, screen divided into boxes, split screens, mirrors, inclusion of the planning in the film, film within the film, 'subjective' images, I-narrations, etc. But it is the chapter on images and sounds that are called 'neutral' which allows Metz to make his point about 'impersonal' speech; for, as he reminds us, there is no 'nobody's shot', no 'objectif' framing ('not from point') that is able to hold, even if the regime he describes as 'objectif-non-conditionné' can be seen to correspond to what we call 'neutre': 'il faut tourner le dos à cette façon de voir, quelque ancienne et courante qu'elle soit, il n'existe pas d'images neutres. Tout élément visuel ou sonore de tout film ... s'est construit sur des choix multiples impliquant une activité ... L'énonciation – à ne pas confondre avec ses marques et ses configurations – est omniprésente et responsable de chaque détail' [we have to turn our back on this way of looking, however old-fashioned or current it may be, as there is no image that is neutral. Every visual and sound element in every film is based on a range of choices which suggest that someone has taken an active role. Utterance – not to be confused with its markings and its configurations – is omnipresent and responsible for every detail] (*ibid.*: 170). In all, whether perceptible or not, whether hidden or not, 'dans un certain sens [l'énonciation] se montre toujours puisque le texte est offert à la vue et à l'ouïe'. This suggestion ties in with the theory of enunciation based on the very idea that subjectivity is manifest also in language, even in the most 'neutral' aspects! But for Metz, 'même si le concept d'énonciation filmique résiste assez bien' the 'énonciateur' does not exist, or rather he is but a personification of the enunciation, of the origin of the text that is 'proféré', and that is offered to the concrete body that is the spectator. That is to say, meta-linguistic and impersonal (necessarily) as it is, 'l'énonciation elle-même n'est jamais anthropoïde, elle reste accrochée au texte' [uttering itself is never anthropoid, it remains tied to text] (*ibid.*: 214). This personification of utterance, possible in a book, is declared impossible in a film by Metz, for its origin is always and necessarily collective and diversified. These points now made, Metz does not however then evacuate the notion of 'sujet' in its psychoanalytical sense. On the contrary Metz considered psychoanalysis an indispensable discipline on which he wrote an important study, which looked at its relations with the 'machine-cinéma' (1977b).

Le signifiant imaginaire

First published in the *Communications* number (1975d) given over to 'Psychanalyse et cinéma', this book (1977b) was to be published under the same title in the 10/18 series with Éditions UGE, but benefiting from three extra chapters: 'Histoire/Discours (Note sur deux voyeurismes)', already published in the collective homage to Émile Benveniste (1975b); 'Le film de fiction et son spectateur (Étude métapsychologique)', which appeared in the same issue of *Communications* (1975a); finally, 'Métaphore/Métonymie, ou le référent imaginaire', not published elsewhere. These texts, which are very important and hard to summarise, still influence contemporary cinema-related research. They include an assessment of Freudian and Lacanian psychoanalysis (on the mirror) with regard to cinema, of the work of Melanie Klein (the notion of the object), as well as an analysis of the different sorts of psychoanalytical studies available on cinema. Metz observes that many of these are often 'des tentatives de diagnostic (nosographique ou caractériel) portant sur des personnes (les cinéastes)' [attempts to provide either nosographic or characterial diagnostics on certain people (film-makers)]. Other psychoanalytical studies of film scripts consider these to be the manifest signifier of a latent discourse to be revealed. Finally, there are the rarer examples, at the time, of psychoanalytical studies of the textual system in its entirety, which look at the relation between script and cinematography in a particular film. Witness, for example, the 'imposante étude' of Hitchcock's film *North by Northwest*, by Raymond Bellour in *Communications* no. 23, called 'Le blocage symbolique' (Bellour 1975). But, for his part, Metz proposed to study 'directement, hors de tout film particulier' [directly, outside of any film in particular], the psychoanalytical implications of the cinematographic so as to 'éclairer en termes freudiens des phénomènes comme le hors champ, le cadrage, le montage court ou le tournage en profondeur' [to explain using Freud phenomena such as the off-screen, framing, the short film or deep-vision filming] (1977b: 179).

We might want to indicate several areas of progress which seem to be crucial, in particular the analysis of the 'l'état filmique', distinct for Metz from the dream state, but which is linked by hidden motivations, the engagement of the unconscious and the relative lowering of vigilance to waking dreaming, to fantasy, more than to dreams, while remaining radically separated from them through the very materiality of the film, of the images and the sounds. Another crucial area is the analysis of the process of identification in the cinema, which is invoked today in order to back up the supposed efficiency of visual communication especially in advertising or politics. 'A quoi s'identifie le spectateur durant la projection du film?' [With what does the spectator identify during the projection of the film?] The character? The actor? These are possible but only in a way that is 'secondaire', in the psychoanalytical sense of the term, that is, after a necessary identification with one's own look which has been confused with that of the camera 'dans un double mouvement projectif et introjectif' [in a double movement of the projective and the introjective]. We are clearly a long way from a simplifying reductionism that is supplied by this psychic phenomenon to a supposed sympathy for one or another character.

Finally, Metz helps us to understand the cinema-machine by the very title of his work: 'Au cinéma comme au théâtre le représenté est par définition imaginaire; c'est ce qui caractérise la fiction comme telle … Mais la représentation … au cinéma est à son tour imaginaire, le matériau étant déjà un reflet …' [In the cinema as in the theatre that which is represented is imaginary; it is this that characterises fiction as such. But representation in the cinema is itself imaginary, as the material is already a reflection]. Metz is looking then for the psychoanalytical implications of an art form 'où tout est absent, où tout est enregistré' [where everything is absent, where everything recorded], where the entire signifier 'est absence' [is absence]. He points out this very absence, redoubling that of the referent, which then acts more to the benefit of the diegesis, tends more to get stuck in it, to be paid into its account by the spectator's belief (1977b: 92–5). It is this absence which reactivates the scopic impulse in a dual act of voyeurism: in order that the film 'ait lieu' [take place], 'je regarde et j'aide' [I watch and I help], 'j'assiste' [I assist], as if able to 'être témoin et être-adjuvant' [to be both witness and counsel], a text both 'exhibitionist', as we watch, and 'cachottier' [secretive] of the 'dispositif' [plan], so that 'l'histoire règne' [the story is in charge]. This absence also feeds the imaginary capacity of the researcher as much as of the spectator, in a way which is more projective than that of identification. Metz's main preoccupation is then to look for 'la constitution psychanalytique du signifiant au cinéma' [the psychoanalytical dimension of the signifier in the cinema] (*ibid.*: 51), to discover by which 'chemins' [routes] the cinema is able to get into the unconscious and to explore the specificity of the mechanisms of identification, of voyeurism, of exhibitionism, or fetishism, which are all in operation. Elsewhere, the aim is to show how the mechanisms of metaphor and metonymy, of displacement and condensation, overwhelm us again within this absence, how the rhetorical categorisations are there, traditionally, in order to highlight 'dans des affinités d'opérations, des parentés dans le travail du sens' [within those operations which have affinities, the deep links that exist in the work on meaning]. Here, and as we have seen elsewhere, we can see one of the characteristics in the work by Metz, which is that of taking seriously previous ideas, even preconceived ones, and then exploring them to the point of rejecting or accepting them: in either case they are modified in a systematic mode of thought that is linked to linguistics and to structuralism, and which privileges the contemporary notion of interaction in all its dimensions.

Teaching and influence

It would be impossible not to mention, by way of a conclusion, the intellectual influence of Christian Metz. This appreciation of his work very consciously targeted from an early stage the educational aspect, but it was soon to spill over into other areas, all testament to a success which worried Metz . Indeed, from 1967 to 1971, he was an adviser for a pilot experiment of 'Initiation à la Culture Audio-Visuelle' organised by the education authority in Bordeaux. He mentions this in the article 'Images et pédagogie', published in the number 15 of *Communications* (1970b), the same number in which appears his 'Au-delà de l'analogie, l'image'. In the former article he reflects on the 'vaste problème des relations entre image et enseignement', of images in teaching in relation to the teaching of the image; that is, crucial problems nowadays now that the question of the multiplication of media and of images seems problematic throughout the world. While all this experimentation was taking place there were all sorts of thoughts, observations or seminars at which Metz was present and which have led to publications in article, journal or report form.[6] Meanwhile there were similar experiments in many educational authorities (such as in the Midi-Pyrenees, or in the Paris region).[7] It seems, unfortunately, that, at the very moment when we find ourselves more than ever 'envahi' [invaded] if not 'manipulé' by images, all the conclusions and educational suggestions emerging from this work have disappeared and have not been taken up in contemporary institutions nor in discussion in the mainstream media, which rely on outmoded ideas, while ignoring totally these pioneering ideas of the 1970s.

For his part Metz recommended that we respect certain stages which are necessary pedagogically speaking; first, we have to 'régresser – c'est-à-dire progresser – d'abord en direction des mécanismes perceptifs fortement codés culturellement' [regress – that is, progress – first towards those perceptual mechanisms that are heavily culturally coded]; then, we need to institute a form of teaching that is 'proprement iconique' [properly iconic], coded in socio-cultural terms; finally, we need to move 'du niveau langagier au niveau méta-langagier' [from the level of language to that of metalanguage], in order to allow students to develop a form of intelligence 'que seule l'école peut développer à grande échelle' [that can develop on a wide scale only by being in higher education] (*ibid.*: 165). This preoccupation with and respect of the intelligence of others, be they pupils, students, colleagues or researchers, was a central element in Metz's approach and which 'contribua à lui donner cette sensibilité de culture-civilité intérieure que sa présence imposait discrètement et péremptoirement à ses interlocuteurs' [helped to give him an inner sensitivity both cultural and civil that his presence would impose discretely and peremptorily on his interlocutors] (Garroni 1994/95).

What is also symptomatic of the personality of Christian Metz is that, as early as May 1975, a special number of the journal *ça cinéma* was given over to him, as a kind of summary of ten years of writings and theoretical progress all crucial in the development of a semiology of cinema. One other summary of the importance of his contribution to cinema and image theory was made in 1989, at a 'Cerisy' conference called 'Christian Metz et la théorie du cinéma', published in the journal *Iris* (Marie and Vernet 1990). Here American researchers, as well as British, Japanese, Italian, Chinese, Danish, Dutch, Uruguayan and French all worked on, and testified to the theoretical importance of Christian Metz for their generation and their work. In the interview with Marie and Vernet at the end of the volume, Metz is keen to end with an idea of Barthes's, 'son seul vrai maître' [his only true master], who had died in an accident nine years earlier. He also tries to replace his own work, with a measured and modest eye, in its general context, while announcing his next book *Le mot d'esprit*, as well as the final stage in his work on enunciation. This last project appeared as a book in 1991, whereas the 'mot d'esprit' work was never to be published, as Metz died in 1993. If the 'galaxie sémiologie' was in the intellectual driving seat of social science research for about a quarter of a century, it was not to be in the 1990s when, as Metz pointed out, the theory was no longer 'à la mode'. Nowadays, not only is semiology no longer 'à la mode', but also, in the words of Christian Metz, 'cela renseigne sur la mode, non sur la théorie' [it tells us about fashion but not about theory] (Marie and Vernet 1990: 276). Then, in *Les Cahiers du CIRCAV* (6/7, 1994–95), there is another homage to Metz with, once again, the respectful participation of forty or so researchers from all theoretical and geographical horizons, who all underline his human, as well as intellectual, qualities. To conclude, it is worth remembering once again Barthes for whom Metz was above all someone 'respectueux des autres' [respectful of others], and also a 'didacticien merveilleux' [wonderful tutor]; in Barthes's words: 'lorsqu'on le lit, on sait tout comme si on l'avait appris soi-même' [when reading Metz you understand everything he says as if you have learned it yourself] (Barthes 1975: 6). So, let's read him and use his work and thought, which today are more relevant than ever.

References

Barthes, R. (1964), 'Éléments de sémiologie', *Communications* 4 (1964), 91–135; reprinted in R. Barthes, *L'Aventure sémiologique*, Paris: Seuil, 1985, 17–84; *Elements of semiology*, trans. A. Lavers and C. Smith, New York: Hill & Wang, 1968.

—— (1975) 'Apprendre et enseigner', *ça cinéma* 7–8 (May), 5–8; 'Christian Metz' (Paris: Albatros); 'To Learn and to Teach', trans. R. Howard, in *The Rustle of Language*, Oxford: Blackwell, 1986, 176–8.

Bellour, R. (1975) 'Le blocage symbolique', *Communications* 23 (1975), 235–350.

Bergala, A. (1975) *Pour une pédagogie de l'audio-visuel*, Paris: La Ligue française de l'Enseignement.

—— (1977) *Initiation à la sémiologie du récit en images*, Paris: La Ligue française de l'Enseignement.

Château, D. and Jost, F. (1979) *Nouveau cinéma, Nouvelle sémiologie*, Paris: UGE, 10/18.

Cohen-Séat, G. (1958) *Essais sur les principes d'une philosophie du cinéma*, Paris: PUF.

Garroni, E. (1994/95) *Les Cahiers du CIRCAV* 6–7, 'La lyre et l'aulos, hommage à Christian Metz', Gerico: Université de Lille III, 105–9.

Marie, M., and Vernet, M. (1990) *Christian Metz et la théorie du cinéma*, Paris: Méridiens-Klincksieck (special number of *Iris* 10, April).

Metz, C. (1964) 'Le cinéma: langue ou langage?', *Communications* 4, 52–90.

—— (1965a) 'Une étape dans la réflexion sur le cinéma', *Critique* 21(214) (Mar.), 227–48; [see 1972: 13–34].

—— (1965b) 'Le cinéma, monde et récit', *Critique* 21(216) (May), 485–6.

—— (1965c) 'A propos de l'impression de réalité au cinéma', *Cahiers du cinéma* 166–7 (May–Jun.), 74–83.

—— (1968a) 'Cinéma moderne et narrativité', in *Essais sur la signification au cinema*, vol. 1, Paris: Klincksieck, 1971, 185–221; 'The Modern Cinema and Narrativity', *Film Language: A Semiotics of the Cinema*, trans. M. Taylor, Oxford: Oxford University Press, 1974, 185–227.

—— (1968b) 'Le dire et le dit au cinéma: vers le déclin d'un vraisemblable?', *Communications* 11, 'Le Vraisemblable' (ed. Roland Barthes), 22–33.

—— (1970a) 'Au-delà de l'analogie, l'image', *Communications* 15, 1–10.

—— (1970b) 'Images et pédagogie', *Communications* 15, 162–8.

—— (1971) *Langage et cinéma*, Paris: Larousse (new edition with new afterword: Paris: Albatros, 1977); trans. C. Umiker-Sebeok, The Hague: Mouton, 1974.

—— (1972) *Essais sur la signification au cinéma*, vol. 2, Paris: Klincksieck; *Film Language: A Semiotics of the Cinema*, trans. M. Taylor, Oxford: Oxford University Press, 1974.

—— (1975a) 'Le film de fiction et son spectateur (Étude métapsychologique)', *Communications* 23, 108–35.

—— (1975b) 'Histoire/discours (Note sur deux voyeurismes)', in J. Kristeva, J.-C. Milner and N. Ruwet (eds), *Langue, discours, société: Pour Émile Benveniste*, Paris: Seuil, 301–6.

—— (1975c) 'Le perçu, le nommé', in *Pour une esthétique sans entrave-Mélanges Mikel Dufrenne*, Paris: UGE-10/18, 345–77.

—— (1975d) 'Le signifiant imaginaire', *Communications* 23, 3–55.

—— (1977a) *Essais sémiotiques*, Paris: Klincksieck.

—— (1977b) *Le signifiant imaginaire (Psychanalyse et cinéma)*, Paris: UGE, 10/18 (new edition with a new preface, Paris: Christian Bourgois, 1984); trans. C. Britton, *Psychoanalysis and Cinema*, Basingstoke: Macmillan, 1982.

—— (1991) *L'Énonciation impersonnelle ou le site du film*, Paris: Méridiens-Klincksieck.

Notes

1 Between 1966 and 1968, working with Émile Benveniste and Algirdas-Julien Greimas, he also participated in founding the Association Internationale de Sémiotique (AIS).

2 See Metz (1965a) (on vol. 1 of Jean Mitry, *L'Esthétique et psychologie du cinéma*) and Metz (1965b) (on Albert Laffay, *Logique du cinéma*).

3 Originally called the École Pratique des Hautes Études (EPHE), the institution in which Metz worked was renamed the École des Hautes Études en Sciences Sociales (EHESS) in 1975.

4 See Barthes (1964).

5 In 'Christian Metz: Entretien avec M. Vernet et D. Percheron', *ça cinéma* 7–8 (1975), 19.

6 See the Centre Régional de Documentation Pédagogique in Bordeaux.

7 See for example, the works by Alain Bergala, *Pour une pédagogie de l'audiovisuel* and *Initiation à la sémiologie du récit en images* (Paris: La Ligue française de l'Enseignement, 1975 and 1977).

Part II
New art histories and genealogies

3

Daniel Arasse's joyful visual science: in the intimacy of history and art

Ralph Dekoninck

The art historian Daniel Arasse (1944–2003) is today known as someone who moved between the worlds of history of art, theory of art and art criticism, so running the risk of blurring traditional disciplinary frontiers; and as one who moved between the Renaissance and the present day, risking anachronism. It is these two points in particular – the question of art, and the question of history – which will be our focus in this chapter, leaving to one side two other dimensions: his role as an intermediary between the circle of specialists and the wider public,[1] and between foreign and French art history.[2]

History of art and theory of art

Arasse may be considered primarily as a historian (2004: 102) and is probably the least theoretical of the thinkers discussed in this volume,[3] even though he collaborated with several of them, notably at the École des Hautes Etudes en Sciences Sociales, an institution he joined in 1993 after having taught at the Sorbonne (Paris I and Paris IV) since 1969. Arasse was a former student of the École Normale Supérieure and carried out his early doctoral research first under André Chastel ('Art and society around Saint Bernard of Siena'). He later changed the orientation of his research, under the direction of Louis Marin, to the relation between history and memory in Italian painting of the fourteenth and fifteenth centuries (*ibid.*: 151–63). Since Arasse never wished to become affiliated to any particular intellectual body, this double direction is evidence of the way in which he was able to work within different disciplinary traditions, operating in particular at the meeting point between two intellectual sensibilities which at that time might have seemed difficult to reconcile: on the one hand, that of a history of art that sought to gain academic recognition and autonomy for itself; and, on the other hand, a history of art opening out to various fields in the social sciences, especially through an interest in semiotics and psychoanalysis. The composition of this double heritage is enough to make of him an unclassifiable figure blurring the boundaries of the history of art in France, divided by diverging traditions (Dekoninck and Roucloux 2012).

While openly acknowledging the debt to a so-called 'classical' history of art, and advocating its empiricism, Arasse nevertheless maintained a critical viewpoint with regard to a certain type of practice of this discipline that is entirely devoted to either stylistic or to iconographic analysis. In particular, his critical position took the form of theoretical thinking whose sole aim was to enrich his historical approach. It is precisely on the problematic issue of the connection of history to theory that Arasse owes most to Louis Marin and Hubert Damisch. Arasse shared their belief that the history of art could not do without a theory of history, just as it cannot hide the theories of art it conveys, whether consciously or unconsciously. Arasse thus inherits from Marin the belief that every work of art is also a theoretical object, both as the construction of a science of art and as an object thinking itself (Marin 1993). It is perhaps in this latter idea, according to which every representation represents itself, that the debt to Marin is seen most clearly. According to Marin, 'the reflexivity internal to the work determines its theoretical dimension' (2006: 17). This idea is shared by Damisch, for whom 'painting not only shows, it thinks' (1987: 406); as such, the art object is a theoretical object, in the sense that it produces its own theory. This topic was previously explored by Pierre Francastel, who was the first to consider the idea of figurative thought at work in painting (2004: 154). Arasse makes this idea his own by stating that 'painting thinks, pictorially' (*ibid.*: 101), while emphasising the fact that this theoretical object can be understood only in its historical context. Rather than opposing history and theory, it is therefore for Arasse a matter of thinking about their connection, but doing so from a historical point of view.

With respect to the problematic of the relation between the historical and the theoretical, it is worth mentioning the example Arasse's analysis offers of *Las Meninas* in a Festschrift for Damisch (2003b). Velázquez's famous painting (Plate 1) offers an extraordinary case study since it has been the object of a large number of historical investigations and has also lent itself to a series of theoretical interpretations, beginning with that offered by Michel Foucault (1966). Foucault saw in *Las Meninas* 'the representation of classical representation', based on the 'necessary disappearance of that which is its foundation' (*ibid.*: 31), that is, the model replaced by the presence of the beholder. Historical research on Velázquez's painting has since been able to show the anachronism of Foucault's reading, which did not take into account, in particular, the private nature of the painting, which was created for a single viewer, none other than King Philip IV. But Arasse asks us to think about the historical efficacy of this anachronism: 'how can a painting created for the private sphere of the sovereign ... found and legitimate a deliberately anachronic interpretation?' (2003b: 17). Answering this question assumes, once the historical conditions of the painting's production have been made clear, that we take into account the effects created by the painting's devices when the painting is no longer viewed in the circumstances that, historically, were foreseen for its reception. So it is not necessarily a matter of questioning the relevance of modern interpretation, but of investigating the fact that certain works may entail an effect which seems to contradict their historical 'truth', whether this truth be identified with the intention involved in their creation or with the immediate context of their reception: 'Everything happens as if, in this case, it was the painting that produced meaning visually, independently of and beyond the ideas that the painter and his client made of it – and long after their death' (Arasse 2000: 189). Arasse thus calls for 'a historical approach to the theoretical effect produced by the devices of *Las Meninas*' (2003b: 23), proof that art, through its works, can think independently of the artist. From this, Arasse then draws the conclusion that 'art does not exist outside of works that enable it to see and that, as such, are historical objects: produced at a given time, transmitted through a series of periods of which they bear the traces, and seen today in a contemporaneity that is anachronic in relation to that of their production' (*ibid.*: 15).

This last quotation sums up the issues that lie at the heart of Arasse's work: art does not exist outside of art works and of history; the works do not exist without a creator and without a spectator's gaze. If there is a method in Arasse's work, it lies essentially in the attention paid to the connection of these three dimensions: the work, the artist and the spectator, as well as to the three sorts of time that link them, with the work serving as the bridge between past and present. 'Analytic iconography' is the name given to this search for the subject in the painting, and that of 'subject' to the focussing on the interrelation of these three important dimensions and of their respective temporality, making each work a unique case (1997a).

Knowledge put to the test in the close-up view

Let us begin with the first point in this triangulation: the work. Arasse defines himself not so much as an art historian as a historian of painting, and more specifically of paintings, of those unique objects of history perceived in history. This insistence on the material uniqueness and on the sense experience of painting gives depth, or even flesh, to what is now, in the era of mechanical reproduction, approached only as images. Among the paintings analysed by Arasse, Italian works from the Trecento to the Cinquecento occupy pride of place, even if his insatiable curiosity also drew him to other periods and other geographical areas: seventeenth-century Holland, with Vermeer; eighteenth-century France, with Fragonard and Greuze; as well as contemporary art with Anselm Kiefer. This preference for Italian art may be explained, in addition to the elective affinities born out of his early contact with this land of the arts, by the foundational dimension of the Renaissance for the history of art, in the double sense of the historical development of art and of the discipline responsible for its study. Hence, for anyone seeking to examine the aesthetic and epistemic foundations of modern representation and of its study, the Italian Renaissance constitutes the origin of its practice and its theory, with practice and theory representing the two sides of the same coin.

Here we touch on a central aspect of Arasse's thought, which never stopped enquiring into the modalities of the connection between seeing and knowing. Knowledge, whether that of the period or that developed by art historians, conditions the perception of works, as do also our contemporary ways of exhibiting and reproducing art. Rather than trying at all costs to abandon these multiple layers of interpretation as well as the technical devices that offer us the works to see, it is necessary to recognise that there is no seeing without knowing, that there is no immaculate perception which might precede knowledge. These layers of commentary have to be considered before attempting to see the paintings in a different way or to see in them for the first time what had remained unnoticed by the discursive frameworks forged by art history. We should note, however, that the un-seen ('in-vu'), in Arasse's sense, is not the invisible, but designates the optical unconscious concealed in the work; that is to say everything that escapes the norm both at the level of the construction of representation (especially through perspective) and at the level of the conceptual and perceptual *habitus* specific to art history. In order to reveal it he calls for a 'microhistory' of art whose operating method is that of the close-up look ('regard rapproché'). However, this does not free him from questioning the evidence of looking and of the visible: what does it mean to look at a work of art? What are we doing while looking at a painting? What are we thinking about? What do we imagine? How can we say to ourselves what we see or sense? And on what do we bring our view to bear? But if the dialectical confrontation of seeing and knowing appears to be central, according to Arasse, the touchstone of the knowledge of the art historian is looking. And it is this test of looking that unleashes enquiry and reflection.

If painting is thus a matter of looking, it will attach itself primarily to the material(s) ('plastique') employed by the work which is seen as a closed, but dynamic and organic, whole. For what matters is not the iconographic content that we might be content to 'spell' with the help of 'bookish erudition', but 'the specific unity of meaning formed by the way motifs have been assembled across the surface of the representation', what Arasse calls the 'figurative framework' (1997a: 13). All the attention of the historian of painting, then, should be brought to bear on the way in which 'form contributes to constituting and transmitting its content' (*ibid.*). But in order to grasp the significant issues of the materials deployed, the look must be directed as closely as possible at the work. Only the exercise of such a close-up look is in fact able to lead to intimacy, which is the ultimate aim of Arasse's method of interpretation. More precisely, intimacy appears as both the object of study and the privileged method of approaching it, the two indissolubly linked to each other.

In search of the intimacy of painting and the painter

Intimacy, as object, is not to be confused with the subject represented. It is not in fact a matter of iconographic content. Thus, if we take the example of Vermeer's paintings (1993), which seem to exemplify best this intimacy, it is access not to the private world of seventeenth-century Holland that interests Arasse but to what is beyond the represented, to what he calls 'the (subjective) inside of the (objective) inside' (*ibid.*: 167) or 'the intimate in the private' (2004: 139). In other words, we need to get to the heart of what these paintings only evoke thematically: the intimate experience that is at the heart of painting as a monument, rather than painting as a document (historical, sociological or cultural), to use a favourite distinction made by Foucault. Vermeer's image in *The Lacemaker* (hanging in the Louvre in Paris) of a woman absorbed in her work, offers a fine example of this perspective. It is not simply a matter of understanding the human theme of the intimate self, but of tracking the intimacy of the painting that allows access, pictorially, to an experience of figured human intimacy; or, to cite Arasse, it is a matter of showing how the painter 'invites the viewer to share the inaccessible intimacy' (1993: 178) of his paintings.

The desire to tie closely together thematic and pictorial intimacy, form and content, is found in Arasse's work on depictions of the Annunciation in the Renaissance (2010), which are also expressions of a mysterious intimacy. The theme of the Annunciation reveals two different and apparently divergent issues: both as the space of the conquest of perspective and as the place par excellence of the expression of the Christian mystery. In this paradoxical confluence of science and religion, where there is a tension between the theme represented and the instrument of its representation, it is more precisely a question of observing the pictorial strategies deployed to give pictorial substance to the Mystery of the Incarnation, an intimate mystery if ever there was one, and which finds no finer expression than in the figure of the enclosed garden of the Virgin. Once again, what matters is not the iconography of the Annunciation as such, but the way in which the Incarnation is itself at work in the painting; this also leads us to ask how painting, literally, gives pictorial substance to thought or how thought is incarnated in painting.

Now, the intimacy that constitutes the main object of the enquiry cannot be better approached than by an intimate relationship with painting. Intimacy, as has been noted, is as much the approach taken by the historian of intimacy as it is their object of study. The historian practices the intimacy of the look in order to penetrate the intimacy of painting. Looking close up involves being attentive to the slightest details in which the intelligence of painting might be expressed (1992: 2004). Whether this is Lippi's vase or the buttonhole he opens up in the Virgin's robe (National Gallery, London), the snail placed at the edge of Francesco del Cossa's painting (Gemäldegalerie, Dresden), Lotto's grasshopper, the eye-shaped navel of Antonello da Messina's *Saint Sebastian* (Gemäldegalerie, Dresden), a baby's hand laid over a balustrade in the oculus of Mantegna's *Bridal Chamber* (Ducal Palace, Mantua); all these details, which do not show us what we should look at but how we should look at what we see, thus appear as the privileged means of access to intimacy.

But this intimacy is not only that of painting. It is also that of the painter in his work, that is to say, the portion of subjectivity he invests in his painting, 'their intimate relation to what they are representing' (2004: 79). The history of the modes of expression of this intimate relation, through which the modern subject is prefigured and configured, takes the form notably of a genetic approach which is interested in 'traces of thought in action' (*ibid.*: 199), which Arasse pursues in relation to the work of Leonardo da Vinci (1997b/2002), but also through the study of all visual anomalies compared to norms and expectations in the Italian painting of the Renaissance. Analytical iconology therefore should not be confused with any kind of 'applied psychoanalysis' that might consist in a deep examination of the artist's psyche through his or her work. Rather, its aim is to reveal the process of figurability at work in the painting, while being particularly attentive to the operation of displacement and condensation, both of which, according to Freud, are characteristic of the dream-work. It is thus not so much the arrangement of figures or their specific meaning that interests Arasse as the advent of thought in the figure, 'what is in the process of figuration, what is at work in order to reach the figure' (1997a: 15). Inspired by the use Marin has made of the term, figurability is thus understood as being the principle which is at work in the representation in order to reach the figure. 'At the level of the individual work, the notion of figurability denotes the singular and intimate guiding principle that works to appropriate the message of the work while secretly modifying it' (*ibid.*).

Anachronism and the intimacy of the spectator

There is no question of subscribing to the theory of the 'Death of the Author' nor to the demise of art whose very existence is characterised, in the view of Arasse, by the survival of its effects today. Indeed, the distinctive feature of art, or rather the specificity of these singular objects that are works of art, lies essentially in the fact that they continue to incite our viewing (1992: 8). Such is the singularity of these historical objects: to be always of the present time and therefore to be by their nature anachronic (2004: 149). And this is where the third subject arises; for the subject in the work does not designate only the investment of its creator but also the involvement of the spectator's subjectivity (including the art historian's), both of them moved by the circulation of pleasure and desire aroused by the work. To this third subject there is a corresponding temporality: the time of present contemplation is the only channel through which one can gain access to the singularity of the work. It is therefore from the present time that the work is viewed and that it touches us: the work of art is 'my contemporary [...] it acts on me, this physical presence matters' (2004: 149). But how can we hold together both historicism and anachronism, both the historicity unique to the work and also our own historicity, the contemporaneity of our view? In brief, how can we conceive of a history of these singularities when they themselves mix together the temporalities that constitute them? 'How can we interpret the exception *historically*?' (1997b/2002: 14). In approaching this delicate problem of putting something unique into historical perspective, a work which furthermore may be thought of as an event that repeats itself at each encounter, Arasse seeks to unravel the plot of the work, which no longer depends solely on its figurative framework but also on the different layers of interpretation aroused by that figurative framework and which have formed deposits over time, enriching or impoverishing the meaning of the work.

The emblematic example might be that of *La Gioconda*, on which Arasse wrote at some length (1997b/2002, 2004). The emotion it continues to arouse derives from both its visual force and the myth that has enveloped it in a series of commentaries and images. To grasp the reasons for the persistence of its effects, it is necessary therefore not only to reconstitute the actions and intentions of Leonardo da Vinci, but also to bear in mind the images of the work forged through the centuries and which now constitute so many layers interposed between the work and ourselves; this is a third dimension to time whose various strata the historian must identify. While this intermediate temporality creates a link between the work and the present-day spectator, the latter in turn invests the work with his or her own intimate experience.

Understanding the still-living effectiveness of a painting therefore assumes a knitting together of these three temporalities that form a single whole and that make art history an art of memory. This art of memory will therefore engage with the role both of the present time and of the anachronism that is constitutive of the work; otherwise it runs the risk of negating its historical depth and its aesthetic specificity. If reconstituting the circumstances (historical, biographical, stylistic), values and conventions that obtained at its creation proves to be necessary to avoid any interpretation 'not founded in history' (2004: 84) – that is to say, any anachronic reading disconnected from historical reality – this is often not sufficient to explain why this work can still affect us outside of its original context and in conditions of exhibition that it did not have initially. From this it follows that the specificity of a work is not reducible to its original historical context.

This specificity results above all, to return to this point, from the material ('plastique') thought that is peculiar to the work of art and from the sense experience made of it, which allows a bridge to be built between the original context and the present day. For it is not a question of approaching the work in order to obtain knowledge of the context, but of using knowledge of the context (as with new viewing conditions offered by laboratory techniques such as X-rays) in order to create in the present day a relationship with the work that is more total, that is to say, more intimate, a relationship whose challenges are at one and the same time aesthetic and cognitive. A proximity that is simultaneously temporal, physical and psychological is thus quite different from either subjective aesthetic contemplation or objective scientific observation; for it is necessary to maintain an equal distance from empathy or projection and from critical and historical distance so as to bring together past and present, a connection that works in two directions: 'the look can touch and be touched' (*ibid.*: 152). Hence the following rich paradox: objectivity, as an approach (historical or not) to art, therefore consists in giving more access to subjectivity, and vice versa. This sharing of perspectives, as we have seen, lies at the foundation of both the object of study (complexity of the work) and of the approach (the viewer's complicity); the method derives, as it were, from the object. It restores intimacy historically by taking shape in it and by taking pleasure in it; for pleasure and knowledge here become one in a bid to arouse the lucid enjoyment of the painting's intimate complexity.

Such a perspective necessarily leads us to reflect on the writing of history. Challenged by the persistent effectiveness of a painting through time, and rather than try to resolve the intrigue at the heart of the depicted story (and at the heart of the many stories that the painting has generated), Arasse the historian must give an account of it in his turn by producing not a history but a story, even a fiction, whose goal is to make us enter into the intimacy of the painting and in so doing to recreate the sensory proximity which was none other than that of the artist to their work, but also that of the narrating historian telling us *stories of paintings*. The aim of all narrative strategies is not only to communicate knowledge but also to enable us to see an incarnated look. Arasse shows himself in the act of seeing in order to restore and share the vivacity of an experience that is at one and the same time emotional and cognitive, created from the feeling of having penetrated the intimacy of the painting's and the painter's thought. While this reasoned sensibility is not to be confused with a form of subjective self-reflexivity, it remains true that this is the most unsettling aspect of his work, but it is also the one that has given Arasse's work a broader audience beyond the circle of specialists.[4] Arasse's writing, with its mixture of rigour and surprise, of the humorous and the serious, reinvents historical knowledge for the benefit of the dialogue with his reader. This is a dialogue he also puts to the test of contemporary art by adopting not the posture of the art critic but by maintaining his role of historian investigating the memory of works in the present day, the past being incorporated within the experience of the present. Convinced of the fact that if we question the past it replies in the present, conversely he sought to show that when we question the present it replies in the past.

Situated under the sign of the singular and of the intimate, of history and of memory, Arasse's work remains fundamentally the work of a historian who never stopped examining the epistemic and aesthetic issues of temporal and psychic distance in relation to the artwork. Speculating simultaneously on the effects of painting and on the effects of historical writing, Arasse succeeded in putting art history to the test of the anachronism constitutive of all artworks and of the fiction constitutive of all historical narration. He thus lies at the origin of a visual, joyful science where the pleasure taken in the interpretation of works invents a mode of writing able to communicate this pleasure of knowledge and this knowledge of pleasure.

Shared perspectives with Damisch, Marin and Didi-Huberman

If we now consider the connections between Arasse's work and other theorists of the visual in France, we cannot avoid noticing a certain community of spirit with Hubert Damisch, Louis Marin and Georges Didi-Huberman, writers who were all colleagues of Arasse at the École des Hautes Études en Sciences Sociales. As we have already shown for the first two of these figures, there is no doubt that Arasse shares many features with them, especially through his thinking on the problematic connection between art theory and art history. A similar concern can be seen in the analysis of the socio-historical conditions of the production and reception of works mingled with the analysis of their specific formal and aesthetic features. For, if the study of works in themselves keeps any historical determinism at a distance, it is no less attentive to the structural relations that link these works to other works or to other cultural phenomena.

Furthermore, the attention brought to bear on their particular processes of figurability is accompanied in these thinkers by a consideration of the rhythm specific to their history. But once again this presupposes not neglecting the interactions of their particular temporality with historical contexts. For these interactions actualise the aesthetic and semiotic potentialities that are specific to them only under the pressure, conscious or unconscious, of the most diverse objectives (whether individual or collective). Through this weaving together of different temporalities a rich reflection on the historicity of the work of art has been set in motion.

If these different temporalities therefore share this same conviction that no history of art can do without a theory of history, they are also aware that one cannot hide the art theories that underlie the practice of art history. Rather than avoiding the question of beauty or abandoning the concept of art in favour of a supposedly neutral concept such as that of the image, it is necessary to recognise, according to this group of thinkers, that art history goes hand in glove with aesthetics and that art is by its nature a theoretical object. If, then, we wish to write art's history, we must know the nature of its status and of its specific forms at each moment of this history. In this way, the term 'artistic production' is to be understood not only in the sense of the making of works of art but in the sense of the production and reproduction of the material, ideological and theoretical conditions of this production and of its effectiveness.

From this point of view, it is no coincidence that these four authors were interested in the Renaissance, a key moment in the constitution of modern representation. They tracked down all the areas of opacity through which representation thinks itself, thereby revealing the dialectic between transitivity and reflexivity which constitutes representation and which allows us to connect the semantic and the expressive dimensions. An enquiry of this nature carried out into the semiotic and aesthetic modalities of figuration naturally led them to question the powers of this visual thought, powers which depend precisely on this unstable play between presence and representation. The interest in the opaque flesh of painting (in opposition, therefore, to the hiding of this dimension by the classical theory of art) thus allows them to understand how matter, form and meaning can be woven together in the cognitive and emotional experience of artworks.

This reflection devoted to the thought and the power of images is accompanied in work by these authors by a critical return to the epistemological foundations of art history, beginning with the heritage of Panofskian iconology, itself the inheritor of a humanist thinking on art that contributed to establishing art as knowledge, with the consequence of a certain reduction of the visible to the legible. Hence the interest they bring to everything that adds to placing classical mimesis in a state of crisis. With regard to this, it is interesting to note that if these authors take the Renaissance as their privileged hunting ground, it is in order to discover at work within it the Christian process of incarnation. From this point of view, it is not surprising that all of them were interested in the theme of the Annunciation, through which something visible beyond all appearance allows itself to be thought. As a counter-model to or model diverging from, that of the classical aesthetic, the Christian paradigm of incarnation, in that it *displays* itself and uses the figurative device of the Annunciation, questions the limits of imitation. Here too, then, it is a matter of thinking of the dialectic between dissimilarity and resemblance as being constitutive of all representation. Resemblance, seen not as a state but as a dynamic and relational process with real and pragmatic effects, must therefore be understood in its relation to dissimilarity, in transparency's relation to opacity: in other words, we must take into consideration the dialectical play from which representation draws all its power. Hence their interest in all figurative processes, that is to say in those visual phenomena, even more than in visible objects, which disturb mimesis while challenging the viewer caught in this game. For it is not possible to distinguish between the image as object, the image as subject and the image as operation of the subject.

In terms of the construction of historical narrative, Arasse shares with Didi-Huberman the idea that 'faced with the image, we are faced with time', that is to say that 'faced with the image, the present and the past are ceaselessly reconfigured' (2000: 9). The classical models of temporality are thus questioned by anachronism, which expresses at one and the same time the *longue durée* of survivals and the discontinuity of historical time. How can the present reconfigure an image of the past, and how can the past survive in a recent image? Such questions derive from the fact that every image is a result of the sedimentation of heterogeneous times. Its meaning is therefore not to be sought only in the time that gave birth to it. We must rather be able to probe the depths of its memory in order to access the multiple stratified times that compose it. In short, the image is a matter of memory more than of history, with history of art transforming itself therefore into a form of an art of memory, in which the historian's own memory is implicated at every point.

Finally, we might say that for Arasse, as for Damisch, Marin and Didi-

Huberman, there is no history of art or theory of art that can dispense with an examination of its objects and their historicity. Furthermore, all four theorists seek to reintroduce presence into representation, presence of painting and of the painter, but also presence of the viewer, including the art historian. Recognising that all historians make theoretical choices, involves a reflexive step that certainly seems to characterise their approach. Another distinctive feature which goes hand in hand with the previous one is their desire to keep together both objects of the past and contemporary theories as well as old theories and contemporary objects, in a constant coming and going. The aim is to find a way to make works from the past speak in their own language while showing how what they say still concerns us today. The connection of theory to history might appear to be one of the prominent features of the work of these visual thinkers, all of them aware of the historical depth at work within images. We may therefore say that history, like the unconscious, is at the heart of their theory of art and of the image, and that their thought is penetrated by the question of time.

References

Arasse, D. (1992), *Le Détail: Pour une histoire rapprochée de la peinture*, Paris: Flammarion.

—— (1993) *L'Ambition de Vermeer*, Paris: Adam Biro.

—— (1997a) *Le Sujet dans le tableau: Essais d'iconographie analytique*, Paris: Flammarion.

—— (1997b/2002), *Léonard de Vinci: Le rythme du monde*, Paris: Hazan, 2002.

—— (2000) *On n'y voit rien: Descriptions*, Paris: Denoël.

—— (2001) *Anselm Kiefer*, Paris: Éditions du regard.

—— (2003a) *Les visions de Raphaël*, Paris: Liana Levi.

—— (2003b) 'L'art dans ses œuvres: Théorie de l'art. Histoire des œuvres', in D. Cohn (ed.), *Y voir mieux, y regarder de plus près. Autour d'Hubert Damisch*, Paris: Rue d'Ulm, 15–27.

—— (2004) *Histoires de peintures*, Paris: Denoël.

—— (2008a) *L'Homme en jeu: Génies de la Renaissance italienne* (1980), Paris: Hazan.

—— (2008b) *L'Homme en perspective: Les Primitifs d'Italie* (1986), Paris: Hazan.

—— (2010) *L'Annonciation italienne: Une histoire de perspective* (1999), Paris: Hazan.

Cousinié, F. (ed.) *Daniel Arasse: Historien de l'art*, Paris: INHA/Les Éditions des Cendres, 2010.
Damisch, H. (1987) *L'Origine de la perspective*, Paris: Flammarion.
Dekoninck, R. and Roucloux, J. (2012) 'Art History in France: A Conflict of Traditions', in Matthew Rampley, Thierry Lenain, Hubert Locher *et al.* (eds), *Art History and Visual Studies in Europe: Transnational Discourses and National Frameworks*, Leiden: Brill, 315–33.
Devant la peinture: Daniel Arasse, special issue of *Esprit* (June 2006).
Didi-Huberman, G. (2000) *Devant le temps: Histoire de l'art et anachronisme des images*, Paris: Minuit.
Foucault, M. (1966) *Les Mots et les Choses: Une archéologie des sciences humaines*, Paris: Gallimard.
'Hommage à Daniel Arasse', *Revue de l'Art* 148(2) (2005), 63–73.
Lafargue, B. (ed.) (2010) *Daniel Arasse: La pensée jubilatoire des œuvres d'art*, special issue of *Figures de l'art* 16.
Marin, L. (1993) 'L'œuvre d'art et les sciences sociales', *Encyclopaedia Unversalis. Symposium. Les enjeux*, t. 2, Paris: 947–71.
—— (2006) *Opacité de la peinture: Essais sur la représentation au Quattrocento*, new edn Cléo Pace, Paris: École des Hautes Études en Sciences Sociales [1st edn Paris: Usher, 1989].
Morel, Ph. (2004) 'Daniel Arasse', *Revue de l'Art* 146, 4.
—— and Bédard, C. (2005) 'Bibliographie de Daniel Arasse', *Studiolo* 3, 7–18.
Sapir, I. (ed.) (2007) *Hommage à Daniel Arasse*, special issue of *Images re-vues* 3, available at www.imagesrevues.org

Notes

1 We should mention Arasse's participation in the 'France-Culture' radio broadcasts; these talks have been collected as *Histoires de peintures* (2004).
2 Through his translations of the works of Erwin Panofsky, Frances Yates, Rudolf and Margot Wittkower, John Michael Montias, Jeffrey Hamburger, Giovanni Tabacco, Wolfgang Prinz, Bram Kempers, Gherardo Ortalli, David Rosand.
3 A more theoretical synthesis, which was started but subsequently interrupted by Arasse's death, was due to be called *L'art dans ses œuvres: Théorie de l'art et histoire des œuvres.*
4 Arasse's death also interrupted the project of writing a novel entitled *The Lost Reflection* (*Le reflet perdu*).

4

Dream perspectives: Hubert Damisch, psychoanalysis and early modern art history

David Packwood

Hubert Damisch can be considered as both art historian and philosopher. He held a professorship at the École des Hautes Études en Sciences Sociales (EHESS) in Paris from 1975 until 1996. Damisch's repertoire is vast; it ranges from art history, architecture, philosophy to aesthetics. As well as studying with French philosophers such as Maurice Merleau-Ponty, Damisch has worked with art historians outside France such as Meyer Schapiro and Stephen Bann. In recent years, with books on the 'Judgment of Paris' and Piero della Francesca, Damisch has explored the relationship between art history and psychoanalysis, the subject of this chapter.[1]

Displacing psychoanalysis

In an interview of 2005, Hubert Damisch contrasted the notion of displacement with invention (Damisch and Bann 2005: 159). Unlike another French thinker – Gilles Deleuze – Damisch said that he did not invent concepts or new interpretations, but displaced continually. More recently, in an unpublished lecture, Damisch used the concept of displacement to interrogate the problem of representation and subjectivity in a series of canonical works including Diego Velázquez's *Las Meninas* (Plate 1), which has provoked many sorties on the subject of art history's relationship with other disciplines such as modern French critical theory, as explained in the introduction to this volume.[2] Drawing on his discussion of *Las Meninas* in *L'Origine de la perspective* ([1987] 1994), Damisch engaged with the problem of the elision of the subject by painting, represented by Velázquez at his easel who fixed the spectator, his model, with the gaze of painting (*ibid.*: 425–39). A noticeable difference between Damisch's earlier discussion of *Las Meninas* and this lecture was the use of psychoanalysis in the latter, specifically the ideas of Jacques Lacan, to articulate a strategy of orientation in which the painting provides an opportunity for a subject to get its bearings. This involved going from the position of a spectator to a looker who desires 'where it is I must go'.[3]

This turn to psychoanalysis to explain difficulties in the field of representation is conspicuously lacking in the literature on *Las Meninas*, even in Foucault's celebrated account, which is surprising since other French philosophers have used psychoanalysis to theorise representation in the seventeenth century (1970: 3–16). For instance, Louis Marin when discussing Nicolas Poussin's *Et in Arcadia Ego* of 1638 chose to use Freud's tenet that all negation was a displaced form of affirmation. Thus, the canvas was simultaneously affirmed and negated, 'technologically and ideologically assumed transparent, a necessary condition of visibility', which helped to define what Marin called the 'plastic screen of representation' (1995: 47). Unlike Marin, Foucault chose not to perceive the mechanisms of representability in seventeenth-century art in terms of the unconscious and the dream. Foucault would never suggest that the initial marks of paint that Velázquez is about to make – or has made – on his canvas could be seen as the equivalent of painting's dream thoughts metamorphosed, or 'translated' into visual images within the representational system exposed in *Las Meninas*. Foucault's reluctance to use psychoanalysis in a discussion of early modern representation probably stemmed from the fact that he distrusted the idea of reducing the imaginative content of dreams to mere images, a reservation he expressed in a lengthy introduction to the Swiss psychoanalyst Ludwig Binswanger's *Dream and Existence* (1954).[4]

Unlike Foucault, Damisch has pursued analogies between the operation of painting and psychoanalytic tropes, although he remains aware of the difficulties of this approach ([1972] 2002: 90; 1984: 32–4). The earliest example of this strand of Damisch's research is detectable in *Theory of/Cloud/*, first published in 1972, in which Damisch suggests that formal procedures of painting can approximate to the operations of dreams, although he takes care to point out that the comparison is not 'well founded' at the level of the function of the painter ([1972] 2002: 90). Later, in *Fenêtre jaune cadmium ou les dessous de la peinture*, Damisch offers a concrete example of this problem in relation to Poussin. One must be careful to distinguish between what Poussin called the 'thought of the picture', and what Freud called the dream thought, or latent content (1984: 35).[5] As Ralph Dekoninck points out in Chapter 3 of this volume, like Arasse, Damisch believes that painting not only shows but thinks, an idea that will be examined in relation to Lacan and perspective later in this chapter.

When formulating rules of engagement with classical painting and its devices, Damisch unapologetically displaces psychoanalysis from its usual medical and forensic contexts into conceptual subdivisions of art history such as perspective, composition and aesthetics, a displacement yielding stimulating results for those who are receptive to Damisch's ideas. This chapter explores Damisch's continual project of displacing psychoanalysis into early modern art history and diverse models of visual theory. The first section explores Damisch's appropriation of Lacan's theory of dreams and its implication for problems of representation, particularly perspective. Next, as a practical application of Damisch's Lacanian orientation towards perspective, the second section considers Giovanni Bellini's unfathomable *Sacred Allegory* in terms of a dream image that enacts Damisch's concepts. The final section analyses Damisch's use of Freud's *Interpretation of Dreams*, as a way of understanding Raphael's *Choice of Scipio*, a 'dream-work' which had generally not been troubled by a psychoanalytic approach until Damisch.

Between Panofsky and Lacan

Far from the materialistic and mechanistic philosophy that underpins most accounts of visual perspective, Damisch chose to view perspective as both model and modality. He was influenced by Panofsky's groundbreaking thesis on the symbolic nature of perspective, which had significantly used Ernst Cassirer's notion of symbolic form, to re-evaluate the perspective concept (Panofsky 1927). Michael Ann Holly has helpfully used Alberti's famous perspective device, the cross-section through the visual pyramid, to explain the concept of symbolic form in relation to perspective. From one side of Alberti's glass we receive information about the world, while the other side ushers in ordering mechanisms produced by the mental processes of the observer. Within this elegant model, the concept of symbolic form becomes the picture plane in the pyramid, mediation between a humanly produced experience and a disclosed reality (Holly 1984: 152).

It is important to note that Damisch's use of the symbolic became increasingly more oriented towards the concept as defined by Lacan. It is a measure of the importance that Damisch attached to Lacan's post-structuralist and anti-humanist conception of the subject which enters the symbolic order of language and narrative that he appended a quotation by Lacan about 'all humanist references to the subject being superfluous' to his book on perspective ([1987] 1994: 56). This use of Lacan seems to function almost as a repudiation of Panofsky's humanism, which is not entirely fair as Panofsky had not divorced science from the humanities in his famous set of essays on the Renaissance, *Meaning in the Visual Arts* (1970: 28ff.). Panofsky was not oblivious to the construction of subjectivity. Within his account of perspective he saw the concept as an expression of the Kantian I and not-I, claiming, in Michael Ann Holly's words, that 'a perspective painting owes its existence to the necessary "distance" between man and objects in the world' (Holly 1984: 149). Panofsky took this further by arguing that perspective was a half-way house between the subjective and objective worlds; it fixed the eternal world in space and extended the sphere of the ego into it (Panofsky 1927: 287). The creation of a distance between subject and object was like the distance that perspective placed between the eye and the world of things (Panofsky 1968: 51).

However, for Damisch, under the influence of Merleau-Ponty, who had also read Panofsky's essay on perspective, the whole issue of subject and object in relation to perspective needed to be rethought. In *Origin of Perspective*, Damisch drew attention to Merleau-Ponty's recasting of the subject; the subject was a 'significant being', secure and confident in its knowledge of its own immanence rather than its relation with the represented world. This anchoring of the subject was seen by Damisch (via Lacan) in terms of the seventeenth-century French philosopher René Descartes's *cogito*. Lacan had used the Cartesian *cogito* as an analogy to seeing with his example of the anamorphic perspective of Holbein the Younger's *Ambassadors* of 1533 (Plate 2). The distorted skull in the foreground of this canonical picture was connected with a different viewpoint than the 'geometral point', the point of perspective, coexistent with a unified and coherent subject. The loss of the geometral point in the distorted skull generated unconscious desire, a structure in which the subject was caught between looking and being looked at – what Lacan called the gaze. To look at Holbein's *Ambassadors* constantly destroys the viewpoint because skull and painting must be viewed separately, a process that negates the field of vision. Associating the obliterated field of vision with the *cogito*, Lacan argued that doubt was an intrinsic quality of orientation within subjectivity: 'I think where I am not, therefore I do not think where I am' (1977a: 166; 1977b: 85–9).

Under the influence of Lacan, Damisch turned to the classical myth of Narcissus who stared at his reflection in a pool. Narcissus was used by Damisch as a way of supplementing a model of vision reliant on a geometral point. Damisch noted Lacan's remark about the geometral aspect of vision reinforcing the idea of the painting capturing the subject, a process having a relation with the subject trapped within a structure of desire ([1987] 1994: 92). Desire in relation to the art of painting was important because, according to Lacan, it urged the artist to 'add something else to the operation of painting' (Lacan 1977b: 93). Damisch saw Narcissus, who was regarded by Alberti as a symbol of the origin of painting, as a concrete example of the subject not defined by optical geometry, but by a circuit of desire in which the subject is lured and attracted by the painting (1966: 64). However, displacing Lacan, Damisch agreed with Merleau-Ponty that what the observer saw was reinforced by a 'complementary vision', Narcissus's reflection, a vision which corresponded to the way that the observer in the world would see the subject looking ([1987] 1994: 46).[6] To clarify, Merleau-Ponty had used the phrase 'palpation of the gaze' by which he implied that the act of looking presupposed a reflection, a contact or 'touching' with the outside world. This concept was important to Damisch because the 'capture' of the subject within this system was helped by perspective.

It is fitting that Damisch chose Narcissus because he provided an example of painting demonstrating its own operability while under scrutiny from all directions. Lacan had used this idea of the subject 'seeing from one point, but being looked at from all sides' which led Damisch to ponder the question of whether a painting could be seen in the same manner (Lacan 1977b: 72). A way of investigating this issue of painting in relation to Lacan's idea of seeing offered itself by an experiment in the Quattrocento. The Florentine architect Brunelleschi painted a small panel which contained a representation of the baptistery of San Giovanni in Florence. The experiment consisted of looking through a small hole in the back of the painting while holding up a mirror in which was reflected the small panel, or *tavola*. Looking through the painting, at the mirror, the viewer did not see the painted sky but a reflection of a reflection since Brunelleschi had covered the painted surface with a layer of silver in which the real sky and passing clouds were reflected. For Damisch, the doubling function of the mirror was an example of *di-mostratio*, with the prefix implying duplication by the agency of the mirror. However, Damisch deduced that Brunelleschi had not used a mirror to paint the panel; the mirror was used in the viewing structure to show the firmament whose appearance in Quattrocento art was considered part of perspective itself since it eliminated the flat golden ground favoured by earlier Renaissance artists such as Giotto. Summing up Brunelleschi's innovation, Damisch claimed, as we will see, that the mirror demonstrates while painting shows, an idea developed from Lacan's discussion of unconsciousness and the waking state.

Dream perspectives

What attracted Damisch to Brunelleschi's use of a mirror within a demonstration of painting was that the Renaissance architect had resorted to artifice, which Damisch identified as a necessary aspect of the perspective regime. Perspective was less about the creation of a mechanism to impose order on the world and could even be defined in the opposite way. In its use of deceptive devices like Brunelleschi's mirror, perspective invited a hallucinatory and disturbing way of apprehending reality. In Damisch's telling phrase, the history of perspective was the 'history of a dream' revealed by such deceiving mechanisms as anamorphosis ([1972] 2002: 135). Such 'dreaming perspectives', to coin a phrase, developed out of Lacan's discussion of anamorphosis and dreams, particularly the distinction between dreaming and the waking state (1977b: 75).

According to Lacan, in the waking state, the gaze is elided as well as the fact that not only does it look, but also shows; the dream, however, just shows (*ibid.*). What Lacan seems to be saying here is that within the dream the subject does not see or even care about the direction in which the dream is proceeding; the subject simply follows and has no sense of where he or she is in relation to the dream because the subject cannot recognise itself in terms of the Cartesian *cogito* within the field of the dream (*ibid.*). He or she cannot say 'I am a consciousness in a dream'.[7] As Martin Jay says, the awakened consciousness functions with a 'looking eye', but in our dreams, 'images show themselves to our unconscious', a condition of not-seeing (1993: 359). This distinction between Lacan's waking and dream state is important to Damisch because he argues that perspective should be seen in terms of the dream state that shows itself of its own accord ([1987] 1994: 97). Yet in that moment of recognition, a 'slippage of the subject occurs', and that is the moment when the perspective image 'demonstrates its presence' (*ibid.*).[8] The Narcissus factor, as defined by Damisch, is triggered. The slippage is equivalent to waking up at the moment of recognition or demonstration in which one sees oneself captured within the mechanism of representation.

Damisch's displacement of perspective from Renaissance art to the field of Lacanian psychoanalysis has not troubled Quattrocento scholars, but against the grain, I will analyse a painting that might be illuminated by the use of Damisch's ideas. The work in question is Giovanni Bellini's *Sacred Allegory* (*c.*1487, also dated 1499–1500; Plate 3), a painting that has strenuously resisted attempts at explanation, and as Oskar Bätschmann notes belongs with that class of indecipherable works that include Giorgione's *Tempesta* (2008: 131).[9] Usually celebrated for what is regarded as a planned and rationalised construction, Bellini's small panel depicts a mountainous landscape below a gloomy firmament in which lurk cumulous clouds. Near to the picture plane, a large checkerboard terrace is populated by religious figures such as the Madonna and St Sebastian, while other smaller genre-like figures are situated at the back of the painting whose middle ground is made up of an expansive blue lake.

My approach to Bellini's *Sacred Allegory* is to consider whether it should be regarded as the depiction of a dream in which Damisch's 'slippage' between showing and demonstrating occurs. In addressing the first part of this question it is important to state that just because there is no recognisable 'iconography of dreams' within the *Sacred Allegory* that does not discount it as a dream image. As Mosche Barasch has said, viewers of classical pictures may not have expected to have seen a sleeping figure, but the 'meaning' of the dream set out before their eyes (1997: 135). Much in the same vein, N. Rasmo has suggested that the panel should be seen as a personal fantasy, a reading rejected by Giles Robertson who sees such figures as a 'floating woman' in the lake not in terms of the dream, but as a painting decision. According to Robertson, Bellini originally intended to give her feet, and if he had wanted to show a floating figure, he would have shown her with feet above (1968: 101). Such details of 'naïve transcendentalism' seem to Robertson be incongruous in a painting planned with 'strict rationality', and therefore out of place within the fantasy or dream that Rasmo believes the painting shows. Yet, recalling Damisch's statement, that the history of perspective is a history of the dream, it seems unwarranted to see geometrical elements such as the checkerboard terrace as irreconcilable with fantasy or dream elements within Renaissance pictures.

Rasmo further argued that the *Sacred Allegory* could have been a *sacra conversazione* commissioned by Isabella d'Este, the Duchess of Mantua. What supports Rasmo's interpretation is that the Madonna and Sts Job and Sebastian are borrowed from a slightly earlier painting, the San Giobbe altarpiece, a canonical example of the *sacra conversazione* in Venice. Ingeniously, Bellini seems to have displaced saintly figures from the San Giobbe altarpiece in order to subvert and unravel the pictorial organisation of the *sacra conversazione.* What results is a dreamland, or to use Oskar Bätschmann's words, 'a capricious fantasy', in which elements of perspectival construction such as the terrace with its marble surround and the clouds with their reflections in the water, float before the viewer's attention rather than direct it to a focal point (2008: 135). The problematic 'floating woman', a floating signifier, has been mentioned, but it is especially the clouds reflected in the lake that invite a free-floating attention on the part of the viewer, rather than a concentrated intellectual looking, if a model in which the painting becomes the 'figure of psychoanalysis' is permitted (Marin 2001: 59–60).

It is difficult to gauge whether the reflections of clouds in the water are of those of the clouds directly overhead since Bellini decided to block out that portion of the sky with mountains whose reflections accompany those of clouds which are not directly overhead. But assuming that the panel has not been cut down, it seems as if Bellini wanted to show the displacement of the clouds, which now having passed, are visible in the wedge of sky towards the back of the picture.[10] Damisch has stated that the clouds in Bellini's paintings were never 'realistic', but components within the model of perspective, 'no more realistic than theatrical clouds' ([1972] 2002: 127). The clouds, an element of the 'perspective code', to use Damisch's term, also recall Brunelleschi's ruse of a mirror-like surface on his panel to record real clouds as they passed by overhead (*ibid.*: 125–6). It will be remembered that Damisch saw this operation, which uses the real clouds to simulate clouds on Brunelleschi's *tavola*, as an irruption of the real world into the realm of representation, what Damisch calls 'both a reflection and a body alien to the representational circuit'. With this idea Damisch's thinking accords with Arasse and Marin, who believed, as noted by Dekoninck, that 'the history of art ... cannot hide the theories of art it conveys, whether consciously or unconsciously' (Chapter 3 in this volume, at p. 76).

The use of such reflections brings us back to dream images and their relation to the specular structure of Narcissus. Such irruptions within the mirroring construction confer, in Lacanian terms, strangeness on the field of perception, an idea appropriate to Bellini's *Sacred Allegory*. If this picture is regarded as a painting that shows, the relationship between the clouds and the mirror of the lake within the *Sacred Allegory* should be viewed as a demonstration. The interaction of clouds and mirror demonstrates, in the sense that Damisch identified it in his discussion of Brunelleschi, which he saw as significant for Quattrocento painting as a whole, including Venetian art. The mirror of the lake demonstrates the sky by the process of *di-mostratio* involving duplication, but within that process, reality intrudes like the waking state penetrating the dream. The spatial and temporal displacement of the clouds, the break in the representational circuit, could be seen in terms of the waking state's intrusion on the dream, the appearance of the model without which the illusion of perspective – the dream content – cannot be sustained.

Dream-works

In his essay on the representation of dreams in the period of late antiquity, Moshe Barasch observes that in seeking to understand dreams in this period we 'remain within the shadow of our own age' (1997: 131). By this he is, of course, referring to the influence of Freud's *The Interpretation of Dreams*, published in 1899, but largely linked with the modern period where it has been mostly influential. As part of the process of displacing Freudian psychoanalysis to earlier periods, in *The Judgment of Paris* ([1992] 1996) Damisch suggests that the division of labour in Raphael's studio legitimates speaking in terms of 'work' in the sense of Freud's 'dream-work', a suggestion that deserves to be absorbed into the literature on Raphael's workshop and the problem of its configuration and organisation (*ibid.*: 90).[11]

Renaissance scholars might consider the use of psychoanalysis anachronistic when interpreting art of this era, although they might do well to heed Lacan who said that the unconscious existed and acted before Freud (1977b: 126). If Renaissance art history focuses on this issue at all, it takes care to differentiate between modern theories of psychoanalysis and period concepts such as *fantasia* (Fermor 1993: 29–37). Despite this understandable caution, the process of dreams has been discussed by some writers, notably Maria Ruvoldt (2004) on the baffling print known as *Raphael's Dream*. Like many Renaissance specialists, Ruvoldt admits to an iconographic approach where the emphasis is always on the 'meaning' of the dream image as opposed to the mechanics of it. Yet, 'meaning' is problematic here since, as Damisch has said, in resorting to iconography when investigating dream images, one runs the risk of performing crude readings in which the hidden text of iconography corresponds to the 'meaning' of the dream buried within the unconscious: 'Here, the position of the interpreter is close to that of the psychoanalyst who must try to discover the grammar of dreams as he proceeds in his or her deciphering, without hope of ever being able to lay bare a system on the basis of which it would then be possible to translate the whole of the dream' ([1972] 2002: 90).

In her discussion of Panofsky's iconographical principles, Michael Ann Holly has noted that the method of moving from the pre-iconographic stage to the iconological one has echoes of the Freudian schema in its descent through deeper and deeper layers of experience and meaning (1984: 167). This link between Freud and iconology had also occurred to Damisch who claims that Panofsky's iconology does not recognise the unconscious explicitly, the implication being that it exists in iconology nonetheless ([1992] 1996: 198). For Damisch, this suggests a project of analytic iconology which opens up interpretation to the unconscious, but as a safeguard against crude psychoanalysis, the interpreter had to consider beauty as part of the mechanism of representation. This explains Damisch's choice of the 'Judgment of Paris' as a subject for analysis in the volume of the same name, whose themes of moral choice and aesthetic inclination, as we shall see, have important implications for understanding Raphael's *Choice of Scipio*, also known as *Allegory* (*Vision of a Knight*) (Plate 4).

Inspired by this displacement of Freudian dream analysis to the interpretation of Renaissance art, it should be possible to start a tentative debate on how Renaissance works of art that contain the iconography of dreams, might be orientated towards work in the sense that Damisch evokes in his reference to dreams. As Freud says, the transformation of thoughts in the unconscious into the dream content is a process that can be considered in terms of 'representability in visual images' (Freud 1976: 459). Retaining an analogy with aspects of art, dream thoughts in the Freudian unconscious might be seen as abstract, colourless and schematic figures that are converted into vivid pictures. Here, the parallel that I am drawing is the relationship between the preliminary monochromatic drawing, and the finished picture in all its coloured glory. But far more suggestive for Damisch than the drawing with its 'first thoughts' is the engraving which the theorist does not see in terms of reproducibility, 'mechanical reproduction' in Benjamin's famous essay, but in terms of invention ([1992] 1996: 86; Benjamin 1970: 211–44). To Damisch, the engraving enacts the function of Freudian representability because it simultaneously bears witness to the dream-work while fixing that stage of the creative process ([1992] 1996: 90). The analogy with representability can be sustained especially as engravings lack colour, a fact that Carl Goldstein explains in terms of reproductive technology since engravings were mainly responsible for denigrating colour, which resulted in paintings being reproduced in black-and-white photographs because they did not do justice to colour in Renaissance art (1996: 84–5).

The problem of colour in relation to the dream-work will have to be put aside for now, but it is significant because it bears on the question of aesthetics and the characteristics of art in Damisch's project of analytic iconology. Rather than analytic iconology being governed by an iconographic code which might help to interpret these dream pictures that appear through the process of representability, the selection of dream thoughts is dependent on aesthetic validation, something not found in the realm of Freudian psychoanalysis, but only in art and aesthetics. An investigation into the 'meaning' of a picture must include an aesthetic dimension since it cannot be an art thought unless it has been 'interrogated', to use Damisch's word, by issues of representation and beauty, which bear upon judgement of taste, as theorised by Kant and implied by Freud ([1992] 1996: 39–51).

Before considering Raphael's *Choice of Scipio* as a 'dream-work', it is necessary to show how this image has been used to reproduce meaning and interpretations by art historians sympathetic to the iconographical method. The history of modern interpretation of this painting begins with Panofsky whose (1930) essay on the *Choice of Hercules* could be seen as the ur-text of interpretation. For Panofsky, this small panel was a variant on the convention known as the *Choice of Hercules*, in which philosophical exegesis and notions of pleasure were united to illustrate moral exempla. Building on Panofsky's foundation, Edgar Wind claimed that the missing text of iconography was the Roman archaeologist Macrobius's *Dream of Scipio* in which the hero was warned against the voluptuous life in a disquisition on philosophy (1980: 81–96). Wind argued that the London panel represented the discipline of the hero who would choose the path of duty, the picture therefore standing for the virtuous nature of the hero. A companion piece, *The Three Graces* (Chantilly, Musée Condé), was thought by Wind to represent liberality, a pictorial counterweight to Scipio's heroic dream.

These canonical readings centre on the allegorical aspect of the image in which the women within the dream form part of a moral structure dependent on the polarisation of virtue and pleasure. The problem of virtue and vice is not irrelevant to modern psychoanalysis since Freud considered how other writers had explored the way the dream is bound up with a working over in the unconscious of the remnants of daily experience, including the way moral nature remains after the daylight hours have dropped away (Freud 1976: 135). The dream in Raphael's painting could be construed as the visualisation of a moral code in dream formation, but our knowledge of how the morality of dreams functioned in the context of the Renaissance is limited. Yet, dream morality in the Renaissance could be connected with *fantasia* that was not only about image creation, but the distinction between virtue and vice (Fermor 1993: 29). Certain stoic and Christian writers used the notion of *fantasia* in relation to artistic invention: an aspect of faculty psychology that was used to guard against the encroachment of vile thoughts which might unseat virtuous ones.

Moral choice within allegory as an expression of the artist's own 'inner world' may have been a convention in this period. In his monograph on one of Raphael's contemporaries, Albrecht Dürer, Panofsky speculated that the artist's print of Hercules, in which the hero is shown between two women, may be an elaborate allegory of Dürer's own circumstances at an early way station in his artistic career (1955: 76). However, the problem with Panofsky's approach towards Dürer's *Choice of Hercules*, and by extension, all works with related subject matter, including Raphael's *Choice of Scipio*, is that it disavows the aesthetic experience. Aesthetics was removed from art history by Panofsky because it was concerned less with the art object as a historical phenomenon, or even the artist who created it. It was instead preoccupied with the effect of art on the beholder, an aspect of interpretation that Panofsky chose to disregard (Holly 1984: 87). Even in problems of interpretation where such notions of beauty and pleasure were involved, Panofsky reduced them to elements of a philosophical formula. And though the embryonic stage of Panofsky's iconographical method involved a consideration of form and shape, he may ultimately be responsible for divorcing style from iconography, and form from content, a schism that bedevils art history to this very day.

An indication of Panofsky's neglect of aesthetic concerns can be seen in his essay on the *Choice of Hercules* where he placed Raphael's colourful panel next to an austere German print of virtue and vice in order to point up iconographical similarities. Yet, qualities such as beauty were ignored in this scenario of moral choice. In commenting on this juxtaposition of Italian and German sources, the Dürer scholar, Joseph Leo Koerner, in a tone very similar to Damisch, reminds us that choice is part of the aesthetic appeal of Raphael's *Choice of Scipio* (1993: 391). Unlike Panofsky, who would use comparative analysis to create a moral polarity, Koerner says that 'hero and beholder together occupy a middle ground balanced by the panel's exquisite compositional equilibrium' (*ibid.*: 392). Thus Koerner links aesthetics with the spectator, and more importantly, stresses that the relationship between dream and dreamer suggests the free play of interpretation in which pleasure plays an important role. This recalls Damisch's point about the use of the dream in German versions of the 'Judgment of Paris' where it is used to conjure up the figures or dream thoughts translated into the condition of Freudian representability ([1992] 1996: 197). Within that psycho-formal structure, figures become interchangeable, and the dreamer in the picture, and indeed the observer of the dreamer's dream outside the painting, do not feel coerced into making choices by creating figures that convey distinctive ideas or themes.

Koerner is surely right when he says that Raphael's painting itself does not join in the psychomachia between virtue and vice. A moral divide in life is not created in the *Choice of Scipio*, but an aesthetic one. This reading challenges those who see the two female visitations as polar opposites with the woman holding the book and sword allegorising moral duty, and the woman with the flower, unbridled pleasure. As Koerner observes, Virtue may look slightly more austere than Pleasure, but she is hardly the ugly, minatory type found in the German engraving that Panofsky used in his iconographic method (Koemer 1993: 392). More significantly, the figure of Pleasure is not entirely given over to voluptuousness as she was in the preliminary drawing for the painting. This finessing of the allegory is visible in the changes between the cartoon and the final painting. In the cartoon Raphael made Virtue's neckline more angular; he also modified the décolletage of Pleasure and gave her a more modest tunic (Plazzota, in Chapman *et al.* 2004: 142). This suggests that Raphael was using beauty as a unifying force rather than something structuring an opposition, a subtlety that an iconographical interpreter working in the Panofsky vein, would, unlike Damisch, discount.

As Damisch's translator John Goodman suggests, this author's circumambulatory style resembles Lacan's circling around a perpetually absent object ([1992] 1996: xvi). The same can be said for the project of analytic iconology. Rather than zeroing in on a hidden text that corresponds to the 'meaning' of the painting, the kind that Edgar Wind insisted on, and Panofsky made a principle of iconographic exegesis, the interpreter in the guise of both psychoanalyst and art historian constantly circles around meaning which is never present or fixed. As Damisch says, psychoanalysis tries to 'make the image disappear from consciousness' but iconology works to impress it on the individual memory, and the collective memory in the form of museums and academic institutions (*ibid.*: 201). If this is doubted, consider how Panofsky's iconographical readings of Renaissance works of art do not disappear but remain in the memory of art history despite the attempts of scholars to submerge these interpretations (Bann 1992).

Conclusion: psychoanalysis encounters art history

Damisch's long engagement with psychoanalysis is far from over. In 1997/2007 he published *Piero della Francesca: A Childhood Memory* in which Freud's infamous monograph of Leonardo is playfully intertwined with Damisch's insights on questions of biography, iconography, style and childhood in Piero's art. Damisch's displacement of psychoanalysis into the sphere of established debates on early modern culture and art-historical problems has become more striking in recent years with the publication of his Piero book and his *Judgment of Paris.* This suggests to me that despite being thoroughly immersed in the debates about art and historiography, Damisch still considers the history of art in terms of a psychoanalytic narrative in which such concepts as perspective and cloud are displaced or detoured into the structural unconscious.

Perhaps this is the ultimate displacement for Damisch, the transversal knight's move into psychoanalysis, a way of encountering art history in terms of Freud and Lacan, and even Foucault whose early text on the phenomenology of dreams is clearly relevant to debates about the unconscious and representation in the seventeenth century (Foucault 1984–85). As Damisch was at pains to point out in his Amsterdam address, it was left to psychoanalysis – in the formidable person of Lacan – to pose the searching question of what a picture is (1977b: 105–19) Despite Lacan's intervention in the 1960s, this movement from psychoanalysis towards art history truly began with Aby Warburg in 1893, two years before Freud started to formulate his theories of dreams (Rose

2001: 15). And, as Damisch has observed, Warburg was guided by a 'principle of structural function' in which systems of thought and traditions of learning were amalgamated to create a European consciousness that drew on the classical past ([1992] 1996: 148). Freud used a similar structural model with his famous superimposition of different strata of Roman eras in *Civilization and Its Discontents* of 1929 to describe the unconscious (1985: 16–18).[12] Yet, Rome had already come to Freud's mind in 1899 with his invocation of Raphael's great Vatican wall paintings when explaining the concept of the dream-work in the *Interpretation of Dreams* (1976: 424). Here, as Louis Rose has said, Freud was confronting problems that had occurred to Aby Warburg, namely how one converts mental processes into visual images, a trans-disciplinary and trans-historical problem that Damisch continues to wrestle with (2001: 78).

References

Alberti, L. B. (1966) *On Painting*, trans. J. Spencer, New Haven, CT and London: Yale University Press.

Bann, S. (1989) *The True Vine: On Visual Representation and Western Tradition*, Cambridge: Cambridge University Press.

—— (1992) 'Meaning/Interpretation', in R. Nelson and R. Shiff (eds), *Critical Terms for Art History*, Chicago, IL: University of Chicago Press, 87–100.

Barasch, M. (1997) 'The Dream in the Art and Lore of Late Antiquity', *The Language of Art: Studies in Interpretation*, New York and London: New York University Press.

Bätschmann, O. (2008) *Giovanni Bellini*, Chicago, IL: University of Chicago Press.

Benjamin, W. (1970) *Illuminations*, ed. H. Arendt, London: Fontana.

Bowie, M. (1987) *Freud, Proust and Lacan: Theory as Fiction*, Cambridge: Cambridge University Press.

Chapman, H., Henry, T. and Plazzotta, C. (2004) *Raphael: From Urbino to Rome*, London: National Gallery Publications.

Damisch, H. ([1972] 2002) *Théorie du nuage: Pour une histoire de la peinture*, Paris: Seuil, 1972; *A Theory of /Cloud/Towards a History of Painting*, trans. J. Lloyd, Stanford, CA: Stanford University Press, 2002.

—— (1984) *Fenêtre jaune cadmium ou les dessous de la peinture*, Paris: Seuil.

—— ([1987] 1994) *L'Origine de la perspective*, Paris: Flammarion, 1987; *The Origin of Perspective*, trans. J. Goodman, Cambridge, MA and London: MIT Press, 1994.

—— ([1992] 1996) *Le Jugement de Pâris: Iconologie analytique 1*, Paris: Flammarion, 1992; *The Judgment of Paris*, trans. J. Goodman, Chicago, IL: University of Chicago Press, 1996.

—— ([1997] 2007) *Un souvenir d'enfance par Piero della Francesca*, Paris: Seuil, 1997; *Piero della Francesca: A Childhood Memory*, trans. J. Goodman, Stanford, CA: Stanford University Press, 2007.

—— and Bann, S. (2005) 'A Conversation', *Oxford Art Journal* 28(2) (2005), 155–81.

Fermor, S. (1993) *Piero di Cosimo: Fiction, Invention and Fantasia*, London: Reaktion.

Foucault, M. (1970) *The Order of Things: An Archaeology of the Human Sciences*, trans. A. Sheridan, London: Tavistock.

—— (1972) *The Archaeology of Knowledge*, trans. A. Sheridan, London: Tavistock.

—— (1984–85) 'Dream Imagination and Existence: An Introduction to Ludwig Binswanger's *Dream and Existence*', trans. F. Williams, *Review of Existential Psychology and Psychiatry* 19(1), 31–78. [first published in 1954]

Freud, S. (1976) *The Interpretation of Dreams*, The Pelican Freud vol. 4, Harmondsworth: Penguin.

—— (1985) *Civilization and Its Discontents*, The Pelican Freud vol. 12, Harmondsworth: Penguin.

Goldstein, C. (1996) *Teaching Art: Academies and Schools from Vasari to Albers*, Cambridge: Cambridge University Press.

Hall, M. *et al.* (2005) *The Cambridge Companion to Raphael*, Cambridge: Cambridge University Press.

Holly, M. A. (1984) *Panofsky and the Foundations of Art History*, Ithaca, NY: Cornell University Press.

Jay, M. (1993) *Downcast Eyes: The Denigration of Vision on Twentieth-Century French Thought*, Berkeley and Los Angeles, CA: University of California Press.

Koerner, J. L. (1993) *The Moment of Self-Portraiture in German Renaissance Art*, Chicago, IL: Chicago University Press.

Lacan, J. (1977a) *Écrits: A Selection*, trans. A. Sheridan, London: Tavistock.

—— (1977b) *The Four Fundamental Concepts of Psycho-Analysis*, trans. A. Sheridan, London: Penguin.

Lucco, M. and Villa, G. C. F. (eds) (2009) *Giovanni Bellini*, Milan: Silvana (exhibition catalogue, Rome, Scuderie del Quirinale).

Marin, L. (1995) *To Destroy Painting*, trans. M. Hjort, Chicago, IL: University of Chicago Press.

—— (2001) *On Representation*, trans. C. Porter, Stanford, CA: Stanford University Press.

Owens, C. (1992) *Beyond Recognition: Representation, Power and Culture*, Berkeley and Los Angeles, CA: University of California Press.

Panofsky, E. (1927) 'Die Perspektive als "symbolische Form"', in *Vorträge der Bibliothek Warburg* 1924–25, Leipzig and Berlin, 1927, 258–330; *Perspective as Symbolic Form*, trans. C. Wood, New York: Zone Books, 1991.

—— (1930) 'Hercules am Scheidewege und andere antike bildstoffe in der neueren Kunst', Studien der Bibliothek Warburg, vol. 18, Leipzig and Berlin.

—— (1955) *The Life and Art of Albrecht Dürer*, 4th edn, Princeton, NJ: Princeton University Press.

—— (1968) *Idea: A Concept in Art Theory*, Columbia, SC: University of South Carolina Press.

—— (1970) *Meaning in the Visual Arts*, London: Peregrine Books.

Rasmo, N. (1946) 'La sacra conversazione belliniana degli Uffizi e il problema della sua comprensione', *Carro minore* 5(6), 229–40.

Robertson, G. (1968) *Giovanni Bellini*, Oxford: Clarendon.

Rose, L. (2001) *The Survival of Images: Art Historians, Psychoanalysts and the Ancients*, Detroit, MI: Wayne State University Press.

Ruvoldt, M. (2004) *The Italian Renaissance Imagery of Inspiration: Metaphors of Sex, Sleep, and Dreams*, Cambridge: Cambridge University Press.

Wind, E. (1980) *Pagan Mysteries in the Renaissance*, rev. edn, Oxford: Oxford University Press.

Notes

1 Preparation of this chapter coincided with an invitation to speak at a symposium on Hubert Damisch at the University of Amsterdam, 27–8 May 2009. My thanks to Sophie Berrebi and Eric van Bruyn for inviting me to participate in this event. Many of the ideas in the 'dream-works' section were presented in a paper given in the presence of Damisch who gave a keynote speech on the subject of 'displacing' at the symposium.

2 Author's notes from Damisch's keynote address 'Displacing' (see n. 1 above).

On the relationship between art history and critical theory, see the excellent discussion in Owens (1992: 89–93).

3 Damisch, 'Displacing' (see n. 1 above).

4 'Psychoanalysis gets only to the hypothetical, thus generating one of the most fundamental paradoxes of the Freudian conception of the image. Whenever analysis tries to exhaust the whole content of the image in the meaning it may secrete, the link uniting image to meaning is always defined as a possible, eventual, contingent one. Why does the psychological meaning take shape in an image, instead of remaining implicit or dissolving into the limpidity of a verbal formulation?' (1984–85: 31–78, at 36).

5 Space precludes me developing Damisch's remarks here. On the 'psychoanalysis' of Poussin, see the 1986 interview with Louis Marin (2001: 59).

6 See Stephen Bann's use of Damisch's ideas on Narcissus (1989: 134ff.).

7 Compare Lacan with Foucault: 'the subject of the dream is not so much the personage who says "I" as the whole dream in the entirety of its dream content' (1984–85: 59).

8 Marin calls this the 'breaking point in the model' (1995: 152). See also Marin's review of Damisch's *Théorie du nuage* (2001: 14–37).

9 For the various interpretations of the picture, see Robertson (1968: 100); Lucco and Villa (2009: 236–7).

10 Robertson says that the picture in its present state seems 'completely coherent' (1968: 100).

11 Scholarship on the problem of Raphael's workshop is sparse, but see Bette Talvacchia, 'Raphael's Workshop and the Development of a Managerial Style', Patricia Emison, 'Raphael's Multiples', and Linda Wolk-Simon, 'Raphael Drawings: Pro-Contra', all in Hall (2005).

12 See Malcolm Bowie's discussion of Freud and the metaphor of archaeology (1987: 18–27).

5

Christine Buci-Glucksmann: the archaeology of shadows or the aesthetics of image-flux

François-Xavier Gleyzon

To understand the work of Christine Buci-Glucksmann is, first of all, to understand the movement intrinsic to every image in all its temporal fluidity. If *image-flux* is a theory of the image, it proceeds above all by apostrophising and by *spatial* contextualisation: 'you imagine . . .', 'You are in London', etc., thus offering to the reader's gaze an aesthetic itinerary in the course of which is displayed not just another *mundus* [world] but also a quite unusual modus operandi [mode] of seeing. Through spaces and points of view that invoke Shakespeare, Mannerism and the Baroque and that circulate up to the era of virtual reality and technology, the question of a 'folie du voir', the contours of which offer a veritable 'cartographie de l'art', may then be posed in a theoretical/conceptual way (Buci-Glucksmann 2002, 2001a). Such would be what Christine Buci-Glucksmann proposes, and, at the same time, the critical stake of this chapter: *a journey of the gaze*, a journey reminiscent of that of Icarus in which the eye takes flight in order to contemplate better and thus direct us to the frontiers, to the limits of the visual. Beyond this limit representation can no longer represent itself, vacillating and then toppling into rhetoric and a quite unusual topology: 'an archaeology of shadows' [*une archéologie de l'ombre*] (Buci-Glucksmann 1988: 23).

But what is an archaeology of shadows? How can we at the same time envisage the ephemeral nature, the wandering and the floating mobility of shadows in an archaeological sense theorised by Foucault, as Buci-Glucksmann suggests? There is a strange oxymoronic polarity of darkness and light, of chiaroscuro: that of the cast shadows which invites us to bring to light a *situs* and the visual mechanisms and inner workings, buried the artefacts of thought. If the archaeology of shadows exhibits and calls into question a well-defined dualism of opposing concepts, it illuminates a creative permutation in the gap created by this conceptual interchange and which will end up, according to Buci-Glucksmann (2008b: 24), in a certain logic of fluidity, in 'a fluid logic of inclusion'. But does the possibility of such a conceptual coupling, not come in the first place from a desire and a will to reform, if not rediscover, the becoming, the fluctuating, in short, the ephemeral? Perhaps we are coming close here to the heart of the philosophy of Buci-Glucksmann (2003a), in which an alternative progression of 'the Aesthetics of the Ephemeral' will be developed. The investigation of them will allow us to make bridges between Western and Oriental thought, through a series of philosophical connections.

The West classifies the ephemeral as that which is vulnerable to the passage of time, a 'melancholic ephemeral' which lives the passage of time as a tragedy in which being is undermined from the inside, emptying itself into death, its body thus turning into a crypt (Buci-Glucksmann 2008b: 15; 2005: 126). As it happens, the ephemeral – *ephemeros* – in Greek philosophy is not time itself but a modulation of time, a mobile image of time in its novelty and fluidity. What concerns us here is the harnessing of invisible forces, of flux and rhythms in the sense that Buci-Glucksmann understands them, and of seizing the moment both present and opportune, or, in other words, the *kairos* (2003a: 28–9). We can read and reread the ephemeral as a characteristic enhanced and rediscovered as a light and floating 'impermanence', an 'affirmative ephemeral' which, beyond all melancholy or Western post-melancholy, receives, in a sort of *ukiyo-e*, the oriental art of the floating world of impermanence in ancient Japan, the suspended and invisible vibrations of time that resound in the moment of actual time (Lafargue 2006: 11). We can see here how Buci-Glucksmann's attempts at making bridges with a philosophy of visual art links up with that of Gilles Deleuze. 'In art, and in painting and music, we are not concerned with reproducing or inventing forms but with harnessing forces. It is even in this respect that no art is figurative ... The task of painting is defined as the attempt to make visible forces which are not' (Deleuze 2002: 57). Thus, *between* the space of the canvas and the space to be represented, the problem is then defined in all its philosophical intensity: 'two spaces therefore and even a space in between, the moment itself when these two spaces merge' (Buci-Glucksmann 1988: 32). At this moment, this ephemeral moment – as unspeakable and intangible as it is infinitesimal *between* two distinct spaces, between a potency of vision in becoming *a virtuality*, and a force (*virtus*) – a vacuum is discernible and may be drawn as an abyss of light and dark, which allows Buci-Glucksmann to underline one of the lessons of painting: 'There could be said to exist there, in painting [. . .] a great lesson of the philosophy of darkness to produce representable visuality (and we know that Leibniz's monads are both centres of perception and of energy): we need that which cannot be represented' (*ibid.*). Thus, from the passage of the invisible to the visible, this affirmative ephemerality, this *nothing*, can be defined as 'an essential vacuum' or 'a shadow', which will be the term chosen by Buci-Glucksmann (*ibid.*: 28) and which will be the condition for the possibility and the emergence of representation while simultaneously trying to conceal it.

Shadow, or 'the essential emptiness' of representation, is connected to a certain mystery in the act of representation that operates in an interval. What is at stake here is a certain transformation–transubstantiation from invisible to visible; and it is moreover precisely this movement of nothingness, this nothing-movement, this nothing-flux as a mediator or interface allowing passage from invisibility to visibility which will be mobilised at an opportune moment, for Buci-Glucksmann, that of the Baroque, with its correlate, Mannerism. Since her three books on Mannerism, devoted to a vision of the Baroque: *Tragique de l'ombre: Shakespeare et le Maniérisme* (1990), *La Raison Baroque* (1984) and *La Folie du voir* ([1986] 2002), we know that the high point of her work as she herself describes it (2008b: 28), could be summed up in 'a History/Story of the Eye' that tries to locate and engage with very particular territories, new places that rhetoric and Baroque art harness and isolate in the praise and glory of nothingness, of emptiness. Buci-Glucksmann (2002: 173–90) will go as far as to endow Baroque writers 'with a rhetorical telescope' capable of delimiting and localising the aesthetics and the figures of nothingness, and this 'in all its forms, in all its languages'. '*Il niente, la nada, le vide,* vacuousness, nothingness, the abyss' (*ibid.*: 173), an extreme obsession, on the part of Baroque writers, with the glory of the figures of nothingness – from Mazzini to Tesauro, Gracián to Menestrier. Mazzini does not cease in his *Treatise on Nothingness* to praise 'the nobility', 'the perfection', the artistry so that 'nothing outside God is more noble and more perfect than *nothingness*' (*ibid.*: 173, 177). Relying on the primacy of this 'economy of nothingness', celebrated previously by Giuseppe Castiglione in his *Discorso academio in Lode del Niente* (*ibid.*: 183), Buci-Glucksmann shows that a split with the Renaissance tradition of epideictic discourse is in operation here, which breaks with the discourse of flattery, praise and encomia analysed by Louis Marin in his *Portrait of the King* (1981: 109–30; 1975: 111), and which preaches vanity, excess, ornamentation by making inappropriate use of everything so as to sublimate the recipient subject/object. For Baroque writers, Buci-Glucksmann shows a different vision of art not dissimilar to that offered by Jacques Lacan (1966: 155), and for whom the linguistic dimension to the Baroque is central: 'All art is characterised by a certain way of organising itself around this void.' And Buci-Glucksmann adds (1988: 34) that, without this nothing, 'without a void there is no aesthetic'. This void, this creative nothingness around which art is organised, will not find a better field of application and explanation than in Shakespeare, in whom she will detect and mobilise in another key moment of her work, the paradigm of an approach to art or, even, art as a thought, a thought of nothingness (1990: 193–209).

'Shakespeare says it all', declares Buci-Glucksmann (2008b: 19) and she shows us, *avant la lettre*, in a subtle way, the turning point at which an aesthetic is articulated between saying and seeing, a latent topology that is ungraspable and inaccessible between opposing rhetorical strategies, *corpora*. The exchange of this *corpora* triggers the tragedy, as the 'mid-point', and tries, as we shall see, not only to construct a strategy of resistance but also to construct 'a floating corpus of absence' (Buci-Glucksmann 1990: 193). In her analysis of *King Lear*, Buci-Glucksmann picks up on the moment, or rather on the decisive *spacing* that leads to catastrophe in the tragedy: the *nothing* of Cordelia's speech during the Love Test, during the laudatory and flattering speeches meant for the ageing father and king.

> KING LEAR: Speak.
> CORDELIA: *Nothing* my lord.
> KING LEAR: Nothing?
> CORDELIA: *Nothing.*
> (I.1.ll.79–86, my italic)[1]

We know that Cordelia's 'Nothing' does not indicate a deliberate holding back, a lack of love or deference towards her father, but marks the true measure of the love she has for him; for how can she truly express and prove her love for the father-king if not in the retraction and the depth of language, that is, in the 'nothing', in the oblivion as infinite as it is sublime and which is catalysed in that tragic moment ('What shall

Cordelia speak? / Love and be silent', I.1.l.59). Buci-Glucksmann (1990: 194) makes the case that the strength of Cordelia's speech, its essence, does not only reside in that rhetorical strategy which consists in saying *everything* without saying *anything*; Cordelia's 'Nothing' is to some extent, as Deleuze states (2003: 301) in a work pre-dating Buci-Glucksmann's *Tragique de l'Ombre*, 'an act of resistance' which is committed first and foremost to turning upside down the rhetorico-scopic and political machinations of her older sisters, Goneril and Regan. Thus, by refusing to follow and to imitate this rhetoric, that is, by breaking King Lear's rhetorical mirror and this rivalry (that game of bids and counter-bids) and therefore by replying nothing to the king's request, Cordelia condemns herself to paternal excommunication: 'Here I disclaim all my paternal care/Propinquity and property of blood' (I.1.l.112).

Buci-Glucksmann will, of course, not stop there. She goes on to give a powerful reading of the origin of tragedy – or the *origyne*, as we shall see later – and of the sequence that she analyses with the tools appropriate for cinematography, that is, segment by segment, frame by frame. In fact, by refusing to accede to the request of the father-king (and refusing to imitate her sisters), Cordelia's act of resistance introduces and generates a clean break, a distancing or an interval, between father and daughter. And it is therefore in this thin disjunctive thread, the line of fracture between father and daughter that an act of aesthetic creation will be carried out. It is this singular pinpointing between these two Shakespearean bodies, these two enunciatory bodies – *corpora* – that Buci-Glucksmann re-examines and relaunches a specific and particular tradition, the only interesting and valid one in the eyes of Aby Warburg, the *Ikonologie des Zwischenraumes*, that is, 'the Iconology of the Interval'. What Warburg ([1918] 2000: 611–14) means by this is certainly the in-between, the gap, the fissure made visible between objects–things–subjects and also the place of void and nothingness, the unassignable, in short, where the image could nevertheless be said to be placed (Didi-Huberman 2000: 114; 2002b: 452–506).[2] But Buci-Glucksmann prefers to place a different emphasis on this *Iconology of Intervals*, an 'Other Internal Elsewhere [. . .] which could be called the Orient or Asia', and in which, progressively disposing of all Western (and therefore culturally determined) philosophical apparatus, she will place the figure of the Japanese concept of *Ma*, the 'mid-point' as intermediate and unstable space at the very heart of her thought:

> The 'mid-point' [...] in Japan is inseparable from a concept of void as 'a middle between nothing and everything' that makes possible the intervals and intervening spaces of *Ma* which is the foundation of any approach to time. For *Ma* is, at one and the same time, interval, void and spacing, 'between' in the strong sense of the word. It separates, joins and installs a breathing, a fluctuation [...] which together begets this relationship of time to infinity which is special to Japan. For the interval institutes both a distance and a dynamic, a void and a plurality of meanings. It is *silence* and the blank of a spacing. (Buci-Glucksmann 2001b: 13, 36)

Ma, the 'mid-point, the distance of an interval, is first and foremost creative' (*ibid.*: 36). This is what the Shakespearean *nothing* offers us: a gap between the father and the daughter, a nothing, that is, a metaphorical silence which, paradoxically, can only make itself heard in and through language ('What shall Cordelia speak? Love and be silent'/'nothing') but it is also an aesthetic *silence.* In the interval of *n*O*thing* (Lear – *n*O*thing* – Cordelia), the mute O could be a drawing of the open mouth and the empty mouth where the image will be attached.[3] It is possible that Buci-Glucksmann's analysis here finds its pictorial equivalent in the *Silence* that Odilon Redon painted. Here silence appears to the onlooker almost as in a dream, a vision. As Buci-Glucksmann is fond of saying, using the celebrated formula of Paul Klee: here 'the picture looks' (2002: 131). *Lightness, indistinct light,* this image shows in a circle an O-space that is both floating and eerie, an 'airy nothing' to borrow a Shakespearean expression (*A Midsummer Night's Dream*, 5.1.l.14), the face of a woman who indicates, by a gesture well known in art, the 'signum harpocraticum', that silence is required (Langedijk 1964: 3; Chastel 2001: 65–90). Thus, it is through this same creative vein, in the ring/circle of this image where the woman appears and where 'a sort of silence [a nothing] gleams in the background' (Klee, in Marin 1971: 83) that Buci-Glucksmann will be able to weave another text around Shakespeare's and to evoke all the literary imaginativeness of Fernando Pessoa and thus render this visible readable – that is, to turn this aesthetic figure into a figure of poetic language – and to do so by borrowing from Pessoa one single and uniquely admirable expression: *Our Lady of Silence* (Pessoa 1982, 1996; Buci-Glucksmann 1990: 197).

Another important turning point for Buci-Glucksmann then is Pessoa. In this fragment of the *Book of Disquietude*, silence is depicted in the features of a woman: 'O Lady of internal silences' – she is a 'body of absence' which is summed up in Pessoa as a 'Splendour of nothing, in the Name [...] of Nothingness/abyss' (1996: 437–8). Attached to this nothing, to this silence, let us not forget, is the large number of O's that pre*figure* as much as they prefix and provide a name for the Lady: 'O Lady', 'O Shelter of all hazy dreams', 'O Running Water of Sad Experience', 'O Litany of Disquiet', 'O Royal Mass of Weariness', 'O Corolla', 'O Holy Fluid', 'O Ascension', etc. (*ibid.*: 438). This plethora of O's will also carry through the metaphorical/metonymic passage from the O of Our Lady of Silence in a series of scattered pearls. In this way, through the metaphor of the necklace that breaks and lets drop a torrent of pearls, of O's, the image of the woman of silence in Pessoa is merely a set of fragments that cannot be reassembled: 'You are nothing [...] your profile is to be nothing and the contour of your body undoes in isolated pearls the necklace of the very idea of contour' (Buci-Glucksmann 1990: 197). But with respect to the necklace which comes undone and disintegrates into a nothing, Buci-Glucksmann will note here its oxymoronic character in which nothing is associated with a necklace of pearls/of ideas through which the braiding of paradoxes constitutes a negative path and will allow access to a sort of visualisation *by default* of the Lady of Silence. It is indeed the string of the necklace, that semantic chain that joins that torrent of silent O's and that leads us to the nothing that Our Lady of Silence embraces and that Pessoa (1996: 441) will continuously name *intersticio* (interstice) or even *intervallo* (interval): 'You occupy the interval of my thoughts, you are the interstice of my sensations.' Interval and interstice are the space, the aesthetic in-betweenness, in which (in an O of silence and of nothing) the vision of this Lady of Silence resides. So it is in the interval/interstice (in this silent nothing) that for Buci-Glucksmann the greatest affinity is produced; it represents in short an artistic correspondence between Shakespeare and Pessoa, and even Redon. But it is also this interval, this spacing or mid-point, which seems to engage a process of aesthetic-cum-iconological materialisation of the discourse on nothing/silence offered to us by Buci-Glucksmann by means of this triangulation, and is even, to borrow a Deleuzian expression, 'une mise en correspondance réglée' ('a measured process of correspondence') (Deleuze 2003: 293).

Let us return for a moment to Shakespeare, to *King Lear*, and to Buci-Glucksmann's analysis, and focus once again on the discourse on *nothing*, which will allow us to identify the origin of the drama of Lear and thus to take note of everything that bursts and flashes like a thunderbolt or lightning, and echoes *between* the two shores/bodies, that is, all the dynamism of the space–time proper to this tragedy. Everything is played out quickly and everything rushes into the interval of *nothing*. But we must not be surprised at such speed, at such a dizzy rate of acceleration, for it is indeed also one of the specificities of the interval, or, according to Deleuze's terminology, of the middle: 'the middle has *nothing to do* with a mean; it is not a centring. It is, on the contrary, all about absolute speed: that which grows, that which lies in the middle is endowed with such a speed' (Deleuze and Parnet 1996: 39). It is in the exchange of the two bodies (or corpora), in the exchange of looks, over and above the interval opened up between Lear and Cordelia, and over and above this nothingness of language perforating the text, that the true and secret apparition will intervene: in the concave pupil belonging to Cordelia, in the setting of her look, the child then becomes something completely other, for 'the child', writes Nietzsche (1977: 54, §4), 'is the unbearable mirror image of original eternal suffering, of the unique foundation of the world' – that of the woman-mother. An apparition as dazzling as it is searing for all is played out in the space (interval) of a look in what we could call *the interval of the original gaze.* Perhaps it is there, in that particular interval, in the very eye of the tragedy, or as Julia Kristeva would say (1983: 42) during a 'hallucinatory *nothing*', that the Origin of the feminine could be said to emerge: *the origyne.*[4] Buci-Glucksmann finds in this interval that perforates language and that degenerates into emptiness, into shadows, the opportune moment to establish her 'archaeology of shadows', at the heart of which we can see 'the arcana of the feminine' (2002: 67), in the wandering and floating, that is, in the sense of Foucault's *archaeology*, 'as at the edge of the sea a face on the sand' (Foucault 1966: 398).

In this way Buci-Glucksmann (1990: 197) positions us before the place of the interval, *between* and *in the middle* of the two bodies (Lear's and Cordelia's) where emptiness and vacuity of shadows act as true breaths, rhythms, flux or dynamic forces, 'a nodal point woven from virtual reality and becoming' which, exactly as in Chinese aesthetics, allows us to seize the 'li', those 'internal laws of things'. This 'li' is where the vision of the female body in a Pessoa or a Shakespeare takes up residence and is crystallised. This floating, wandering female body which only emerges through an 'archaeology of shadows' and which is born from nothing, from emptiness – O – refers us back, as Buci-Glucksmann indicates, to that specific phenomenon of *Das Ding* inherent to art. Taking her cue from Lacan (himself reinterpreting Freud), Buci-Glucksmann points out to us that *Das Ding* is that thing, that body, that 'true buried secret', 'lost maternal thing', 'prehistoric and unforgettable other', 'empty body of the ghost of a pale incubus'. This thing-body is a 'mute reality', 'outside signifier' (Lacan 1966: 155; in Moscovi and Rey 1988: 36). We only need go a little further in Buci-Glucksmann's analysis to find in this elusive female body the pure event of the gaze – so important for Aby Warburg – and which he designated as *Ninfa*. Didi-Huberman draws our attention to this female body inasmuch as it is based and unfolds into a *modern* destiny in the sense understood by Baudelaire and Benjamin:

> *Ninfa* traverses the objects of Warburgian art history like a veritable 'enigmatic organism'. The impersonal heroine of the *aura* – that distance which moves the event of our looks – she moves constantly between air and stone, effluvia and paralysis: fleeting like a wind, but pale and tenacious like a fossil. A reducible heroine of disquieting strangeness, she gives us 'prior resemblances' [*arrière-ressemblances*] wherein all times, all of a sudden, begin to dance together. And wherein all her possible incarnations come to mix with one another as in a dream. (Didi-Huberman 2002a: 10–11)

But Buci-Glucksmann will not name this body, 'this enigmatic organism'. She prefers to retain a nameless depth. Perhaps the female body remains this forever barred subject, the *S* as Lacan defines it (1966: 805), a subject that finds itself barred by the vector of language or discourse and thus consigned to emerge only in the vanguard of the text. Thus the feminine – *surreptitious*, *different* and *transient* – is for Buci-Glucksmann a veiled shadow, an abyss, a gulf and a vacuousness, but also an original matrix, in short an 'indefinable power of the foreign female', as Maurice Blanchot put it (in Buci-Glucksmann 2002: 67). In relation to the female question here, all Buci-Glucksmann's work devoted to Mannerist and Baroque space–vision will undergo a sort of mutation–translation, for, as we have seen, 'the Baroque will become *modern*' (*ibid.*: 50). A whole scenography of the 'female body as interpretative principle of modern allegory' can now be drawn and reconstructed, instituting a regime of feminine imaginary proper to modernity or to 'the original historical form of the 19th Century' in which Benjamin and Baudelaire will both come into play (*ibid.*: 75).

But the apparition of the female body in its modern meaning is nonetheless only an event of the gaze. Thus Buci-Glucksmann does not hesitate to borrow from Deleuze his definition of the event as a spatio-temporal dynamism and an identity of the form of emptiness: 'Events are like crystals, they only come into being and grow by and in their edges' (Deleuze 1969: 83; Buci-Glucksmann and Wright 1999: 2). Just as in Shakespeare, as we have established, the origin of tragedy emerges in the event of the gaze of a female body taking place at the mid-point between two luminal bodies, in empty shadows, where tragedy will be established in the fall that it provokes, as Pessoa declares: 'You are woman before the fall' (in Buci-Glucksmann 1990: 200). In 'this event site' of the in-between (to use an expression by Alain Badiou), Buci-Glucksmann questions 'the event as [...] a site in time – in other words, the event [...] in the singularity of time' (1996: 110; Buci-Glucksmann and Wright 1999: 3). It is 'modernity' [which] reinvents the poetic interval of a distinct newness, of the "always new" proper to the present, by the allegorical distance of a past that is present [...] of a creative absence of form' (1990: 200). And the flows, respiration, rhythms, swarmings and turbulence at the heart of this in-between position us at the mid-point of time and help us finally to *see* the event in time, as Gilles Deleuze suggests (1985: 109), as through a crystal: 'the crystal reveals a direct image-time [...] Time must be split into two dissymmetric streams, one of which conveys the whole of the *present* and the other preserves the whole of the *past*. Time consists in this scission and this it is, it is time *that we see in the crystal*. The crystal image was not time, but we see time in the crystal.'

We know that, from her *Folie du voir* onwards, the philosophy of Deleuze has been a factor in Buci-Glucksmann's work. But such an understanding of time, at the heart of intervals, of interstitial spaces and spaces *between*, which shows itself through the crystal, allows Buci-Glucksmann to make time emerge from the angle of an *encounter*, that is, of the event as a moment seen from the angle of an entropic eye, namely 'an event which represents time, at the junction of time where different times coexist and meet' (Buci-Glucksmann and Wright 1999: 2).[5] As she notes after Benjamin, it is precisely this encounter, this dialectic, which mobilises and animates the concept of the image of the modern female body or even 'the original phenomenon of [modern] history'.[6] In her chapter on 'Walter Benjamin and Baroque reason' (2002: 47; 2003a: 14–15), she picks up on that dialectical image proposed by Benjamin as *pure happening*, a veritable *flash* emanating from a system that is both temporal and visual. Thus, with respect to modernity, 'the dialectical image is an image that dazzles', wrote Benjamin in his *Fragments* on Baudelaire in 1939 ([1938–39] 1982: 240). As it does in Benjamin's Paralipomena of the theses *On the Concept of History* in 1940, the image will be the moment of a lightning flash, a ball of fire shaping itself on the horizon (Benjamin 1991: 348). Such is the power of the image of modern space: a power which illuminates the original (*origynal*) phenomenon of history but which, as Buci-Glucksmann points out, once made visible, the thing/subject/object illuminated and presented is condemned to fall and disappear into darkness and pours forth into the emptiness of night:

> The authentic image of the past only appears in a *flash*. It is an image which springs up only to be eclipsed forever in the moment that follows. The motionless truth that merely keeps the researcher waiting bears no relationship to this concept of truth as far as history is concerned. It leans rather on the lines of Dante that says: 'it is a unique irreplaceable image of the past which vanishes with each present which has not been able to recognise itself as its aim'. (*ibid.*: 342)

Or as Benjamin wrote: 'We must not say that the past illuminates the present or the present illuminates the past. An image, on the contrary, is that in which the past meets up with the present in a *flash* to form a constellation' (1989: 491; Buci-Glucksmann 2003a: 14–15). But let us leave the flash suspended for a moment longer, to use a Proustian expression – 'Isolate, immobilise the duration of a flash, a brief length of time in its pure state' (in Blanchot [1959] 1971: 23). For it is at the moment of that flash – the dialectical image of the modern par excellence – that the Female will be seen, 'the most precious treasure' in the eyes of the moderns, as Buci-Glucksmann points out quoting Benjamin (2002: 52). In addition, the poem 'À une passante', in *Les Fleurs du mal* by Baudelaire ([1857] 1975: 92–3), is an emblem of that peculiar vision of the woman who appears suddenly only then to disappear in the city of Paris in a flash:

> Un éclair... puis la nuit! – Fugitive beauté
> Dont le regard m'a fait soudainement renaître,
> Ne te verrai-je plus que dans l'éternité?
>
> Ailleurs, bien loin d'ici ! trop tard ! jamais peut-être !
> Car j'ignore où tu fuis, tu ne sais où je vais,
> Ô toi que j'eusse aimée, ô toi qui le savait.
>
> [A lightning flash... then night! – Fleeting beauty
> By whose gaze I was suddenly reborn
> Will I see you no more before eternity?
>
> Elsewhere, far from here! Too late! Perhaps never!
> For I know not where you flee, you know not where I go
> Oh you whom I would have loved, oh you who knew it too.]

It is by going through the crowded streets of Paris that Baudelaire's *flâneur* will enjoy this sublime and sublimated vision of the female. But in Baudelaire's imaginary world, woman unfolds into ambivalence, while carrying strangeness and blackness; and she persists in retaining her female body even when it is in rags like 'la mendiante rousse' ['the red-haired beggar woman'] 'whose dress through its holes/ lets us see her poverty/ And beauty [. . .]' (*ibid.*: 83–5), or even when it is the prostituted body, as shown in the poem 'Allégorie' ['Allegory'], or, a little later, in the hysterical female bodies exhibited by Charcot, photographed at la Salpêtrière; for Baudelaire this body will not cease to evince wonder: 'With *jouissance* I claim my right to be hysterical' (in Buci-Glucksmann 2002: 52).

Modern woman emerges thus in a flash. 'The face of Modernity strikes us down with an immemorial gaze', wrote Benjamin (*ibid.*: 83). Is the flash of this female apparition, which comes to lodge in the eye of the *flâneur* only to sink subsequently into obscurity, not also the *scotome scintillant* [glittering scotoma] (Charcot 1890: 76), like the patient struck down by lightning? We know that Charcot, fascinated by this case of lightning and thanks to his scopic keenness always to look closer, asked his patient to reproduce in detail what she had seen in her eye, that is, the exact form of the *flash*. The representation based on a sketch by the patient is surprising from many points of view, since this 'scotome scintillant' portrays the flash as a true spiral: a multi-centred spiral which seems to roll up from bottom to top and to be repeated in the eye. The eye of moderns could be said to be that of a journey in which – in a flash – the bedazzlement of the female body pours out into obscurity; that is, we are talking here about an eye-spiral.

It is at the heart of this eye-spiral that Buci-Glucksmann, in another part of her work and still possessed of that *folie du voir*, will concentrate her efforts. Likewise, in her *Philosophie de l'ornement* (2008a: 32), she will trace in the feminine curves of Klimt's *Fulfilment* all the intricacies of spirals: 'joining life to a female eroticism in which fluid bodies flirt with adornment as an aesthetic principle of composition'. 'Dynamic and energetic, this line-flux, both open and closed, is like an immense eye slipping into infinity', she wrote of the spirals of the artist Pascal Dombis or of the *Spiral Woman* by Louise Bourgeois (Buci-Glucksmann 2009: 5–6). Still inhabited and caught by the spiral in all its forms and sizes, Buci-Glucksmann, quoting the work of Michel Serres in *L'œil cartographique de l'art*, went on to describe it as 'a thing which experiences irregular alternations of ascent and descent, of advancement and retreat. Its evolution is represented by a carefully composed vibratory movement' (1996: 106). But as Buci-Glucksmann accurately points out, the spiral calls – in order to be contemplated and measured in all its aesthetic economy, on the scale and amplitude appropriate to it – for another 'morphological operator' (*ibid.*: 107), for the cartographic gaze of Icarus. We must therefore, according to Buci-Glucksmann, deterritorialise ourselves and grasp for a moment that folly proper to the vision of Icarus – that plunging, overhanging and panoramic gaze.

However it is soon clear that Icarus's vision works along the vertical axis and participates in a double perspective of height and depth, of elevation and therefore of falling. Icarus's fantasy is here nothing other than a 'falling upwards', 'a fall into the sky', that is, a desire as intense as it is burning to go there, 'to rush still higher into the sky and yet where the sky really appears as an upside-down abyss [...] an abyss that is earthly then' (Bachelard 1943: 125). It is here in this dynamic that the image of the tellurian and the aerial comes together, and, between these two poles, Man is the hyphen, the cosmic vertical vector. The great spiral of the celebrated land artist, Robert Smithson, *Spiral Jetty*, obeys this peculiar command of the gaze exemplified by Icarus. For 'only the Icarian gaze of aerial photographs taken from a helicopter or a plane can restore the economy [of the spiral]' (Buci-Glucksmann 1996: 107). Smithson's spiral will, from this point on, for Buci-Glucksmann, take on all its cosmic amplitude, thus becoming that eye of the cosmos, the eye of the cyclone 'fallen asleep on the pale violet sheen of the lake in the infinite shimmering of its salt crystals' (*ibid.*). Smithson's cosmic eye-spiral also brings to mind Van Blime's *cosmic art* analysed by Buci-Glucksmann (2006: 9) which sets out a whole 'cosmogenesis' of the universe in which everything is flux, image-flux or even harnessing the forces, the coloured energies of time (as shown in the paintings *Summer* or *Winter*), of sky and earth (*Sky and Earth*), of ascending and descending rhythms (*Blue Note* or even *Verdi and Debussy*).

From the immemorial time of the first neolithic spirals carved on earth and stone, through the cosmic art of *Land Art*, from Van Blime to the virtual images of the technological era, the nomadic, convoluted, rolled up, curved lines of the spiral bear witness to a certain cosmic flux, to an urge going back on itself in a cycle that represents eternity. An image of time, the spiral could be said to rediscover in a floating lightness that gentle music of the ephemeral, namely an affirmative ephemeral, an impermanence, as pointed out at the beginning of the chapter. These precise and floating lines in the Universe, this structural fluidity, this hypnotic and rhythmic whirlwind are not to be understood as a loss of being and meaning, like the melancholic ephemeral of the West, but imply a conception of art which could be summed up in a formula by Paul Klee (2008b: 17): 'becoming is our only eternity'. However, in this becoming-eternity of the spiral where the focal point, the eye-centre, shows itself as a concentration or an expansion of possible spheres of energy, that is, in the spiral part of the idea of wandering, of flight and of emptiness, 'the point shifts when we want to discover its centre. Where therefore is the central point, the axis, the pole, the dominant interest, fixed positions, absolute structures or the sought-after aim? The mind is always pushed back towards the periphery on unpredictable trajectories that make one dizzy' (Buci-Glucksmann 1996: 94, quoting Robert Smithson).

In the mid-point – *Ma* – of the spiral we are pulled into a storm of conflicting forces, of convergences and divergences, only to be marginalised outside of any representation and within a topological limbo of shadows as strange as it is veiled; and this spiralled point of emptiness is this point on no longer to be understood as nothingness, emptiness, hole or void but as a corridor or network leading towards 'the beyond of the borders of the visual', 'towards that painful point [...] where representation can no longer represent itself and [then comes] to tip over into an "archaeology of shadows"' (Buci-Glucksmann 1988: 22–3).

References

Bachelard, G. (1943) *L'Air et les songes*, Paris: José Corti.

Baudelaire, C. ([1861] 1975) *Les Fleurs du mal*, in *Œuvres Complètes*, vol. 1, C. Pichois (edition), Paris: Gallimard.

Benjamin, W. ([1938–39] 1982) 'Zentralpark. Fragments sur Baudelaire', in *Charles Baudelaire: Un poète lyrique à l'apogée du capitalisme*, trans. J. Lacoste, Paris: Payot, 209–51.

—— (1989) *Paris: capitale du XIXe siècle*, Paris: Cerf.

—— (1991) 'Paralipomènes et variétés des thèses sur le concept d'histoire', in *Écrits français*, Paris: Gallimard, 348–9.

Blanchot, M. ([1959] 1971) *Le Livre à venir*, Paris: Gallimard.

Buci-Glucksmann, C. (1984) *La Raison Baroque: De Baudelaire à Benjamin*, Paris: Galilée.

—— ([1986] 2002) *La Folie du voir: De l'esthétique baroque*, Paris: Galilée.

—— (1988) 'Une archéologie de l'ombre. Foucault et Lacan', in Moscovi and Rey (1988: 20–37).

—— (1990) *Tragique de l'ombre: Shakespeare et le Maniérisme*, Paris: Galilée.
—— (1996) *L'œil cartographique de l'art*, Paris: Galilée.
—— (2001a) *Cartographie de l'Art*, Paris: Galilée.
—— (2001b) *L'esthétique du temps au Japon: Du zen au virtuel*, Paris: Galilée.
—— (2002) *La Folie du voir: Une Esthétique du Virtuel*, Paris: Galilée.
—— (2003a) *Esthétique de l'éphémère*, Paris: Galilée.
—— (2003b) *Modernités Chinoises*, Paris: Skira.
—— (2005) *Au-delà de la Mélancolie*, Paris: Galilée.
—— (2006) *Van Blime: Un art cosmique*, Paris: Éditions Cercle d'Art.
—— (2008a) *Philosophie de l'Ornement: D'Orient en Occident*, Paris: Galilée.
—— (2008b) *Une Femme Philosophe: Dialogues avec François Soulages*, Paris: Galilée.
—— (2009) *Pascal Dombis, Image-Flux*, Paris: Galerie RX.
—— and Wright, S. (1999) 'Vers une architecture icarienne', in *Parachute: Contemporary Art Magazine*, 1–7.
Charcot, J.-M. (1890) *Œuvres Complètes, Leçons sur les maladies du système nerveux*, t. 3, Paris: Progrès Médical/Lecrosnier et Babé.
Chastel, A. (2001) *Le geste dans l'art*, Paris: Liana Levi.
Cixous, H., [1998 (1975)], *Souffles*, Paris: Éditions des Femmes.
Deleuze, G. (1969) *Logique de la sensation*, Paris: Minuit.
—— (1985) *Cinéma 2: L'Image-temps*, Paris: Minuit.
—— (2002) *Logique de la Sensation: Francis Bacon*, Paris: Seuil.
—— (2003) 'Qu'est-ce que l'acte de création?', in *Deux Régimes de fous*, Paris: Minuit, 293–302.
—— and Parnet, C. (1996) *Dialogues*, Paris: Champs Flammarion.
Didi-Huberman, G. (2000) *Devant le temps*, Paris: Minuit.
—— (2002a) *Ninfa Moderna: Essai sur le drapé tombé*, Paris: Gallimard.
—— (2002b) 'Le montage Mnemosyne: tableaux, fusées, détails, intervalles', in *L'Image survivante: Histoire de l'art et temps des fantômes selon Aby Warburg*, Paris: Minuit, 452–506.
Foucault, M. (1966) *Les Mots et les choses*, Paris: Gallimard.
Greenblatt, S. (1997) *The Norton Shakespeare*, New York and London, Norton.
Kristeva, J. (1983) *Pouvoirs de l'horreur: Essais sur l'abjection*, Paris: Seuil.
Lacan, J. (1966) 'Subversion du sujet et dialectique du désir', in *Écrits*, Paris: Seuil.
Lafargue, B. (2006) 'Le chemin des églantines et le chemin des cerisiers

(Avant-Propos)', in *Figures de l'art N° 12: L'art de l'éphémère, Marincazaou-Le Jardin Marin*, November, Pau: Presses Universitaires de Pau.

Langedijk, K. (1964) 'Silentium', *Nederlands Kunsthistorisch Jahrboek* 15, 3.

Marin, L. (1971) 'Textes en représentation', in *Études sémiologiques, Écritures, peintures*, Paris: Klincksieck, 61–83.

—— (1975) *La Critique du discours*, Paris: Minuit.

—— (1981) 'Les Tactiques du Renard' and 'Les Stratégies Raciniennes', in *Le Portrait du* Roi, Paris: Minuit, 109–30.

Moscovi, M. and Rey, J.-M. (eds) (1988) *L'Écrit du temps* 17 (winter), Paris: Minuit, 20–37.

Nancy, J.-L. (2003) *Au fond des images*, Paris: Galilée.

Nietzsche, F. (1977) *Œuvres philosophiques complètes*, vol. 1, *La Naissance de la tragédie. Fragments posthumes. Automne 1869–Printemps 1872*, ed. G. Colli and M. Montinari, Paris: Gallimard.

Pessoa, F. (1982) *Livro de desassossego*, vol.2, Atica: Lisbon.

—— (1996) *The Book of Disquietude*, trans. R. Zenith, Manchester: Carcanet.

Warburg, A. ([1918] 2000) *Gesammelte Schriften, I-2. Die Erneuerung der Heidnischen Antike.* Kulturwissenschaftliche Beiträge zur Geschichte der europäischen Renaissance, eds. H. Bredekamp and M. Diers, Berlin: Akademie Verlag.

Notes

1 Unless indicated otherwise, quotations from Shakespeare's work are taken from Greenblatt (1997).

2 On the subject of Warburg's concept of the iconology of intervals, see his atlas of images *Mnemosyne.* This is a system of images and photographs of works of art stuck onto a dark background whose juxtaposition and ordering create thin black lines and open up a whole (phenomenological) iconology of what takes place and lies 'in between', that is, an iconology of intervals: 'Truth lies in the middle' (for 'middle', read 'interval'), wrote Warburg ([1918] 2000: 611–14). For further discussion of the atlas, see Chapter 11 in this volume.

3 As an echo to Ian James's chapter on Jean-Luc Nancy in the present volume (see Chapter 9), it is worth mentioning that the rien/*nothing* uttered by the voice evokes an image, 'a sound image', O, as Jean-Luc Nancy describes it with the use of another word taken from French, 'sOnOre' (sound): 'I hear you. I can close my eyes and say again in a voice [. . .] that is silent what you

have just said. Does it follow for as much that the text read out excludes all imagery? I am not sure of that. The voice that speaks has its own shape, its sound image. See for yourself: if I say "sonore", are you left without an image? Do you not discern a *round shape*, "o", "o"?' (Nancy 2003: 123).

4 The term, as is well known, is taken from Hélène Cixous (1998: 13) and made up of the words *origin* and *gyné* ('woman', in Greek).

5 See also her 'entropic eye' (Buci-Glucksmann 1996: 95–113).

6 The expression 'the original phenomenon of history' (*das Urphänomen der Geschichte*), taken up by Buci-Glucksmann, comes from Benjamin (1989: 491).

Part III
Representation, mediology and sociology

6

Louis Marin's theories of representation: between text and image, from visuality to figurability

Agnès Guiderdoni

To what extent can we define Louis Marin as a 'visual thinker'? This question arises when considering the career of someone who explicitly inscribed his work in the wake of structural linguistics and whose thought on representation is that of a philosopher. Marin was certainly a *critical* thinker. Being a critic, taking a critical position before a work of art, could be a defining feature of his thought and methodology: within the objects that he studied, Marin was always concerned to track down the markers of their own critique, producing distancing effects and giving them the status of representations. These markers also circumscribe the range of these objects, the presuppositions on which they are based, their 'aura', their persuasive power, even their ideological and political violence.

Marin was not an art historian. The fields that Marin has explored are impressively diverse: language and the philosophy of language, painting both old and new, autobiography, portraiture, description, speech in New Testament narratives. A similar diversity can be found in the disciplines he covered: linguistics, semiotics, theology, philosophy, anthropology, rhetoric, art and institutional history. Of the many artists and writers that he analysed, mention should be made of the mathematician and philosopher Blaise Pascal, the painters Nicolas Poussin and Philippe de Champaigne, the writers Michel de Montaigne, Charles Perrault, and Stendhal, and the Jansenist 'Port-Royal' grouped around Antoine Arnauld and Pierre Nicole.

Marin may be a 'visual thinker' but he started in linguistics and moved towards the philosophy of language. This was a deepening rather than a widening or an extension of his research. Indeed, it is essential to stress that Marin never engaged in any linguistic annexation of the many non-verbal objects that he studied. In the first instance, he used the formal model offered by linguistics – mainly Émile Benveniste's linguistics – in order to point, steadily and precisely, to the resistances of the visual, variously called 'gap', 'play', 'interplay', 'articulation', 'work', 'force' – all the differential *loci* thanks to which the objects studied retain their significant peculiarity, in this case, their visual feature, their visibility or rather their figurability: 'Un discours sur l'œuvre de peinture est-il possible? [. . .] Peut-il y avoir un métalangage verbal sur le langage de la peinture? Le langage est-il l'interprétant général de tous les systèmes signifiants?' [Is a discourse on a work of painting possible? [. . .] Can there be a verbal meta-language of painting? Is language the general grid of interpretation for all signifying systems?] ([1977] 1987: 26). Marin is first and foremost a thinker of representation, in all its dimensions, be it verbal, visual or musical, who approached a wide variety of objects as a philosopher (Marin 1990).

Historical overview of Marin's thought

Marin's writings span from 1969, the date of his edition – or rather selection, with an introduction – of Blaise Pascal's *Pensées*, to his *Lectures traversières* of 1992, the year in which he died. Several of his major studies were published posthumously, either from unfinished manuscripts such as *Des Pouvoirs de l'image: Philippe de Champaigne, ou, la présence cachée*, and *Sublime Poussin*, or as collections of earlier articles gathered by other scholars, such as *De la Représentation*, *Pascal et Port-Royal*, *L'Écriture de soi* and *Politiques de la représentation*. This output may be divided into three periods. The first part runs from the *Pensées* selection to *La Critique du discours* (1969–75). In this inaugural period of his work, Marin develops the two threads that will be woven throughout the rest of his research, that is the philosophy of language, mainly from biblical and sacred narrative (either directly or mediated by other authors such as Pascal, Arnauld, and others), and the issues posed by images, found mainly in the figurability of Biblical narrative and the subsequent powers – political, ideological – pertaining to images. Through the *Études sémiologiques* (1971a), *Sémiotique de la passion* (1971b) and above all the groundbreaking *Utopiques: Jeux d'espaces* (1973), Marin analyses the structuring category of 'space', as opposed to 'place' or '*locus*', as a system which develops into an essential feature of his methodology of understanding the visual, both in works of art and in verbal texts. *La Critique du discours* here appears as both a conclusion and a transition. Several key concepts, or rather tools, are already present in this work, such as the 'gap' or 'interval', the 'play' (in the double sense of the word, relating to game and mechanical play) (see also *ibid.*: 10), the 'shifts', the 'opacity' (of the sign) and the 'neuter' as a category of transfer of signification, again also exploited in *Utopiques* as the 'instrument of the conjunction of opposites' (*ibid.*: 20–50).

A second period opens in 1977 with *Détruire la peinture* and extends to *Le Portrait du roi* (1981), during which Marin sets out a new way of understanding the full political power of images as well as deepening his conception of the relationship between the verbal and the visual. In *Études sémiologiques*, he had tried to transfer the tools of structural linguistics and semiotics from the text to the image in order to build a 'pictorial semiology', allowing him to decipher 'cette énigmatique opération de lire le visible et de voir l'intelligible: c'est-à-dire, le sens de la peinture' [this enigmatic operation to read the visible and to see the intelligible, that is the meaning of the painting] (1971: 99). But he had also quickly noticed the shortcomings of this method (*ibid.*: 43). Hence the opening question in *Détruire la peinture*: how do we speak about an image? In the texts of this second period, Marin builds on the indeterminate, unspecified and undecidable parts of images and texts, their inner contradiction: to destroy representation by means of representation (1977), to underline the impossibility of representing oneself as another in *La Voix excommuniée* (1981a) and to highlight the absence/presence at work in the irreconcilable dialectics of a portrait (1981b). *La Critique du discours* and *Le Portrait du roi* frame Marin's thought at this point in his career: while the former sets out the epistemological and philosophical bases, the latter explores the visual possibilities of these foundations and their political impact.

The third and final stage in Marin's intellectual trajectory extends from *La Parole mangée* (1986) to *Lectures traversières* (1992) and other works published after his death, which, though posthumous, nevertheless were overseen by him, texts such as *Pouvoirs de l'image* (1993) and *Philippe de Champaigne* (1995a). *Sublime Poussin* (1995b) may also be placed in this category with the reservation that Marin had left only a draft of the book; the published version of which consists of earlier articles. The 'visual thinker' certainly emerged, as Marin gradually began to focus on visual arts more specifically, in books in which his conception of the visual crystallised. He broadens his historical field in *Opacité de la peinture* ([1989] 2006), devoted to Quattrocento painting and architecture. In his three main final works – *Opacité de la peinture, Des Pouvoirs de l'image* and *Philippe de Champaigne* – Marin draws together the conclusions and consequences from his previous research, leading him to concentrate more explicitly on the processes of transformation of the figure (transfiguration, defiguration, and so on), and outline a definition, *en puissance*, of figurability.

It is clear that Marin, in his first set of studies, was concerned with the production of meaning. He worked initially in accordance with the structural linguistics of Benveniste (Marin repeatedly undertakes 'structural analysis of the narrative'), but also those of Saussure and Jakobson whose work occupied a prominent place among the founding works of structuralism by Claude Lévi-Strauss. Following this, semiotics as proposed by Greimas and Charles Sanders Peirce provided Marin with an intellectual framework with which he combined what he gleaned from Panofsky's iconology (1990). Already in *Études sémiologiques* (1971a), he had set out to elaborate 'a semiology of mimesis'. To a lesser extent, Marin was also indebted to Roland Barthes's narratology, writing (in 1982) a text on him shortly after his death (1999: 3–13), and to the work of Gérard Genette. Both these thinkers' theories were concerned with the functions, uses and effects of language and were the toolbox from which Marin was keen to borrow, as he did quite freely but always with a concern for methodological rigour. Indeed, the relationship between language and thought was his first and most pressing concern as a scholar, as shown in his reading of the *Port-Royal Logic* [*La Logique ou l'art de penser*]: 'une des plus fortes réflexions sur les rapports du langage et de la pensée… un des textes essentiels de la philosophie de la linguistique' [one of the most powerful reflections on the relationship between thought and language … one of the essential texts of linguistic philosophy] (Arnauld and Nicole 1970: 8). His exhaustive investigation into the image and the visible must be seen in this perspective.

In terms of historical sources, from the beginning of his work, and throughout his career, there is the nourishing source of the French seventeenth century, and in particular Pascal together with the Jansenist 'Port-Royal' group, as well as the Bible and other religious narratives. Taking his cue from Foucault's views on the history of Western epistemology, Marin identifies the seventeenth century as the period in which representation emerges and as a moment of the development of a general and reasoned theory of the sign and of discourse, as well as a critical and theoretical reflection on visual and verbal expression (2005: 77). The ideas of the Port-Royal group, as Foucault argues (1966: 57), were crucial in this, and which Marin explored in his first writings and to which he kept returning. However, he did not restrict himself to Foucault's notion of the 'classical age', but included also a reflection on the Baroque.[1] In doing so, he offered an original view of the historical and cultural period known as the French seventeenth century.

It is worth mentioning, briefly, the original way in which Marin designed the table of contents of his books, as it is revealing of the way in which he transmitted his ideas and his awareness of the pregnant nature of the representational process in any discourse, even if an academic one. *Le Portrait du roi* is organised as if it were a performance with three entries and interludes, framed by an overture and a finale, as a way of staging the complex play of the representation of the king. *Détruire la peinture* – the most puzzling of all his books – does not follow the usual patterns of a scholarly study and seems at first sight to develop almost randomly, while in fact Marin leads his reader through his complex thought as if it operated 'in transit' between two paintings and two places.[2] As in a detective story, he patiently gathers, as he goes along, the clues needed to corroborate his argument. The work, the outcome of a series of seminars and lectures, retains some of their features. *Des Pouvoirs de l'image*, meanwhile, alternates 'glose' and 'entreglose', each devoted to a different text. This construction establishes a dialogical relationship between the texts, which are all case studies, each throwing light on a new facet of Marin's argument. In all these cases, representation is clearly his focal point and his thought should be broached first from this point of view.

A thinker on representation

Marin's work on the *Pensées* and the *Port-Royal Logic* led to what can be considered as his foundational study, *La Critique du discours*, in the sense that it contains all the main ideas, both methodological and theoretical, regarding his conception of representation, and of the way the verbal and the visual are linked, or rather the way the visual as 'figurable' necessarily emerges from the verbal. He explores these ideas in subsequent works, from *Le Portrait du roi* in 1981 (7–22 and 263–90) to *Opacité de la peinture*[3] in 1989 and *Philippe de Champaigne, ou, la présence cachée* (1995a: 85ff.). Indeed, the founding paradigm of Marin's understanding of signs of any kind as representation is the representational theory of language and its use in the *Port-Royal Logic*, which he studied at length in *La Critique du discours*. He consistently, almost obsessively, used it in order to understand the dialectical tension between *signum*, *res* and idea (1975: 47). The semiotic process is then understood through the concept of representation: the idea represents the thing in our mind, and the sign, expressed or oriented towards other minds, is the representation of this idea. The sign is therefore a squared or four-way representation, and this representation of representation is the signification of the sign (*ibid.*: 60; [1989] 2006: 65). This equivalence between sign and representation is essential to understanding the rest of Marin's thought.

Marin has given a very precise definition of representation in several instances (see, for example, 1981: 9–11; [1989] 2006: 66–8; 2005: 71–3). There is a remarkable stability in this definition which seems to have formed around 1980. 'To represent' has two different meanings, depending on the value granted to the prefix 're-'. The first meaning is 'to take or fill the place of' (*OED*), where the prefix has a substitutive value and where the representation produces an effect of presence – hence its power – instead of the presence itself. It is the realm of make-believe, 'to do as if', and therefore the transitive moment of the representation, or transparency, when the sign as an object fades before the effect of presence of the represented thing. In this case, the representation represents something. The second meaning is 'to make present, bring to view' (*OED*) and also to 're-present', that is 'to expose before our eyes, to show, for example a passport, a legal document', where the prefix has an intensive value and where the representation repeats the presentation and produces what Marin calls a 'subject effect' ('un effet de sujet'). After the power of the presence effect, the subject power institutes the representation as a subject or as its own subject of presentation. In this case, the representation presents itself as representing something in its own right, pointing then to its reflexive dimension, or its opacity. To sum up, representation holds a double power: one that makes something present in our imagination, and another that constitutes its own legitimate and authorised subject (2005: 73). Both aspects are present in any representation, and the quality of the tension between them determines the signifying depth of the work as well as its *virtus* or power. This two-sided definition of representation accounts for all kinds of media and is non-exclusive. Marin thus applied it to the theatre and to performance (for example, 1981: 236–50; 1993: 133–58; 2005: 173ff.), to gardens, landscapes, cities and maps (for example, *Utopiques*, which includes a study of Disneyland topography; 1981: 209–35; 2005: 247), to architecture (2006) and of course to painting and literature. However, it seems that pictorial representations for Marin are representations taken to an extreme as he suggests in the following: 'All representation – *and the representation of painting first and foremost* – presented itself as representing something' (1988: 9, my italic).

In so far as representation implies a tension between transitivity and reflexivity in its effects, it means that, in the process of signification, it takes a third party into account: the reader and/or the viewer. In *Détruire la peinture*, Marin sets out the three poles of representation (conceived then as a thing being shown in representation): 'moi comme *res cogitans* ou sujet de représentation, le procès de représentation, relation "spéculaire" avec la chose, l'idée dans laquelle la chose est présente à la pensée' [myself as *res cogitans* or as the subject of representation, the process of representation, and the 'specular' relation with the object whereby the object is present in thought] ([1977] 1987: 28). Representation obviously engages, in the first place, with subjectivity as if it were a kind of 'lens' both to produce and perceive the work of art. In this respect, Marin was particularly interested in the representation of the self and the (human) figure, mainly as autobiography and self-portrait.

Methodology

What Marin offers, initially, to the student is a methodology, a specific approach to texts and images, across canonical disciplines and generic borders. He usually proceeds by way of case studies, but in so doing builds a model of thought, not a model of *exempla*. Each case study does not exemplify his thought, but constitutes its core. He never proceeds by theory being confirmed by examples, but by the case study both *being* the theory and the *articulation* of theoretical issues. The object becomes a 'theoretical construct' [*objet théorique*]. This has clear parallels with the procedures adopted by the cinema theoretician Christian Metz and the art historian Hubert Damisch (see Chapters 2 and 4 respectively in this volume).

First step: hybrid objects

Marin was fascinated with what he called 'objets hybrides, *concrétions des interférences entre le texte comme écriture et le tableau comme figure*' [hybrid objects, *the concretions of those interferences between the text as writing and the picture as figure*] (1971a: 10, my italic). In other words, he did not mean to examine the relationship between image and text as a juxtaposition of two heterogeneous objects, nor even their alleged complementarity or rivalry, nor their possible exchange of content, but rather the manner in which they mutually generate each other in their effects on the reader and viewer. In a text aptly entitled 'Transparence et opacité de la peinture... du moi' (1999: 127–36), Marin explains that he wants to participate in the 'dialogue entre l'art des images, du visuel et du visible qu'est la peinture, et la science [...] du signe, du discours, de la lettre et de l'écriture, de la littérature en un mot [...] double peinture en face à face ou en miroir, d'un unique *objet*, une peinture d'images et une peinture de mots, celle du sujet [...] du sujet écrivant et peignant, écrivant avec des images et peignant avec des mots' [dialogue between on the one hand the art of images, of the visual and of the visible that makes up painting, and, on the other, the science [...] of the sign, of discourse, of the letter and of writing, of literature in short, that is [...] a double painting as a face to face or as if in a mirror of a unique object, a painting of images and a painting of words [...] that of the writing and painting subject who writes with images and paints with words] (*ibid.*: 128). In this respect, text and image are like two sides of the same coin; they are only separated by a thin and almost intangible frontier, and constitute the essence of figurability, which can be deployed both in a text (as in Stendhal's or Montaigne's writings) and in a picture (as in Champaigne's or Quattrocento paintings). Here Montaigne's writing is a case in point (1981a: 133–56; 1999: 113–36; 2006: 63) as is also the analysis of the account of the siege of Ghent given by Racine as Louis XIV's historiographer (1978: 93–105). It seems that images and texts cannot be thought of separately because they necessarily refer to each other. *Des Pouvoirs de l'image* is a striking case since there is no discussion of paintings or sculptures per se but rather a reflection on the image as it emerges from the text, as it permeates and subverts it, as it organises the text and gives it its final meaning. The texts are concerned with actual images, either explicitly with their own powers (La Fontaine, Rousseau) or more subtly with the power that they bestow on the text. Hence the plan for this book proceeds by 'glose' and 'entreglose' – gloss of the text, in search of the absent image, whose absence is the motor of the text and the source of its power (1993: 21–2). Hence also the importance of ekphrasis, as a meeting point between narrative and icon, and the importance of questioning the process of depicting images.

Second step: depicting images

Why do we need to speak about images? How do we describe an image? How then do we *account* for an image? Why do we want to describe it? These are the questions with which Marin started his reflection on images. Indeed, images, in their radical strangeness and singularity, should be or are by nature *alien* to verbal description or narration. This is how Marin opens *Détruire la peinture*:

> Comment trouver le chemin de l'œuvre de peinture? Et pourquoi parler du tableau s'il suffit, pour accomplir la finalité de l'acte de peindre, d'y prendre plaisir ou jouissance? [...] Non pas signifier ou expliquer le tableau, mais indiquer le difficile chemin vers la porte sacrée ouverte pour Enée par la Sibylle? ([1977] 1987: 17)
>
> [How do we find the way into a work of painting? And why do we speak about a painting if in order to accomplish the finality of the act of painting all we need to do is take pleasure in it or be thrilled by it? [...]. How do we not so much signify or explain the picture but rather show the difficult route to reach the sacred door opened for Aeneas by the Sibyl?]

In a text dated 1968 and published in *Études sémiologiques* (1971a), Marin presented his undertaking as paving the way for a new science of reading images, based on verbal linguistics and semiotics. He aimed to build a 'semiology of mimesis' or a 'pictorial semiology', 'une sémiologie picturale' (*ibid.*: 17–43). Another text of the same year asked, 'How to read a painting?' (*ibid.*: 89–99), and concluded that the meaning of painting was in the enjoyment of the gaze, which reads the visible and sees the intelligible (*ibid.*: 99). Marin comes back to this issue in 1977 in *Détruire la peinture*, especially following Poussin's injunction to Chantelou in connection with his painting *La Manne* [*Israelites Gathering the Manna*]: 'Lisez l'histoire et le tableau, afin de connaître si chaque chose est appropriée au sujet' [read the story and the picture so as to see if each object is appropriate to the subject] (*ibid.*: 41), and again in 1983 (1995b: 11–34) and 1987 (1994: 251–66). From 1968 to 1987, we can see the transformation of 'description' (depiction), into 'descriptibilité', and a similar metamorphosis of the tools to account for the discourse *of* the painting: visible becomes 'visibilité', figure, 'figurabilité', 'énoncé', 'énonciabilité', etc. The addition of the suffix expresses the idea of a process in construction, one non-yet achieved, what Martin calls the 'markers of virtuality' (1994: 260) thanks to which the reading of the painting does not freeze the meaning, nor, above all, the evocative and moving power of the image. Under these conditions, a reading will not exhaust its meaning, nor annihilate the fascinating – in the fullest sense of the word – power that it is supposed to exert on the viewer, nor preclude the emergence of a virtual narrative in the viewer's mind. It will deploy all its 'virtualities'. In fact, the visual is not commensurable with the verbal, but they entertain a relationship of necessity. Marin finally declares in *Philippe de Champaigne*, written in the 1990s, that the painting, 'l'artefact de la visualité', can hold mysteries and secrets beyond language, discourse and text, and beyond any conceptual knowledge of the work (1995a: 17).

Third step: uniqueness and peculiarity

This incommensurability points to the uniqueness and peculiarity of any one work of art, a feature which was an important concern of Marin, as he explains in an article of 1990, 'L'œuvre d'art et les sciences sociales'. In this text, he gives instructions for his own methodology:

> Œuvre(s) d'art et sciences sociales, tout au plus un domaine ouvert, mais dont l'ouverture ne signifierait pas la dispersion, voire la dissipation de ses objets, l'incertitude de ses limites et de ses frontières, l'opportunisme de ses principes et le caractère hétéroclite de ses méthodes; dont la cohérence cependant ne tiendrait pas à un système unitaire et à la méthodologie qui en serait issue, mais à quelques décisions opératoires, heuristiques, à valeur théorique et à puissance pratique. (*ibid.*: 948)

> [Work(s) of art and social sciences – this remains at most an open domain – but opening them up would not entail a form of dispersion nor a dissipation of its objects, not even an uncertainty as to limits and boundaries, nor an opportunism in its principles nor a heteroclite set of methods; the method's coherence is however not linked to the use of a unitary system nor to the methodology that emerges from it, but to a number of operative, heuristic decisions that have theoretical value and practical strengths.]

The two extremes that beset the critic and between which we should navigate are autonomy on the one hand, and dissolution on the other. In other words, the critic should strike a balance between making use of a variety of disciplines and theoretical tools first, and then focusing exclusively on an artistic work of art. In order to keep its peculiarity and to help resist (scientific) reduction, Marin suggests that we consider works of art plastic, musical or verbal, as signifying sets [ensembles signifiants] in the semiotic and semantic, as well as the aesthetic, pathetic and affective, senses. Moreover they should be envisaged in their proper contexts – historical, material, intellectual and spiritual – in order 'to aim for the unsurpassable singularity of the work' (*ibid.*: 948–9).

Fourth step: the 'theoretical construct' ('objet théorique')

Retaining and stressing the singularity of each work of art consists in setting it back in its context and circumscribing its exact place between external determinations and its inner logic. It also means that the last word goes to the work itself and it is the job of the critic to find a way in the peculiar discourse of the work, within the tension that is organised by this discourse of the work between history and theory: 'How then does an ancient text "become" a theoretical construct?' ([1989] 2006: 23). This is the question which the first chapter of *Opacité de la peinture* attempts to answer, and where we find the best explanation of what a theoretical construct is and how it emerges from the *œuvre*.

The theoretical construct consists, first, of identifying the specific theory of the studied object, the theoretical discourse that it contains, as a kind of set of instructions to guide the attention of the reader and viewer. This leads us to investigate the conditions of application of contemporary theory to objects in the past. Marin advocates an acknowledged 'anachronism', which the critic will use, aware of the epistemological shift that is achieved: 'Texte passé et théorie contemporaine se trouvent déplacés: l'un, hors de l'altérité de son histoire dans l'anachronisme de propositions théoriques impensées; l'autre, hors de l'achronisme [*sic*] supposé de ses propositions et de ses thèses dans l'historicité d'un développement virtuel' [Texts from the past and contemporary theory find themselves out of place: the first are forced out of their discrete historical context by being exposed to anachronistic theoretical propositions unknown at the time; the second is taken out of the supposed achronism [*sic*] of its propositions and of its theses, into the historicity of its virtual development] (*ibid.*). The possibility, one should even say the freedom, is then given to critics to open up their toolbox to a vast array of new conceptual tools which will allow them to put forward hypotheses about past objects that have been unthinkable until now. In return – and the trade-off is essential here – contemporary theory will feed on the historical determinations with which it is confronted, and develop in new directions.

Second, the 'theoretical construct' should be understood as part of Marin's definition of representation. Given that we are looking for the inner theory of the studied object, and given the double nature of representation described above, as both transitive [transparent] and reflexive [opaque] 'l'objet théorique se construira dans une œuvre déterminée à partir de l'ensemble des énoncés qui en réfléchiront l'énonciation' [the theoretical object will be constructed in the specific work starting from that set of utterances which reflects its act of utterance] (*ibid.*: 24). The theoretical construct should be found mainly in the opacity of representation, where it 'exhibits' itself as representing something and designates the conditions of its existence and the key to accessing its meaning. Here Marin identifies a specific type of 'text' that uses by essence the 'exhibition' – 'monstration' in French – as its primary mode of signification: 'il s'agit du *texte iconique* [...] dont toute la finalité s'épuise dans la présentation ou l'ostentation. [...] Parce qu'iconique, ce texte se trouve donc, en quelque sorte, contraint de *se montrer montrant*' [we are talking about the *iconic text* [...] whose finality is exhausted by its presentation or ostentation. Because it is iconic, this text therefore finds itself, in some sense, constrained to *show itself showing*] (*ibid.*: 25–6). He continues:

> Enfin, et c'est ce trait qui le constitue dans sa singularité d'objet théorique, ce texte iconique prend, pour thème de sa représentation, les conditions et les diverses modalités, à la fois générales et historiquement déterminées, de la discursivité. (*ibid.*: 26)
>
> [Finally, and it is this trait which constitutes it in its singularity as a theoretical object, this iconic text takes as the theme of its representation the conditions and diverse modalities, both general and historically determined, of discursivity]

Visuality is space and place

In Marin's thought, visuality is not obviously and not only what is seen. There exist visual objects, visual texts, visual representations, and they all are to be seen, watched, gazed upon. But this does not constitute their visuality as visibility, guiding the direction of the gaze and articulating their meaning. The fact that they are visual – that is, apprehended through sight – does not make them essentially visible. Visuality as visibility should be constructed through various concepts which are all related to the original definition of representation and building a possible theoretical construct for each different object.

As already mentioned, one of the last studies that Louis Marin published in his lifetime is entitled *Lectures traversières*, in which he uses the name of a Parisian street, La Rue Traversière ('crossing street' or 'street that runs across'), as 'l'emblème "itinérant" de [mes] parcours, à travers les textes, parcours qui ont tenté de mimer par l'écriture, et en s'écrivant, diverses réponses à ce que les grammaires latines nomment la quatrième question du lieu: *Qua?* à travers?' [the 'itinerant' emblem of [my] journeys across texts, journeys which have tried by way of writing, by writing themselves, to mime diverse replies to what Latin grammars call the fourth question of place: *Qua?* Across?] (1992: 12). Spatiality is certainly the first point of entry into Marin's visuality, and it should not be taken metaphorically. Indeed space and place, *locus*, *topoi* are the framework within which he has developed all his concepts and methodology, from (proper) names of places in evangelical and literary narratives, drawing up 'topiques' (1971b, 1973, 1981a) and moving to the 'space of representation' and the organisation of places in pictorial representation. An object is indeed visually perceived first of all as occupying a certain place, within a certain space (1981b: 225–8), and the space can be outlined and traversed [parcouru] thanks to the various places which function as markers in the text. In *Sémiotique de la passion*, Marin conceived of 'la scène du récit comme réseau des lieux dans les noms qui les indiquent' [the site of the narrative as a network of places in the names that indicate them] in order to find the meaning of narrative (1971b: 14). In a similar way, when Poussin requests that Chantelou put a frame around *Israelites Gathering the Manna*, Marin reads in the painter's letter the description of a theoretical and complex operation that institutes the painting as 'an object of vision and reading'. Framing the painting will delimit a new space whose unique function will be to show forms and colours: 'espace de représentation dans lequel l'objet comme figure, l'espace comme lieu figuratif peuvent être connus et lus. Le cadre marque donc la possibilité d'accession au regard, de l'objet lisible' [the space of representation in which the object as figure and space as figurative place can be identified and read. The frame marks out therefore the possibility of the look having access to the readable object] ([1977] 1987: 45).

Moreover the operators that he uses in his analyses are spatial: gap, hinge, threshold, border, *liminal*, edge. This is also the case with the concepts that he ends up with, such as utopia and figure. Finally, the overarching conceptual spatiality is representation as a performance.

Figurability

It is precisely in the specificity of its definition – through space, place, opacity, transparency, point of view, all concepts which construct the text as visible and the image as legible – that visuality still seems inadequate in the end to account for Marin's thought. Another concept keeps creeping in insistently in his writings, that of figurability, a concept used to study 'hybrid objects' and 'interferences' within these objects. All Marin's works are suffused with figurability, but this notion acquired greater density and pre-eminence from the 1980s onwards (1988; [1989] 2006: 159–201; 1993: 233–60; 1994: 62–70; 1997: 267–84; 1999: 113–36).

Where does the 'figurable' emerge? The nexus between the philosophy of language, present in the *Logique*, and Marin's later studies of the visual as figurability, is the crucial point of application of the *Logic*'s philosophy: '*Hoc est corpus meum*', 'This is my body', the liturgical phrase for consecrating the Eucharist, which founds the possibility of constituting a body, therefore a figure, first in the linguistic, then the visual realm. From this sacramental word, as it was harnessed by the Port-Royal group in the *Logic*, Marin draws his theoretical and dialectical model of relationship between sign (*signum*), thing (*res*) and word, that is, a somewhat paradoxical model of absence associated with visibility, versus presence associated with invisibility. This makes for an early definition – in Marin's career – of figurability, even though the term itself does not appear explicitly:

> On peut alors poser les premiers éléments du modèle théorique: l'opposition du mot-signe et de la chose-signe est construite elle-même par une double opposition que l'on peut résumer dans les catégories de la *présence* et de *l'absence* et de la *visibilité* et de l'*invisibilité*: *par rapport à ce dont le signe est la représentation, le mot est le signe d'une présence, mais qui est sans rapport visible avec ce qu'il représente. La chose, de son côté, est le signe d'une absence, mais qui a un rapport visible avec ce qu'elle représente.* Ainsi, tout le modèle théorique du mot et du signe se trouve soutendu par une métaphysique de la présence et de la visibilité, le jeu distinctif entre l'un et l'autre pôle du modèle provenant d'un mouvement de compensation entre présence et invisibilité d'une part, absence et visibilité d'autre part. (1975: 59–60)

> [The opposition of the word-sign and the thing-sign is constructed by a double opposition that can be summed up using the categories of presence and absence, and visibility and invisibility: with regard to what the sign is the representation of, the word is the sign of a presence, but without any visible relation with what it represents. As for the thing, it is the sign of an absence, with a visible relation with what it represents. Therefore, the whole theoretical model of word and sign is underlain by a metaphysics of absence and presence. The distinctive play between the two poles of the model comes from a compensatory shift between presence and invisibility on the one hand, and absence and visibility on the other hand]

This early, but foundational, definition comes into its own in the study on the Annunciation paintings in *Opacité de la peinture* in 1989 and in a 1987 article 'Figurabilité du visuel: La Véronique ou la question du portrait à Port-Royal' (1997: 267–84). Here Marin assembles the pieces of the paradigmatic puzzle of modern representation, in which artists strive to figure the 'infigurable' as much as to express the 'ineffable'. Figurability defines the potentiality of the appearance of either the image within language, as in Montaigne and Stendhal (1999), or language within the image (1977 [1987], 1995a, [1989] 2006), and in which autobiography and self-portrait are both emblematic practices and genres of figurability operating at the point of juncture between text and image. Rather than a concept, figurability is a modality of actualisation of a work of art, together with other related so-called concepts such as virtuality, potentiality, 'enonciability', 'nominability', 'descriptibility', and so on (1994: 260). These modalities are the various facets of the work of art understood as a process of enclosing all potentialities ('en puissance') as it is being seized or read by the reader and viewer, 'imminence simultanément d'une venue *et* d'un effacement' ['imminence simultaneously of something happening *and* of something fading'] in the perceiver's space, or as Marin puts it, 'dans la dimension du regard' [in the dimension of the gaze] (1988: 13). Figurability is therefore what underpins the power of an image: 'Travail de la figurabilité, par lequel l'œuvre ne cesse de révéler sa présentation et grâce auquel les figures, loin de se fixer [...] loin de se représenter, ne cessent de renvoyer à la "virtus" de la présentation de l'œuvre, à la puissance (critique) de sa fondation' [The work of figurability, through which the work keeps revealing its presentation and thanks to which the figures, far from becoming fixed [...] far from representing themselves, keep referring to the power of the work's presentation, to the (critical) power of its foundation] (*ibid.*; see also 1993: 9–22).

A peculiarity of Marin's readings is to take literally what others would deem to be simply metaphors in a text. In so doing, he pays attention to otherwise unnoticed dimensions of texts, especially the power of these texts in the reader's mind, how the text takes shape and figures in the reader's mind. In other words, Marin was above all concerned with the mechanism of transformation – transfer of forms, of signs and therefore of signification and its force – between outer and inner representation. It could be compared, if a little subversively, to the 'idols of the mind' imagined by Francis Bacon in his *Novum Organum*, in the sense that these inner representations have the power to slant our opinion, to shape our apprehension of the world and of ourselves, to make us construe a received representation and finally to incite us to action. This peculiar approach to texts led Marin to examine the way an image emerges from a text and conversely the way a text is summoned by looking at an image. These symmetric processes of 'trade', exchange, and dialogue between text–image–reader–viewer are processes of figurability. Here we come close to the exact moment at which it seems almost impossible to determine, in the course of this process, what pertains to the verbal and what to the visual. This part of Marin's thought is certainly the most original and incisive, but also the most unsettling as it transcends our usual intellectual categories. Positioned on the edge of texts and images, scrutinising thresholds of all sorts and what could be termed representation-in-between, the inchoative – a term he used himself on several occasions (1988: 13; 1993: 259; [1989] 2006: 197) – could be the mode of Marin's thought and his main intellectual (pro)position: a thought in process and in progress, for minds on the move.[4]

References

A comprehensive bibliography of works by and on Louis Marin can be found in Giovanni Careri and Xavier Vert, with the assistance of Cléo Pace, *Louis Marin: Le pouvoir dans ses représentations*, exhibition catalogue, Galerie Colbert, 29 May–26 July 2008, Paris, INHA, 2008, 78–95. Further information can be found on the website www.louismarin.fr

Arnauld, A. and Nicole, P. (1970) *La Logique ou l'art de penser contenant, outre les règles communes, plusieurs observations nouvelles, propres à former le jugement*, intro. L. Marin, Paris: Flammarion; *Logic or the Art of Thinking: Containing, besides Common Rules, Several New Observations Appropriate for Forming Judgment*, ed. J. V. Buroker, Cambridge: Cambridge University Press, 1996.

Bacon, F. (1994) *Novum Organum, with Other Parts of The Great Instauration*, trans. and ed. P. Urbach and J. Gibson, Chicago, IL: Open Court.

Foucault, M. (1966) *Les Mots et les choses*, Paris: Gallimard.

Marin, L. (1971a) *Études sémiologiques: Écritures, peintures*, Paris, Klincksieck.

—— (1971b) *Sémiotique de la passion: Topiques et figures*, Paris: Aubier Montaigne/Le Cerf/Desclée de Brouwer; *The Semiotics of the Passion*

Narratives, trans. A. M. Johnson, Jr., Pittsburgh PA: Pickwick Press, 1980.
—— (1973) *Utopiques: Jeux d'espace*, Paris: Minuit; *Utopics: Spatial Play*, trans. R. A. Vollrath, Atlantic Highlands, NJ: Humanities Press International, 1990.
—— (1975) *La Critique du discours: Études sur la* Logique de Port-Royal *et les* Pensées *de Pascal*, Paris: Minuit.
—— (1978) *Le Récit est un piège*, Paris: Minuit.
—— (1981a) *La Voix excommuniée: Essais de mémoire*, Paris: Galilée.
—— (1981b) *Le Portrait du Roi*, Paris: Minuit; *Portrait of the King*, trans. M. M. Houle, Minneapolis, MN: University of Minnesota Press, 1988.
—— (1986) *La Parole mangée et autres essais théologico-politiques*, Paris: Klincksieck; *Food for Thought*, trans. M. Hjort, Baltimore, MD and London, Johns Hopkins University Press, 1989.
—— (1987) *Détruire la peinture*, Paris: Flammarion [1st ed. Paris: Galilée, 1977]; *To Destroy Painting*, trans. M. Hjort, Chicago, IL: University of Chicago Press, 1995.
—— (1988) *Jean-Charles Blais: Du figurable en peinture*, Paris: Blusson.
—— (1990) 'L'œuvre d'art et les sciences sociales', *Encyclopaedia Universalis: Les Enjeux*, vol. 2, 947–71.
—— (1992) *Lectures traversières*, Paris: Albin Michel; *Cross-Readings*, trans. J. M. Todd, Atlantic Highlands, NJ: Humanities Press International, 1998.
—— (1993) *Des Pouvoirs de l'image: Gloses*, Paris: Seuil.
—— (1994) *De la Représentation*, Paris: Seuil/Gallimard; *On Representation*, trans. C. Porter, Stanford, CA: Stanford University Press, 2001.
—— (1995a) *Philippe de Champaigne, ou, la présence cachée*, Paris: Hazan.
—— (1995b) *Sublime Poussin*, Paris: Seuil; *Sublime Poussin*, trans. C. Porter, Stanford, CA: Stanford University Press, 1999.
—— (1997) *Pascal et Port-Royal*, Paris: Presses universitaires de France.
—— (1999) *L'Écriture de soi: Ignace de Loyola, Montaigne, Stendhal, Roland Barthes*, Paris: Presses universitaires de France.
—— (2005) *Politiques de la représentation*, Paris: Kimé.
—— ([1989] 2006) *Opacité de la peinture: essais sur la représentation au Quattrocento*, new edn Cléo Pace, Paris: École des Hautes Études en Sciences Sociales [1st edn Paris: Usher, 1989].
Pascal, B. (1969) *Pensées*, introduced and selected by L. Marin, Paris: Didier.

Notes

1 See for example Marin (2005: 200), on the specificity of the Baroque theory of political power, through representation.

2 I am referring here to the 'Postface by way of an introduction', which starts thus: 'Le texte qu'on va lire – et que je viens d'écrire – *transite* entre deux tableaux, les *Bergers d'Arcadie* de Poussin et la *Tête de Méduse* du Caravage, entre le Louvre et les Offices. Il a mis dix ou quinze ans pour faire ce chemin et il n'a pas fini de le parcourir' [The text we are going to read – and which I have just written – *transits* between two paintings, Poussin's *Arcadian Shepherds* and Caravaggio's *Head of Medusa*, between the Louvre and the Uffizi. It took my text ten to fifteen years to make this journey and it is not over yet] ([1977] 1987: 7).

3 The *Logique* is presented here as 'l'ouvrage qui, au cours du XVIIe siècle, résume toute une histoire de la sémiotique en Occident, en parachevant dans le champ de l'*épistémé* cartésienne la tradition augustinienne [...]' [the work which, during the seventeenth century, summarises a whole history of Western semiotics, by intercalating the Augustinian tradition into the field of the Cartesian *épistémé*] ([1989] 2006: 65).

4 I am most grateful to the editors of this volume, Nigel Saint and Andy Stafford, for their help and support in the final stage of this chapter.

7

Transmission versus communication: Régis Debray's mediology

Andy Stafford

Novelist, short-story writer, dramatist, journalist, essayist and political adviser, these are not the epithets nor activities we might normally associate with a book on theorists in French of visual culture. Yet Régis Debray – like his intellectual forbear Jean-Paul Sartre – has also been, in his long career, an astute critic of visual and more recently media culture. A philosopher and historian of the visual, whose work on specific and discrete areas such as 'mediology' (his own neologism) and communication studies have allowed him to become the very intellectual of the media that he had analysed in 1979, Debray has also seamlessly moved between a university career and a political advisory role on third-world matters. Formerly a Guevarist revolutionary, imprisoned in 1967 in South America in Bolivia's clampdown on Che's allies and released thanks to President Charles de Gaulle, Debray has managed since to combine a left-conservative republicanism with a liberal humanist sense of justice, a left conservatism belonging to a 'réactionnaire de gauche' (Mehlman, in Spoiden 2007: 102). Despite this, it seems clear that there is a deep ambiguity, even ambivalence in Debray's thought that is best illustrated by a photo-essay he wrote in 1994, *L'Œil naïf*, an anthology of essays alongside a series of photographs. Any reservations concerning the comfortable manner in which this photo-text operates the inter-medial potential of image-text (see Stafford 2010: ch. 3) may however stand at odds with the overall positive approach to Debray's mediological work that this chapter adopts.

Debray is certainly not afraid to tackle some fundamental human activities within image culture. Thus communication – as a key human act – is relativised by Debray's theory of transmission: 'Communiquer est le *moment* d'un processus plus long et le *fragment* d'un ensemble plus vaste [...] communiquer consiste à *transporter une information dans l'espace*, à l'intérieur d'une même sphère spatio-temporelle' [Communicating is the *moment* of a longer process and the *fragment* of a much larger whole [...] communicating consists of transporting information across a space within the same spatio-temporal sphere]; as opposed to 'transmettre', which is '*transporter une information dans le temps*' [*to transport information across time*] (2000: 3). As is clear from this division, Debray's understanding of transmission is a historical, tradition-linked, even historicist one. Debray's division of time (diachrony) as the key to transmission, from space (synchrony) as the key to communication has a bearing on his account of the image in today's globalised world, in which, ironically, '[l]e partage du passé commun devient de plus en plus malaisé, au fur et à mesure que la mise en commun de l'information se trouve facilitée' [the belief in a shared history becomes less and less assured at the same as the sharing of information has become much easier] (*ibid.*: 6). The idea that the world is getting synchronically smaller in the technological age and yet the past (or lost world) is getting (diachronically) larger certainly fits with theories of 'glocalisation' and with the postmodernism of the 1990s during which Debray is writing (for a more sustained analysis of this phenomenon, see the Chapter 12 on Baudrillard in this volume). Though globalisation was overstated during the 1990s (and its strengths underestimated), Debray's aim is to use 'transmission' – the overall, wider culturally specific tradition(s) and socio-economic and ideological condition(s) in which communication takes place – to try to bridge the gap between a growing past time and a shrinking geo-cultural global space, for (and in) which the image becomes a key testing ground.

Image and origins

Debray's most sustained treatment of the image is in his seminal 1992 essay *Vie et mort de l'image: Une histoire du regard en Occident*, and is typical of what W. J. T. Mitchell has called the 'Pictorial turn' (1994: 11–34).[1] Not only does this work pave the way for his more recent work on God, religion and society – a 'theological' turn (Bradley 2006) in which 'religion' is seen as that which 'nous relie' (as Debray tells us etymologically), and as the 'symbolique' that brings us together (as opposed to its antonym, the dia-bolique, the devilish which divides us (*ibid.*: 82)) – *Vie et mort de l'image* is also an impressive history of the genesis of the image in anthropological culture, not dissimilar to Vilém

Flusser's work on the origins of the photographic image ([1983] 2000), and which is considered also in Arthur Bradley's chapter on Bernard Stiegler in this book. However, Debray's point is slightly different from Flusser's. Debray wishes to redress the imbalance between painting on the one hand, discussed and aestheticised endlessly, and on the other the modern techniques of image-creation (photography, cinema, digital images) whose aesthetic status is rarely linked to technical questions (1992: 164–5). What, to Anglo-Saxon academics, looks like a form of Cultural Studies becomes for Debray a discussion of the transmission of images. Using death as the key element in the desire to represent human reality in the image, Debray paints a wide social and cultural fresco in which human beings' attachment to others is both palliated in loss and absence and in which also its victims are remobilised and reanimated by visual presence. This dialectical approach then allows him to investigate the material and bodily reality behind the image; and though keen to get past both semiology and semiotics, which he sees as having failed to account for a material reality of the image, Debray nevertheless sees, potentially, the ability of Saussurian thought to cover this material aspect to the image: 'La sémiologie, pour se comprendre, serait-elle contrainte un jour de revenir des faits de langue aux faits d'image, et donc à la charogne humaine?' [Won't semiology one day have to come back from language to the realities of the image, and therefore return to the realities of human flesh, if, that is, it wants to be understood'] (30). However, rather than semiology *tout court*, Debray's argument is trying to address, implicitly, or redress the imbalance brought about by post-structuralism's tendency to promote the written text over the visual image. But Debray's distance from semiology is not simply a representational but also a methodological question. Put simply, Debray's work is far more interested in widening the analysis, from communication to transmission.

Transmission as symbolism

Debray's first job is to show how communication is, has been and can be thwarted and that non-communication is part of humanity's panoply of rebellious acts: 'Il y a quelque chose de profondément subversif à ne rien vouloir exprimer' [There is something profoundly subversive in not wanting to express anything at all] (1992: 68). Interestingly here Debray does not take Barthes's semiological turn (whereby even to thwart communication is still a form of communication).[2] Rather than opting for the pan-communication route (humans are, for Structuralists, 'sign machines'), Debray wants to leave behind the notion of the image as expressive, in order to look at its symbolism – the condition(s) and the function of transmission –, to come to the important conclusion: 'le visible n'est pas le lisible' [the visible is not the readable] (*ibid*:. 72): 'Si l'image était une langue, elle serait traduisible en mots, et ces mots à leur tour en d'autres images, car le propre d'un langage est d'être passible de traduction' [If the image was a language, it would be translatable into words, and these words would then be themselves translatable into other images, because the property of all languages is that they are susceptible to translation] (*ibid*:. 77). Avoiding poststructuralist suggestions on written language having any superior role in relation to visuality, on writing over orality, Debray stresses that it is art criticism which has lost its way in the twentieth century:

> De littéraire et poétique qu'elle était au début, la critique d'art moderne est devenue, vers sa fin, conceptuelle et philosophique [...] la vogue du tout-symbolique dans les sciences sociales a coïncidé avec une désymbolisation en profondeur des arts visuels. (73)
>
> [Moving on from its literary and poetic beginnings, modern art-criticism has become, in its later days, conceptual and philosophical [...] the vogue for pan-symbolism in the social sciences happened at the same time as the overall desymbolisation in the visual arts.]

Blaming pansymbolism on semiology, Debray argues that the 'motivated' nature of the image was soon subsumed within the arbitrary paradigm of (Saussurean) linguistics. In a manner not dissimilar to the opening of Marcel Proust's *Contre Sainte-Beuve* (1954: 43–50), Debray argues that the 'confection' [making] of the image has become 'un acte intellectuel' [an intellectual act] rather than one that is 'sensible' [linked to the senses]; the multimedia age, instead of highlighting 'des textures, des reliefs et des palettes' [textures, reliefs, colours and tastes], is busy transforming 'figures en idéogrammes' [figures into ideograms] (1992: 75). Thus Debray brushes aside what is rather a straw man, the idea that the image is a language. But he retains the crucial 'relais' ([intermediary] to borrow Roland Barthes's photo-text metaphor) of the image's potential to communicate, though he insists that this is an activity of the viewer rather than of the image itself and then underlines that *radical* plurality of meaning resides, not (as poststructuralists would have it) in the written text, but in visuality:

> Une image est un signe qui présente cette particularité qu'elle peut et doit être interprétée mais ne peut être lue [...] Apprendre à « lire une photo », n'est-ce pas d'abord apprendre à respecter son mutisme [...] On ne peut faire dire à un texte tout ce qu'on veut – à une image oui. (*ibid.*: 78–9)
>
> [An image is a particular type of sign which can and must be interpreted but cannot be read [...] Surely learning to 'read a photo' is first and foremost respecting its silence [...] We cannot make a text say what we want – we can with an image.]

This 'ventriloquist' dimension to the image/viewer relationship leads then to a 'polysémie inépuisable' [inexhaustible polysemia], and to the conclusion that 'il n'y a pas de perception sans interprétation', and, by the same token, that 'une image n'est ni vraie ni fausse, ni contradictoire ni impossible' [there is no perception without interpretation; [...] an image is neither true nor false, neither contradictory nor impossible] (*ibid.*: 80).

The image then, symbolic not diabolic, is, in origin, that which brings us together as humans, and its transmission cannot be decoupled from human religiosity: 'L'erreur du jour', declares Debray, 'consiste à croire qu'on peut faire une communauté avec des communications' [Our basic error today is that of believing that we can make communities with communications]. Indeed, continues Debray, Walter Benjamin's 'aura' of the image has not so much abandoned us in the modern world of the infinitely-reproducible image, rather it has become 'personalised' within community (*ibid.*: 82). We will come back to his critique of Benjamin in a moment. In Debray's view, the sacred nature of the image (its religious and symbolic origins) has been slowly transferred to the maker of the image; and the artist who creates an image has overtaken the symbolism of that image whereby its (growing) 'personnalisation' increases its 'désymbolisation'. This is the nub of Debray's argument: 'moins l'image est médiumnique', he argues, 'plus elle se fait médiatique'; and, by the same token, 'moins un art transmet, plus il "communique"' [the less an image is concerned with its medium, the more it becomes mediatised; the less art transmits, the more it is 'communicating'] (Debray 1992: 86; and 1997).

Mediology... or 'middleology'?

> C'est le genre de question que se pose un médiologue:
> pourquoi y eut-il un communisme français et non anglais?
> [This is the type of question a mediologist asks: why has
> communism been French traditionally and not English?]
> Debray in 'Lettre à un ami anglais sur une entreprise des plus bizarres' (1998: 340)

> S'il fallait donner à tout prix une définition
> [de la médiologie], je parlerais d'une discipline
> traitant des fonctions sociales « supérieures »
> (religions, art, politique, idéologie, mentalités)
> dans leurs rapports avec les structures de transmission,
> dépendantes elles-mêmes du développement
> technologique (supports, réseaux, vitesses,
> types de traces utilisées).

> [If I really had to give a definition of mediology, it would
> be: a discipline concerned with 'higher' social functions
> (religions, art, politics, ideology, mindsets) and how they
> are linked to those transmission structures which themselves
> are dependent on technological developments (materials,
> networks, speeds, trace types used).]
> Debray interviewed in 2007, in Spoiden (2007: 118)

The 'complexe médiologique' which results from this new form of analysis of transmission is the result of a clear development in the way Art has fared over the modern period: 'L'art s'est conquis contre *l'aliénation*, s'est grandi dans *l'autonomie*, est mort d'*auto-référence*' [Art has overcome *alienation*, grown in *autonomy*, and died of *self-referentiality*] (Debray 1992: 93). Such is the personalisation of the artistic image in our modern, mediatised world, such is the 'désacraliastion' [loss of sacredness] of the visual object in favour of the creator of it, that Art has ironised its status into a form of narcissism: 'A trop se mettre en abyme, on y roule' [By looking too much inside we have fallen in] (*ibid.*: 91). Barthes's 'Death of the Author' is then (to parody this textualist metaphor) Debray's 'Triumph of the Visual Artist'. For Debray, it is precisely the ambiguity in, the game of slipping between, conceptualism and materialism that defines the modern age of the image; and added to the 'désacralisation' of the image and the concomitant promotion of the sacredness of the artist, Debray's critique of the mediological age is possibly a pessimistic one: '[L]a complète privatisation du regard, évidemment mortelle à la magie des images, l'est peut-être aussi, finalement, à l'art tout court' [The complete privatisation of the look, which is obviously fatal for the magic of an image, may be fatal also for art in general] (*ibid.*: 98). Is this not a different version of the (positive?) view in the 1990s that aesthetics was dead and regretted by some (Jimenez 1997)? It would be, were it not for the powers attributed to mediology, which Debray defines as a battle against a marked Western tendency, 'la coupure de l'esthétique et de la technique' [the split between aesthetics and technology] (*ibid.*: 163). Here is Debray's main aim: to use 'inter' (that is, interdisciplinary) study to unite History of Art, semiology, iconology and the history of mentalities, with mediology as the 'détection des traits d'union' [way of finding the links] between the technical, political and mystical dimensions of image culture (*ibid.*: 146–8). Debray argues then that our ability to read an image, the 'voit double' [double vision] of the human mind, is a part of humanity's specificity (*ibid.*: 154).

At the same time, mediology is a religion-inspired but materialist attempt to understand the visual image and visual culture: 'à quelles conditions matérielles et sociales un héritage est-il possible?' [which material and social conditions make inheriting possible?] (2000: 20). Mediology operates especially by considering the institutionalisation of the image: 'indispensable: la place du moment institutionnel dans tout processus de transmission' [indispensable in any transmission process is locating the moment in which it is institutionalised] (*ibid.*: 8), which, in the digital age, predicts Debray in 2000, will see the return of the 'editor' whose job will be (and, now, is, it seems today) to sift information on the web (*ibid.*: 8, n. 1). This institutional dimension in 'transmettre' functions so as to 'ordonne[r] et subordonne[r] l'école à l'enseignement, le musée à l'exposition, la bibliothèque à la lecture, l'atelier à l'apprentissage, le labo à la recherche, l'église au culte, etc.' [order and subordinate school to teaching, museum to exhibition, library to reading, studio to apprenticeship, laboratory to research, church to service, etc.]. Put another way, mediology considers the way institutions, such as the Church, negotiate new technology and changes within social mores: how, in image terms, to '"épouser l'époque"' [connect with the times] (*ibid.*: 9). This leads Debray to make a key ideological distinction between communicating and transmitting: 'Pour communiquer, il suffit d'intéresser. Pour bien transmettre, il faut transformer, sinon convertir' [To communicate, it is enough to raise interest. To transmit properly, it is necessary to transform if not convert] (*ibid.*: 12). Adapting André

Malraux's idea that the twenty-first will be the century of religion, Debray's aim is to display and assess the degree of religiosity (belief, confidence, faith, fundamentally human, in a pale reflection of Marx's *zoon politikon*), as can be found in the way we commune with visual images; he aims to indicate thereby our specificity as humans in transmitting, as opposed to simply sending messages which many animals do (*ibid.*: 17), again, with an implicit reference towards Marx's example of bees building intricate hives but without any notion of human architecture.

Art history and three different 'regards'

L'IMAGERIE A POUR . . .	EN LOGOSPHÈRE (après l'écriture) RÉGIME IDOLE	EN GRAPHOSPÈRE (après l'imprimerie) RÉGIME ART	EN VIDÉOSPHÈRE (après l'audiovisuel) RÉGIME VISUEL
PRINCIPE D'EFFICACITÉ (OU RAPPORT À L'ÊTRE)	PRÉSENCE (transcendante) L'image est voyante	REPRÉSENTATION (illusoire) L'image est vue	SIMULATION (numérique) L'image est visionnée
MODALITÉ D'EXISTENCE	VIVANTE L'image est un être	PHYSIQUE L'image est une chose	VIRTUELLE L'image est une perception
RÉFÉRENT CRUCIAL (SOURCE D'AU-TORITÉ)	LE SURNATUREL (Dieu)	LE RÉEL (La nature)	LE PERFORMANT (La machine)
SOURCE DE LUMIÈRE	SPIRITUELLE (du dedans)	SOLAIRE (du dehors)	ÉLECTRIQUE (du dedans)
BUT ET ATTENTE DE ...	PROTECTION (et salut) L'image capture	DÉLECTATION (et prestige) L'image captive	INFORMATION (et jeu) L'image est captée De l'HISTORIQUE au TECHNIQUE (Temps ponctuel)
CONTEXTE HISTORIQUE DÉONTOLOGIE	De la MAGIE au RELIGIEUX (Temps cyclique)	Du RELIGIEUX à l'HISTORIQUE (Temps linéaire)	AMBIANTE (gestion techno-économique)

IDÉAL ET NORME DE TRAVAIL	EXTÉRIEURE (direction théologico-politique)	INTERNE (administration autonome)	JE PRODUIS (un événement) d'après Moi (mode)
HORIZON TEMPOREL (ET SUPPORT)	JE CÉLÈBRE (une force) d'après l'Écriture (canon)	JE CRÉE (une œuvre) d'après l'Antique (modèle)	L'ACTUALITÉ (innovation) Immatériel (écran)
MODE D'ATTRIBUTION	L'ÉTERNITÉ (répétition) dur (pierre et bois)	L'IMMORTALITÉ (tradition) souple (toile) PERSONNELLE =	SPECTACULAIRE = Griffe, Logo, marque (De l'entrepreneur à l'entreprise)
FABRICANTS ORGANISÉS EN ... OBJET DU CULTE	COLLECTIVE = ANONYMAT (Du sorcier à l'artisan)	SIGNATURE (De l'artiste au génie) ACADÉMIEÆ ÉCOLE	RÉSEAU→ PROFESSION LE NOUVEAU (Je vous surprends) MÉDIA/MUSÉE/MARCHÉ (arts plastiques)
INSTANCE DE GOUVERNEMENT	CLÉRICATURE → CORPORATION	LE BEAU (Je vous plais)	PUBLICITÉ (audiovisuel)
CONTINENT D'ORIGINE ET VILLE-PONT MODE D'ACCUMULATION	LE SAINT (Je vous sauvegarde) (1) CRUCIALE = L'Empereur (2) ECCLÉSIASTIQUE = Monastères et cathédrales (3) SEIGNEURIALE = le Palais ASIE–BYZANCE (entre Antiquité et chrétienté)	(1) MONARCHIQUE = ACADÉMIE 1500–1750 (2) BOURGEOISIE = SALON + CRITIQUE+ GALÉRIE Æ 1968 EUROPE–FLORENCE (entre chrétienté et modernité) PARTICULIER: la Collection	AMÉRIQUE–NEW YORK (entre moderne et postmoderne) PRIVÉ/PUBLIC: la Reproduction
AURA TENDANCE PATHOLOGIQUE	PUBLIQUE: le Trésor CHARISMATIQUE (anima) PARANOÏA	PATHÉTIQUE (animus) OBSESSIONNEL PLUS QUE L'IMAGE La vision contemple	LUDIQUE (animation)

VISÉE DU REGARD RELATIONS MUTUELLES	À TRAVERS L'IMAGE La voyance transite L'INTOLÉRANCE (religieuse)	LA RIVALITÉ (personnelle)	SCHIZOPHRÉNIE SEULEMENT L'IMAGE Le visionnage contrôle LA CONCURRENCE (économique)

Figure 1 Régis Debray, 'Les trois âges du regard' (1992: 292–3)

Other areas that Debray's 'philosophie du regard' [philosophy of the visual] is keen to challenge, as shown in the Figure 1, are the breaks and continuities placed within the image in history, necessarily in art history. Here he introduces a new historicism to his brand of cultural studies of the image (1992: 210). His theory is a powerful one and leads to a diagram of what he calls the 'trois âges du regard' [three ages of the visual] (*ibid.*) and which we might say operates by a series of displacements.[3] Debray is more positive here, seeing the invention and then the socialisation of writing as openings that allow the image to be freed from the 'trivial' act of communicating (*ibid.*: 302).[4] The first of his three eras of the image in human society – the 'logosphère' which followed the discovery of writing – *pushed* the image into the 'régime idole'. Next, after the discovery of Gutenberg and printing, we enter the age of the 'graphosphère' in which visual phenomena are shunted into the 'régime art'. Finally, Debray underlines the advent of the 'audiovisuel', the 'vidéosphère' of the 'régime visuel', which (in our adopted metaphor of 'displacement') hints that there is an element of reconciliation between the 'sphère' and the 'régime' not seen in the previous two eras.[5] However (and it is a big 'however'), Debray is keen to dispel any hint of harmony in this synthesis. If the image during the 'logosphère' era is one of '(transcendent) presence', becoming one of '(illusory) representation' during the 'graphosphère', then the fate of the image in the contemporary era of the 'vidéosphère' is to be both of these, that is a 'simulation (numérique)' [digital simulation]. Whereas the image had moved from being an 'être' [being] to become a 'chose' [thing], it is now 'virtuelle', a 'perception': hence Debray's view of the moves from magic to religion in the first era, from the religious to the historical in the second, and from the historical to the technical in the last, contemporary phase.

The schema adopted by Debray for the image and its transmission across human history is a tight if not persuasive one, which finds echoes not only in postmodern theory but in much wider notions of post-history of the image. It is worth spending a bit more time fleshing out

Debray's schema of the image's function and conditions of transmission. The schema invites consideration also of the political economy of the image, allowing three different values to operate within each of the three phases (1. Celebration; 2. Creation; 3. Production). Here Debray takes the historical aspect in Walter Benjamin's theory of *aura* to task. He suggests that, far from 'aura' being part of a continuum since the earliest stirrings of human-created culture (becoming debased in the era of mechanical reproduction), Benjamin failed to see that 'aura' belonged to his (that is, Debray's) first era only. In other words, the mechanical reproduction brought into the political economy of the image by photography that Benjamin saw as crucial in debasing the image and leading to its 'desacralisation' in the twentieth century, is, for Debray, something which took place long ago, during what he calls the era of 'idoles'; thus, the aura of 'real presence', of 'authority' and of 'immediate incarnation' had already disappeared (*pace* Benjamin) with the Renaissance (*ibid.*: 1992: 172), a point also made by Jean Baudrillard. Photography, in Debray's history, merely added a further degree to this 'désacralisation' and 'sécularisation' of the image, begun in the fifteenth, not the nineteenth, century (as Benjamin had maintained).[6] This analysis is part of what Debray calls a 'matérialisme religieux', in which the image is seen in its socio-economic, political and symbolic economy. Debray's rare examples of those texts and theorists who have managed to place the visual image within a history of transmission – what we, Anglo-Saxons, would locate in the cultural-studies approach – come, in the contemporary period for Debray, from Barthes's *La Chambre claire* (for the family album), from Deleuze's *Image-mouvement* (on the American thriller) and from Lyotard in his 1985 Pompidou exhibition 'Les Immatériaux' on hologrammes. In the same vein, Antoine Hennion's work on mediation in music is also cited (*ibid.*), as is Bernard Stiegler's anthropological work on Leroi-Gourhan ('La technique a inventé l'homme autant que l'homme la technique' [Technology invented man as much as man invented technology] (*ibid.*: 178; see Chapter 13 in this volume): thus, for Debray, '[l]e *quoi* et le *comment* du transmettre vont ensemble' [the *how* and the *what* of transmitting go together] (*ibid.*: 180). In this optic Western dualism now appears inferior to (say) Asia's monism; for example, calligraphy as practised outside of the West can be seen as a technical–aesthetic complex in which the body's material action inflects the image, thereby providing a counter-example to Debray's belief that the image is split in today's world between its technology and its aesthetics.

This argument seems to allow, however, precious little by way of a discussion of aesthetics as such. If, for Debray, the West has consistently failed to integrate 'la technique' with 'l'esthétique', and is proud of this 'coupure' [split] (*ibid.*: 163), he can see this in the way the influential, New York art dealer extraordinaire, Leo Castelli, rereads Kant in the twentieth century. Thus, Debray points to the sharp contradictions of Art in contemporary culture – specialists claim that aesthetic value is indefinable in a work of art and yet they have never fought shy of deciding ('trancher') who is a good and who is a bad artist (*ibid.*: 191). Debray's conclusion is that Castelli has understood (and implicitly, benefited from) this gap between philosophy of art and living art, and that, with his failure to define the 'beau' in relation to either technique or a theology of the image, Kant is the 'anti-médiologue par excellence' (*ibid.*: 197), and, consequently, Duchamp becomes the first mediologist: 'Le médiologue', summarised Debray, proceeding to quote Confucius, 'est donc cet imbécile qui lorsqu'on lui montre la lune regarde le doigt' [the mediologist is therefore that fool who when shown the moon looks at the finger] (*ibid.*: 199).

It is important to stress that, although disagreeing with Benjamin's historical framework, Debray still seems to end up with similar conclusions. This can be seen in his view of the image's mobility in the digital age: 'Une image voyage mieux qu'un texte [. . .] Elle saute des frontières et arrive où on la veut – mais dans quel état?' [An image travels better than a text [. . .] It jumps over frontiers and arrives where it will – but in what state?] (*ibid.*: 348). The main problem for Debray is that his argument and overall theory risk, unwittingly it would seem, falling into the 1990s trend of denigrating aesthetics (Jimenez 1997), as he repeats the standard critique of the time that the avant-garde in general has lost its romantic notions of rebellion and curse, in favour of recuperation ('moyen d'insertion et de promotion sociales' (*ibid.*: 215) [a way of fitting into, and getting on in, society]); in an orgy of constant newness (Octavio Paz's 'tradition of the new'), the only rule, argues Debray (*ibid.*: 220), is to be 'résolument a-moderne' [resolutely a-modern]. It is as if to concentrate on transmission is to bracket aesthetics, at a time when aesthetics was due for a bit of redefining (if not defending).[7] That said, one could argue that Debray's bracketing of aesthetics merely allows us to reconstruct aesthetics in the light of his mediological theories: the suggestion that having no theory of transmission means having no (decent) aesthetic theory, seems to be a fair conclusion.

'Videosphere' and TV culture

The final section of Debray's volume, *Vie et mort de l'image*, is appropriately on the 'videosphere', which for Debray represents the end of the 'société du spectacle' theorised by Guy Debord in 1967, rather than its apogee (1992: 362). Thus 1968 is the start of this new videosphere period of the image, according to Debray: no longer '*devant* l'image' [*in front of* the image] (as we were for Debord), we are, in this new videosphere, '*dans* le visuel' [*in* the visual], in which 'le son coule' [sound flows] and sound has perhaps 'coulé l'image avec lui' [sunk the image with it] (*ibid.*: 383). The 'passivity principle' that sound invites now contrasts with the 'autonomy of vision'; sound is on the side of '*pathos*', and the image on the side of the '*idea*' (*ibid.*: 383–4). Far from any of the three ages identified by Debray being able to escape various paradoxes, the video age, argued Debray, again, following Baudrillard in his work on America (1986), has its own: 'Après la notion de progrès rétrograde et celle de mondialisation balkanisante, nous devons admettre la réalité d'un autre paradoxe: la société électronique comme société primitive' [Following on from the notions of retrograde progress and of balkanising globalisation, we must accept the existence of another paradox: electronic society as a primitive society] (1992: 412). Here Debray puts forward distinctly Baudrillardian arguments (such as, the visual being interested only in itself nowadays (*ibid.*: 416–19); see also Paul Hegarty in this volume, Chapter 12), as he refers explicitly to Baudrillard's infamous view on the (first) Gulf War of 1991 against Iraq as having taken place in the media only (*ibid.*: 419). The televised world is such that, if once one had felt alone in the community culture of going to the cinema, now one feels like the whole world while at home alone in the front of the television (*ibid.*: 426). We will return to Bernard Stiegler's critique of 'télécratie' in relation to 'démocratie' (2006) in our conclusion. It is not far for Debray, parodying Barthes in the 1970s ([1978] 1995: 803), to say: 'ce n'est pas le langage qui est fasciste, mais le visuel' [it is not language that is fascist but the visual] (1992: 434), allowing Debray to emit one of his trademark schematic (though not unhelpful) maxims in order to set out his critique of television culture:

> Penser c'est dire non. Bon gré mal gré la télé dit *oui* au monde tel qu'il va ; le cinéma, « oui mais » ; la peinture lui disait oui, jusqu'à Manet. Depuis, et c'est encore sa force propre, elle lui dit plutôt *non*. (*ibid.*: 440)

> [To think is to say *no*. By and large TV says *yes* to the world as it is; the cinema, '*yes but*'; and painting said *yes* up until Manet. Since then, and this is its own strength, painting has said instead *no*.]

The proliferation of television images, suggests Debray, might destroy the Image (as Luther thought printing would lead to superficial readings of the Bible; 1992: 455). Furthermore, Debray, writing at a time when France's main television channel, TF1, was being privatised, does not stop to wonder whether it is the political economy of television transmission that counts: who 'controls' television? He prefers to see a battle between visual and written: 'L'image mange économiquement la lettre comme le gros poisson le petit' [In economic terms, the image eats the letter, rather like the big fish the little one] (*ibid.*: 462). Using a populist, tokenistic form of republicanism, Debray berates television for trying to satisfy everyone. This is not democracy, says Debray: reminding us that Hitler was elected democratically, he tells us (highly undialectically, I would add) that 'la démocratie n'est pas la loi de la majorité [...] mais le respect des minorités' [democracy is not the law of the majority [...] but the respect of minorities] (*ibid.*: 464). Thus, this republican stalwart, who has recently suggested forcefully that the Muslim woman's full 'voile' [veil] could be a barrier to democracy and republican citizenship (2004), a view that became part of French law in 2010, does not spot the contradiction in his argument: 'L'impérialisme de l'image renforce la normalisation majoritaire' [The imperialism of the image reinforces majority normalisation] (1992: 464).

Other political contradictions now emerge in Debray's critique of today's televisual culture. Not only does he miss (ignore?) the revolutionary potential of the image and of the audiovisual today (and we will return to this in a moment), Debray fails also to foresee the return, in France in 1995, to militant syndicalism, the very social phenomenon that (as he predicted in 1992) would succumb to the stay-at-home in front of the television culture, allowing only the bosses out onto the streets (*ibid.*: 467). 'Il serait naïf', argues Debray as tries to calm us, 'de voir dans l'empire vidéo la *cause* d'une crise du politique' (*ibid.*: 468), but it is 'aussi bien' an 'effet' [It would be naive to see in the video empire the *cause* of a crisis in the political, but it is also the effect]. The 'also' here seems to betray a causal link between the saturation by television images and (a perceived) political demobilisation of the masses in 1990s France. Looking like a 1980s style critique in the vein of Neil Postman (1985), a pessimism roundly criticised by Pierre Bourdieu (1996), Debray's reticence with regard to contemporary audiovisual culture means that he becomes immune to political events. Indeed, we must ask: what was the first political act of the anti-Ceausescu movement in Romania in 1989, or of the protestors more recently in Tunisia and Egypt? To seize the main television station. Indeed, surely to say that TV is biased, as Debray does (1992: 473), is not really a mediological issue.

This is not to say that Debray is blind to important developments. His view that 'la communication rassure, l'information dérange' [communication reassures, information upsets] (*ibid.*: 478) looks like the radical graffiti written across Parisian walls in 2003, 'médias partout, information nulle part' [media everywhere, information nowhere]. Following his three eras of intellectuals, Debray now sees a new intellectual emerging, the 'journaliste-télé' [TV-journalist] (*ibid.*: 482), whose role is to provide an 'effet de réalité' in television which 'finit par déréaliser l'actualité' [ends up derealising the news] (*ibid.*: 487), as he echoes a point made more recently about photo-journalism's perceived corruption by scoop in the 1990s (Rouillé 2005: ch. 4). In other words, the global reach of television is no guarantee of democracy: '"L'œil écoute" mais n'entend pas l'œil de l'autre' ['The eye listens', but does not hear the eye of the other] (1992: 494). The 'déclin des grands récits' [decline of grand narratives] (*ibid.*: 497), says Debray in distinctly postmodernist terms, is a function of this television era. Here Debray is merely substituting mediological fetishism for technical fetishism, in which content (ownership, control) is a given. Debray declines then to see the revolutionary potential of the image and of the audiovisual in today's world.

Conclusion

> An image is dialectics at a standstill.
> (Walter Benjamin, cited in Cadava 1992: 102)

It is clear that, in writing about the image in 1992, Debray was reacting to semiology and to its perceived superiority, and which has been more maturely critiqued by others (Rouillé 2005: ch. 6). However, in his critique of photo-journalism Rouillé is keen to suggest alternatives that show that 'making photographic images politically', to quote Thomas Hirschhorn's important distinction over 'political art', becomes a new optic for the photographic artist during the 1990s (*ibid.*: 538). Though he is someone who practises its inter-mediality with written language (Debray 1994b), Debray's account in *Vie et mort de l'image* of the image as origin and function of transmission makes no attempt to link text and image, which semiology, though unsatisfactory, had had the virtue to consider. Debray's bracketing of language, text and communication may be a tactical one, but it has negative, strategic effects on the power and persuasiveness of his argument. Debray even draws an analogy between how the written displaced the oral to create national identities and how the standardisation of viewing has lead to the end of national imaginaries (*ibid.*: 141); but he does not stop to consider orality, writing and visuality in a triadic and (partly) antagonistic relationship.[8] Indeed, Debray's insistence on the power of the image over the written – 'l'image est plus contagieuse, virale que l'écrit' [the image is more contagious, viral than the written] (*ibid.*: 126) – is the basis of his liberal–humanist version of the dialectic in which he uses history (origins, religion, the symbolic) to point to an equilibrium (albeit not a structuralist one) of the image in society and in human communities generally. To show the function of an image, its place as and within transmission, is at once to illustrate its power and at the same time to show how it is (potentially, that is once 'cured', returned to its sacred, non-personalised form) a force for progressive democracy. It is finally a 'soft' republican dialectic (hence the 'middleology' of our third intertitle above) that Debray uses to consider the image (at least in relation to writing), and one which allows, potentially, for a 'renversement' [overturning] of the terms. So writing is 'critique', whereas the image is 'narcissique'; the former wakes us up, but the latter 'peut endormir' [can send our brains to sleep]: 'la lettre redresse, l'image allonge' [writing makes us sit up, the image lies us down] (*ibid.*: 155). It is precisely this which makes the image an important battleground: 'Le secret de la force des images', argues Debray in a neat critique of the Lacanian view of the unconscious being structured like a language, 'est sans doute la force de l'inconscient en nous (déstructurant comme une image plutôt que structuré comme un langage)' [The secret force of images is perhaps the unconscious force inside us (unstructured like an image, rather than structured like a language)] (*ibid.*: 156).

This view inevitably raises the thorny question of 'intention' on which both structuralism and poststructuralism had stumbled in relation to the image. Does Debray's 'transmission' argument, especially its critique of semiology and the *arbitraire* applied to the image, help us to get round the dead-end of intentionalism?[9] In a sense it does (though perhaps unsatisfactorily), in that the image's ultimate intention is shown to be a communal one that brings people together, and the meaning(s) generated by it in (or supplied to it by?) the viewer is (are) dependent upon the context in which it is viewed. This may look like an overturning of the poststructuralist insistence upon written text as radically plural, and a challenge to the ensuing view of image as an (inferior) form of communication, but this would be to miss the text-image dimension that semiotics introduced in the 1960s. Nevertheless, Debray's method allows him to look widely and suggestively at visual culture, as in his recent reading of *One Hundred Paintings and the New Testament* (2004).

The other thorny area of Debray's mediology is a political one. A mediologist, as concerned with transmission, has difficulty articulating the concept of bias, as Debray is tempted to do at various stages (1992: 473). The question: 'is TV "biased"?' is surely one that requires a political economy of communication that must involve a 'hard' (not 'soft') dialectical answer: television is able to be considered to be biased *because* historical materialism (fore)sees/hopes for/ bases it arguments on the belief in, the transformational category of media (and of the 'image'), with workers seizing, one day, democratic control of the means of transmission (witness, for example, the 'interim' group of media workers who, in 2007, invaded France's main television stations and, briefly, controlled national television news). Alternatively, or *as well*, it is precisely *because* of the 'capitalist' bias in media that Marxism works towards a transformational category with which to explain the image. Either of these (image considered within a transformational category, or image as a form of ideological persuasion and control) is possible in a historical–materialist account of the image; even both, dialectically, at the same time. Neither Debray's nor Stiegler's critique of television, beholden as they are to a liberal–individualist (that is, bourgeois) republicanism (that of the 'citoyen), is able to deal with a collective challenge to the question of who controls the image. A collective approach to the image in contemporary society, materially and historically informed, represents a dialectically materialist (as opposed to the Stalinist 'dialectical–materialist') view of media and of the image, in contradistinction to Debray's religious materialism.[10] Given that Debray's final chapter in *Vie et mort de l'image*, 'Douze thèses sur l'ordre nouveau', seems to be parodying Marx's 'Twelve Theses on Feuerbach' (1992: 489–506), it is not unreasonable to suggest that Debray's own religious-materialist critique of the image is very little different from what Ludwig Feuerbach was writing in the 1840s.[11] This religious materialism has allowed Debray to make interesting forays into visual culture in relation to religion (2003), but it is not a dialectically materialist approach. In this chapter we have refrained, largely, from relating Debrayist 'transmission' to his politics of republicanism. Our main aim has been to highlight the way in which Debray appears in no way surprised that the 'basculement de civilisation' [the big shift in civilisation] – in the change from grapho-to-video spheres (1992: 74–5) – has affected today's lay society. His approach is indicative of the stiff technologism of his arguments, as undialectical as it is useful, tactically, to consider them.

References

Barthes, R. (1978) *Leçon* (conférence inaugurale au Collège de France), republished in *Œuvres complètes*, vol. 3, Paris: Seuil, 1995, 799–814.

—— (2002a) *Comment vivre ensemble: Cours et séminaires au Collège de France (1976–1977)*, texte établi, annoté et présenté par Claude Coste, Paris: Seuil/IMEC.

—— (2002b) *Le Neutre: Cours au Collège de France (1977–1978)*, texte établi, annoté et présenté par Thomas Clerc, Paris: Seuil/IMEC.

—— (2003) *La Préparation du Roman I et II*, suivi de *Proust et la Photographie: Examen d'un fonds d'archives photographiques mal connu* [1979–80], texte établi, annoté et présenté par Natalie Léger, Paris: Seuil/IMEC.

Baudrillard, J. (1986) *Amérique*, Paris: Grasset.

—— (1991) *La Guerre du Golfe n'a pas eu lieu*, Paris: Galilée.

Bourdieu, P. (1996) *Sur la télévision*, Paris: Liber/Raisons d'Agir.

Bradley, A. (2006) 'Derrida's God: A Genealogy of the Theological Turn', *Paragraph* 29(3), 21–42.

Cadava, E. (1992) 'Words of Light: Theses on the Photography of History', *Diacritics* 22, 3–4.

Debord, Guy (1967) *La Société du spectacle*, Paris: Gallimard.

Debray, R. (1979) *Le Pouvoir intellectuel en France*, Paris: Ramsay.

—— (1987) *Les masques: Une éducation amoureuse*, Paris: Gallimard.

—— (1992) *Vie et mort de l'image: Une histoire du regard en Occident*, Paris: Gallimard.

—— (1994a) *Manifestes médiologiques*, Paris: Gallimard; trans. E. Rauth, *Media Manifestos*, London, Verso, 1996.

—— (1994b) *L'Œil naïf*, Paris: Seuil.

—— (1996) *Loués soient nos seigneurs: Une éducation politique*, Paris: Gallimard.

—— (1997) *Transmettre*, Paris: Odile Jacob; trans. E. Rauth, New York: Columbia University Press, 2000.

—— (1998) *Par amour de l'art: Une éducation intellectuelle*, Paris: Gallimard.

—— (2000) *Introduction à la médiologie*, Paris: Presses Universitaires de France.

—— (2003) *L'Ancien Testament à travers cent chefs-d'œuvre de la peinture*, Paris: Presses de la Renaissance; trans. Benjamin Lifson, *One Hundred Paintings and the New Testament*, London: Merrell, 2004.

—— (2004) *Ce que nous voile le voile*, Paris: Gallimard.

Flusser, V. ([1983] 2000) *Towards a Philosophy of Photography*, London: Reaktion.

Jimenez, M. (1997) *Qu'est-ce que l'esthétique?*, Paris: Gallimard.

Lombardo, P. (1989) *The Three Paradoxes of Roland Barthes*, Athens, GA: University of Georgia Press.

McKinnon, A. 'Opium as Dialectics of Religion: Metaphor, Expression and Protest', in Warren Goldstein (ed.), *Marx, Critical Theory and Religion: A Critique of Rational Choice*, Amsterdam: Brill, 2006.

Mehlman, J. (2007) 'Du tour néo-conservateur dans la pensée française: Réflexions d'un ami américain', in Spoiden (2007: 101–13).

Mitchell, W. J. T. (1994) *Picture Theory*, Chicago, IL: Chicago University Press.

Postman, N. (1985) *Amusing Ourselves to Death*, London: Methuen.

Proust, M. (1954) *Contre Sainte-Beuve*, Paris: Gallimard.

Rouillé, A. (2005) *La Photographie: Entre document et art contemporain*, Paris: Gallimard.

Spoiden, S. ed. (2007) *Régis Debray et la médiologie*, Amsterdam: Rodopi.

Stafford, A. (2010) 'My Favourite Piccies: Sequencing, Structuring and Essayism in Photo-Anthologies by Régis Debray and Denis Roche', in Stafford, *Photo-texts: Contemporary French Writing of the Photographic Image*, Liverpool: Liverpool University Press, 71–83.

Stiegler, B. (2006) *La télécratie contre la démocratie*, Paris: Flammarion.

Notes

1 *Vie et mort* was made into an 'Arte' documentary by Pierre Desfons in 1995, and a later version (2002) contains interventions by Sebastiao Salgado, Jean-Luc Godard and Jean Clair, suggesting a similarity with John Berger's seminal 'Ways of seeing' in Britain (1972), though the latter was a television series that was subsequently turned into a book.

2 'Nonsense' is still a meaning, not a 'non-sense', for Barthes; interestingly, Barthes ended up seeing silence and exemption from meaning as radical in the 1970s (see Barthes's 'Collège de France' lectures in particular, 1976–80 (Barthes 2002a, 2002b and 2003); Lombardo 1989: 22–6).

3 *Vie et mort* was presented as Debray's (delayed) doctoral thesis, at Paris Sorbonne-I in 1993. Though not translated in its entirety (despite being announced), four key sections from *Vie et mort* have been published in English: 'The Image vs. Language' ('La transmission symbolique', Chapter II), in *Common Knowledge* 4(2) (fall 1995), 18–31; 'The Three Ages of Looking' (ch. VIII), *Critical Inquiry* 21(3) (spring 1995), 529–55 (translated by Eric Rauth) which contains also Debray's brief view of the link between visual culture and his (former) revolutionary politics; 'Le mythe de l'art' (adapted from 'La spirale sans fin de l'histoire' and 'Une religion désespérée', chs V and IX) appears as 'Images, not signs', in Debray (1994a/1996), 131–67.

4 As a good French republican thinker Debray likes his classical, three divisions; and here the three philosophers of subjective time are Hegel for entropy (or rise and fall), Bergson for the 'négentropique' (or climbing back up the flow, attuned to newness, innovation, discovery, invention) and Vico for the astronomic (or dusk means dawn, time as cyclical) (1992: 222).

5 Debray will reuse the displacement metaphor to explain how photography became 'artistic' in the 1970s; that is, once video had exploded onto the visual scene, photography could open up its options and become more interested in its status as Art (*ibid.*: 407).

6 However, according to Eduardo Cadava (1992: 93), Benjamin seems to be saying the same thing: the loss of *aura* is progressively intensified with the arrival of photography.

7 Bernard Vouilloux refers to the 'contemporary art polemic' in his interview in this volume (see Chapter 14, p. 303).

8 To be fair, however, Debray does make indirect asides about the status of text and image in gallery exhibitions, implying that contemporary artists play on the fact that they know that their 'raptus d'extase' will be matched by 'la préface de Derrida dans le catalogue' (1992: 96).

9 For Debray, while painting 'relève de l'icône' [belongs to the iconic], photography is 'de l'indice' [indexical]; therefore, outside of composition (focussing, fixing in time, framing), '"Le crayon de lumière" est aveugle: il n'a ni code ni intention' ['the pencil of light is blind': it has neither code nor intention] (*ibid.*: 371).

10 The extent to which a 'transformatory' category in the critique of the image can be traced in work by French-speaking Marxist thinkers such as Badiou, Hadjinicolaou, Jimenez, Lecercle, Noël, Palmier, Rancière or the Moroccan theorists of the journal *Souffles* (especially Laâbi and Serfaty) is a moot point.

11 See McKinnon (2006).

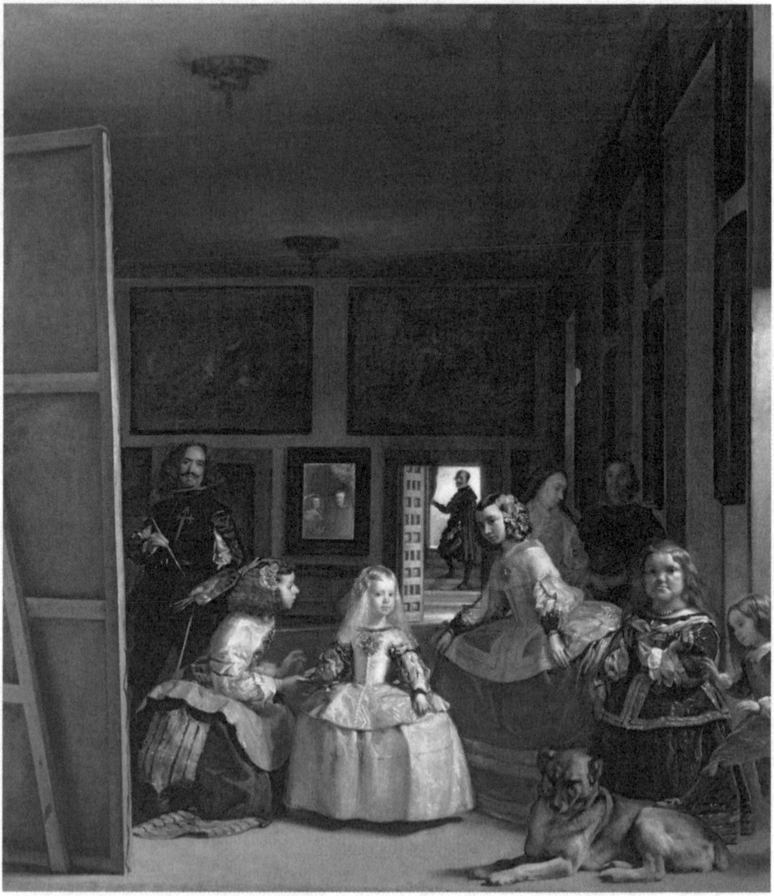

1 Velázquez, *Las Meninas*, *c.*1656

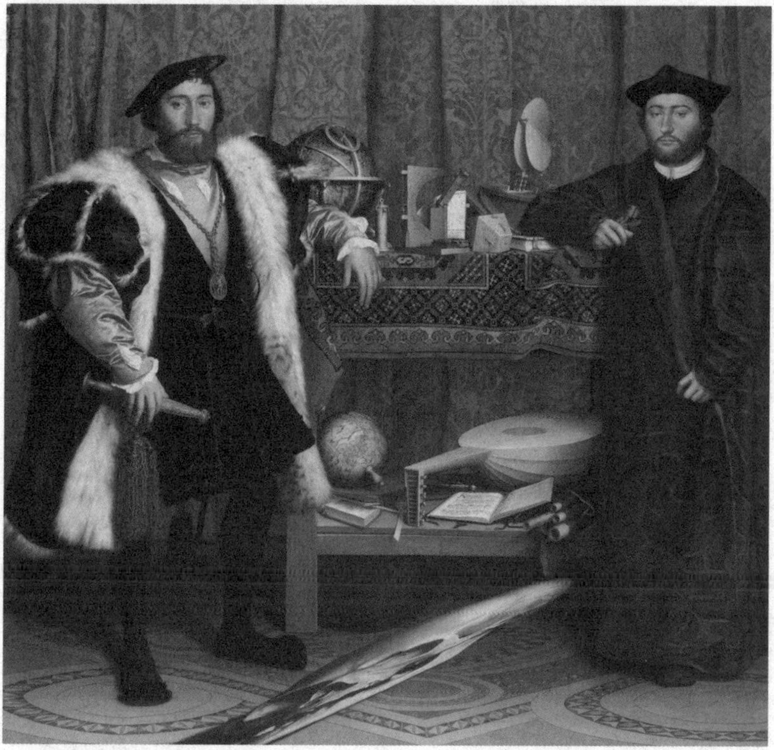

2 Hans Holbein the Younger, *The Ambassadors*, 1533

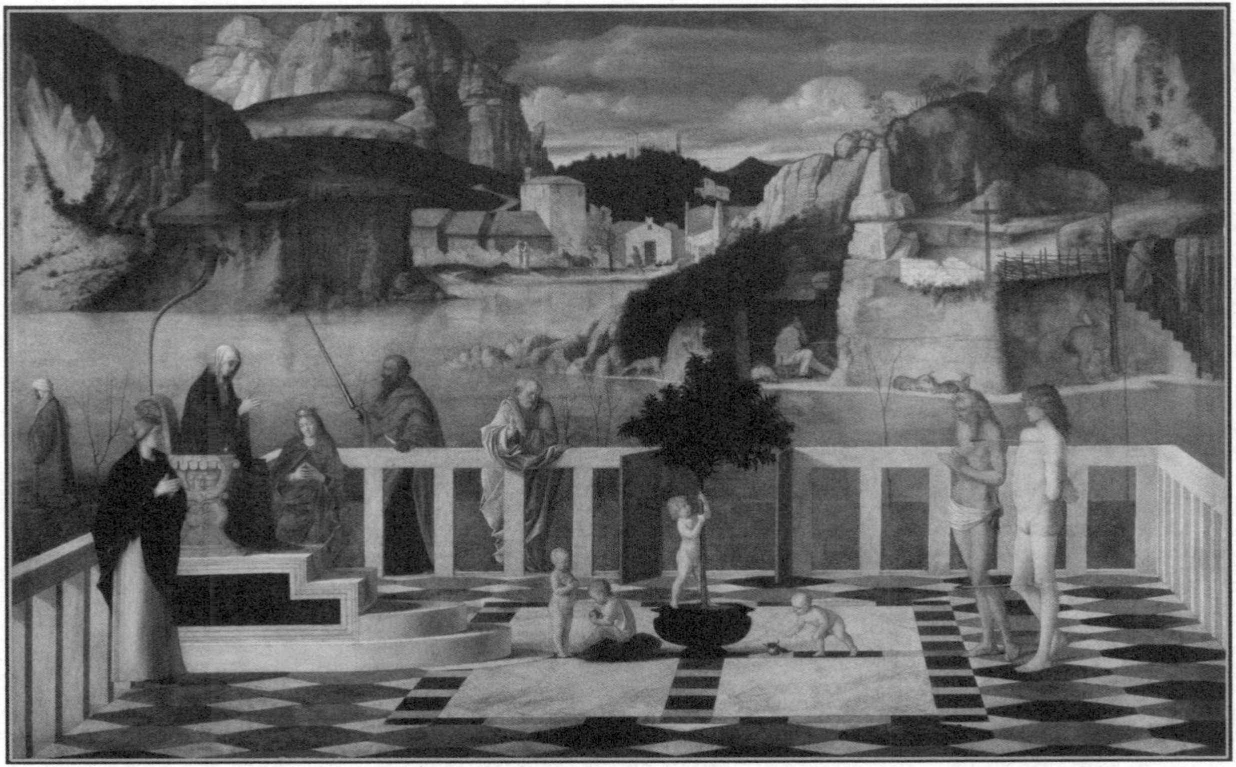

3 Giovanni Bellini, *Sacred Allegory*, *c.*1487

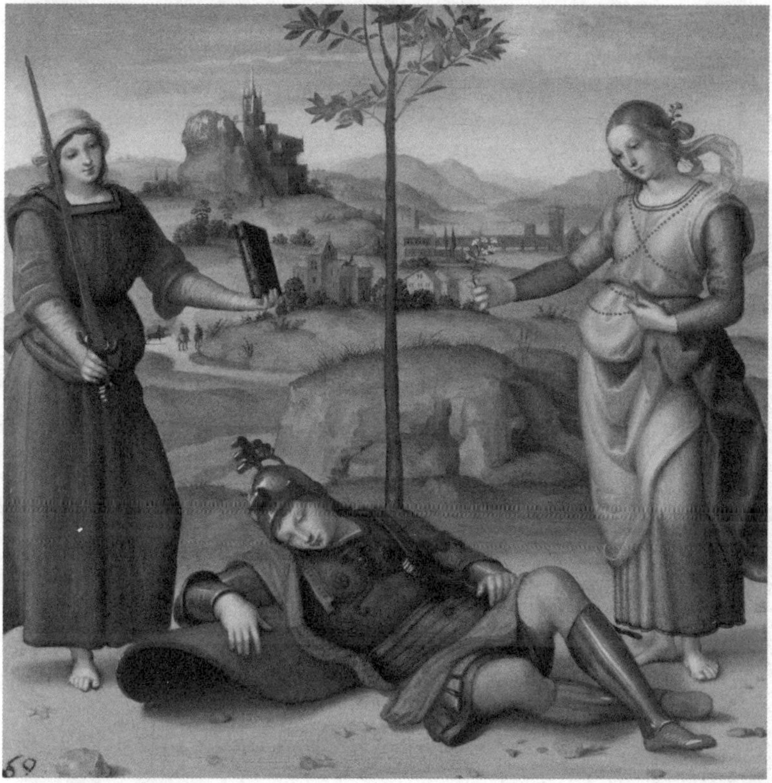

4 Raphael, *An Allegory* ('*Vision of a Knight*'), *c.*1504

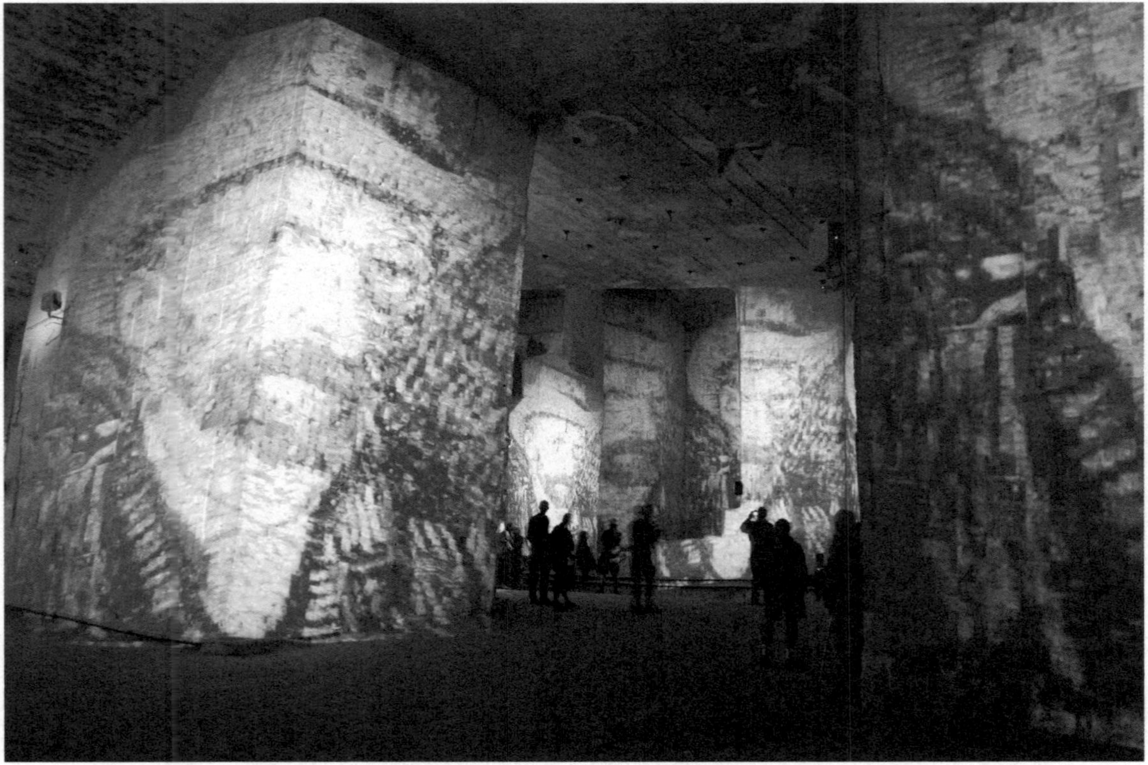

5 Régis Prevot, *Cathédrale d'images: Van Gogh, Les Baux de Provence*, 2008

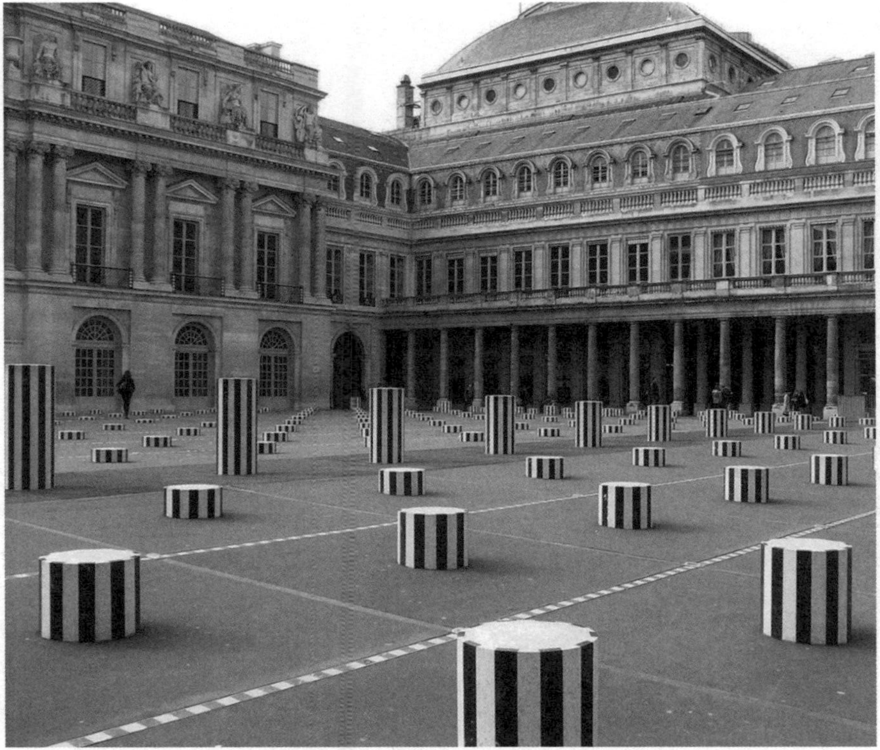

6 Daniel Buren, *Les Deux Plateaux*, 1985–86

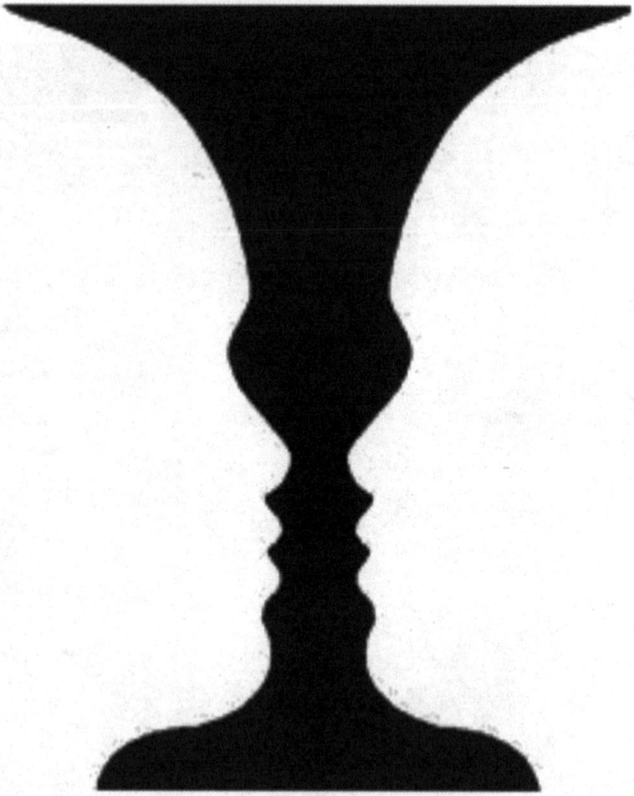

7 Gestalt psychology: figure and ground

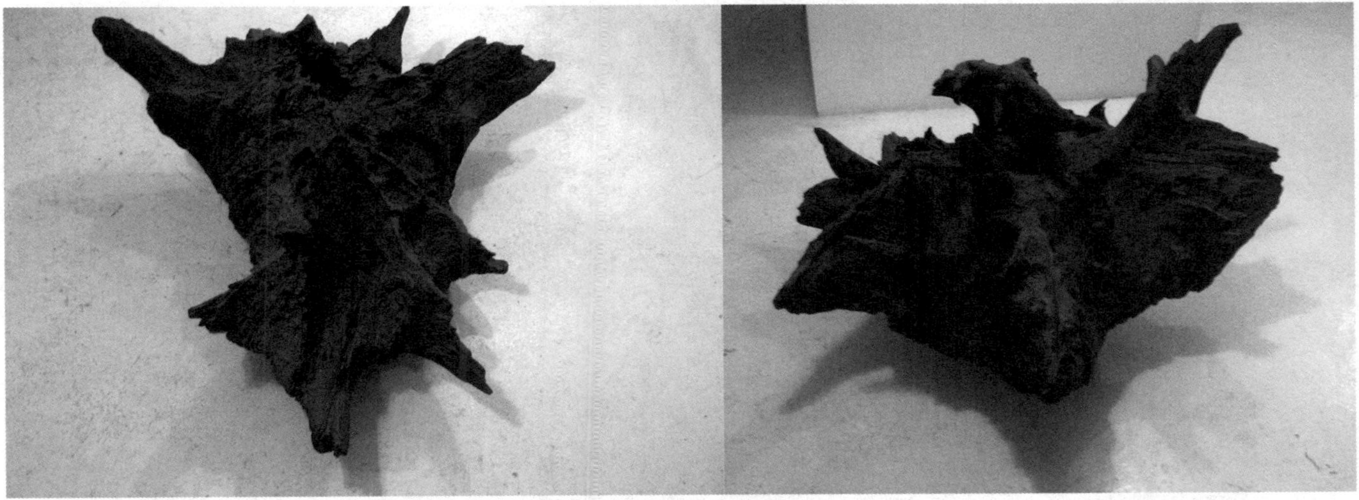

8 Pascal Convert, *Untitled* (Verdum tree stumps), 1996

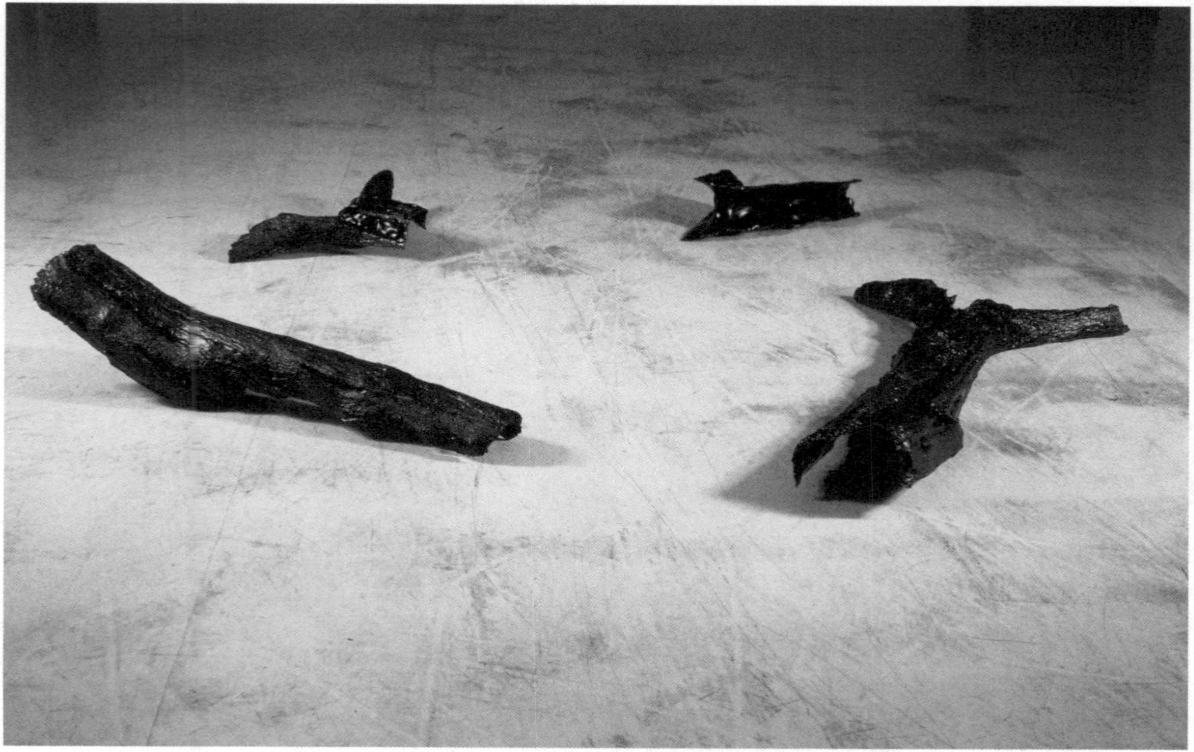

9 Pascal Convert, *Imprint* (Atomised cherry-tree from Seiju-Ji Temple, Hiroshima), 1997–98

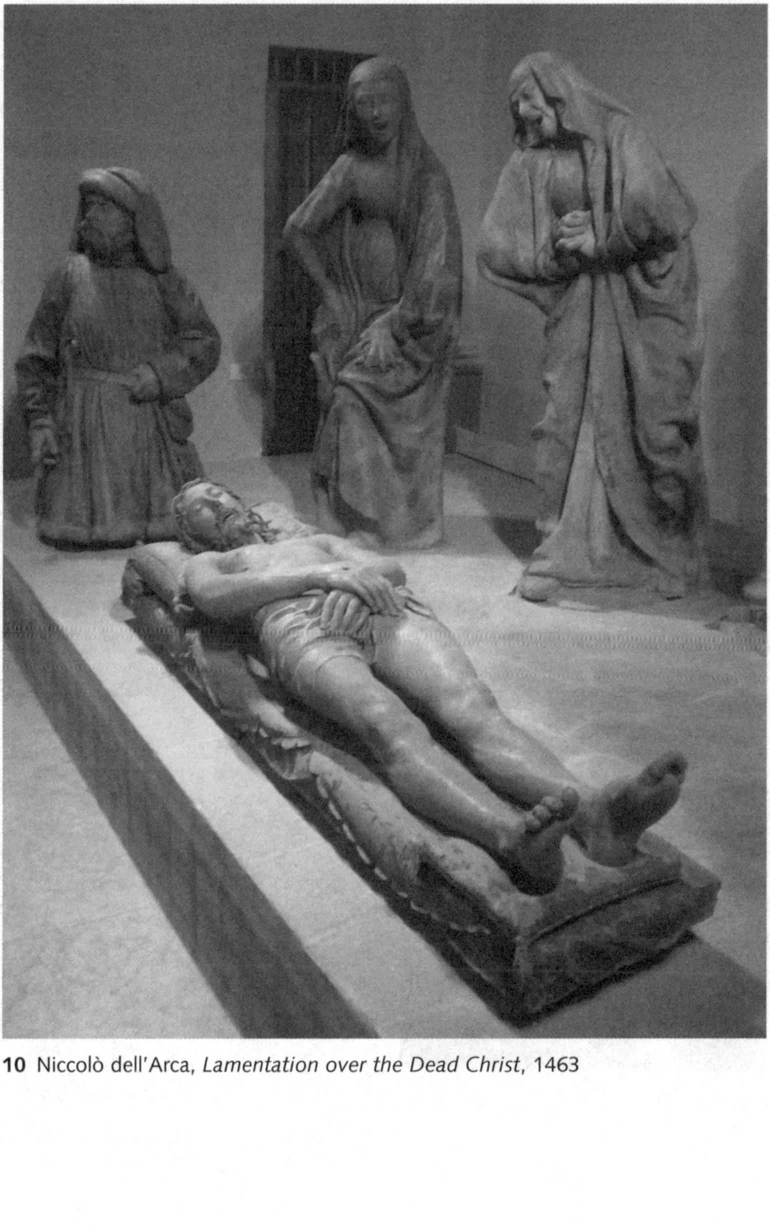

10 Niccolò dell'Arca, *Lamentation over the Dead Christ*, 1463

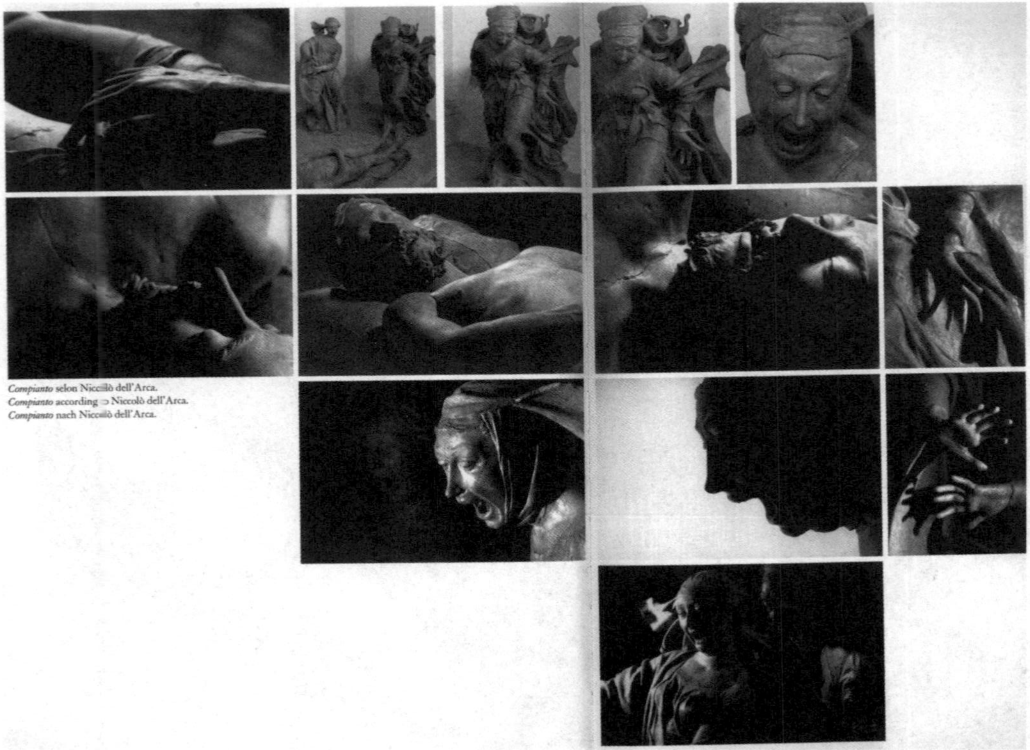

11 Georges Didi-Huberman, *Sketch for an Atlas: Compianto according to Niccolò dell'Arca*, 2007

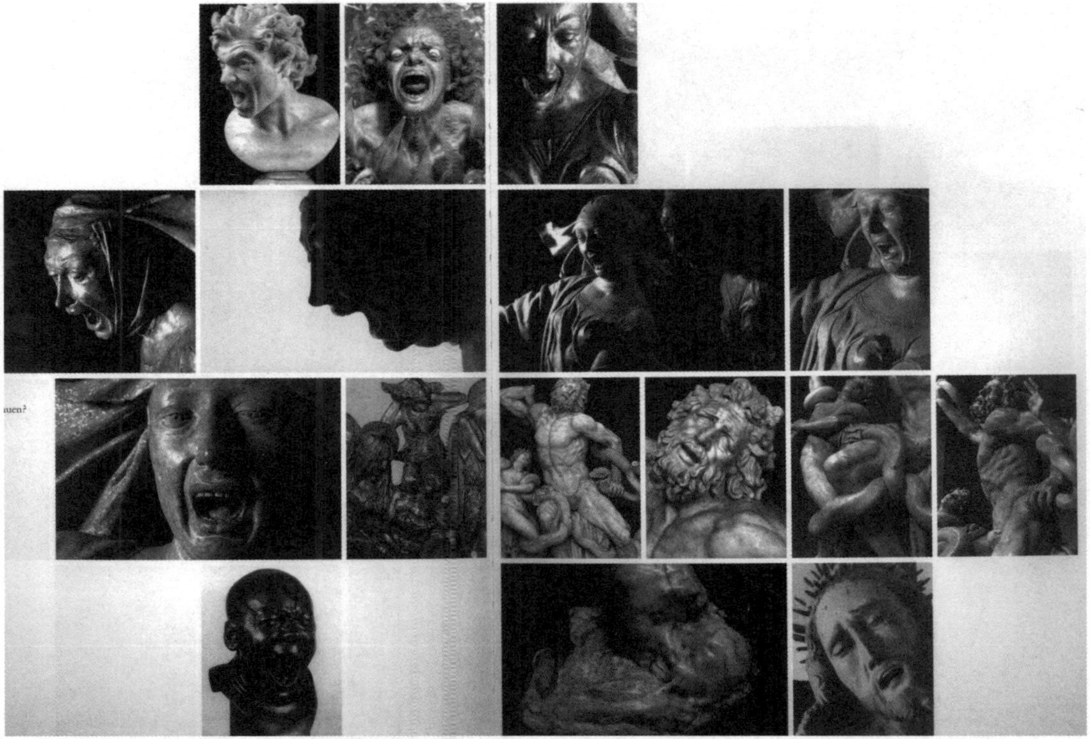

12 Georges Didi-Huberman, *Sketch for an Atlas: Sculpting the Cry?*, 2007

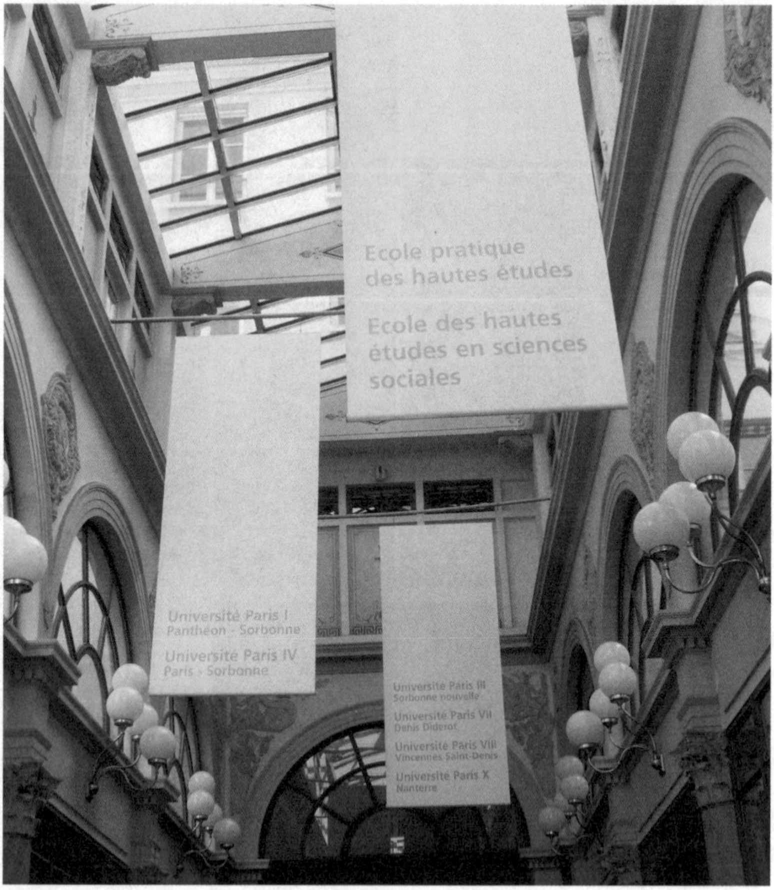

13 Galerie Colbert, Paris, 2011

8

Value, meaning, method: Nathalie Heinich's sociological perspectives on visual culture

Shirley Jordan

In the foreword to her 1998 study *Le Triple jeu de l'art contemporain* (hereafter *The Triple Game*), Nathalie Heinich draws attention to what her analysis lacks: this is a book on art without illustration, evaluation or opinion (1998a: 9–14). How then does Heinich mediate the visual for us? In fleshing out an answer, this chapter first examines in broad terms the specificity of her sociological approach. Thereafter it is divided into two sections: an appraisal of her analysis of the Van Gogh cult, to which she refers as an 'anthropology of admiration' (1996a); and an assessment of her thinking on contemporary art, the *avant-garde* and the phenomenon of rejection.

Questions and thinking tools

Heinich's writing on the visual takes us from the classical to the contemporary periods and covers a wide spectrum of artistic expression, including Impressionism, symbolism, cubism, Surrealism, abstraction, conceptual art, land art and body art. Her principal concern is the sociology of reception, which means that she places not art works but viewing subjects at the centre of her preoccupations: not a Van Gogh self-portrait but the hagiographic impulse that is sustained by it; not Duchamp's notorious *Fountain* (1917) but the disturbance it provokes. In so doing, she raises fundamental questions about the values we attribute to visual art and artists and the spaces and structures we forge for them. These spaces and structures may be physical, intellectual, affective, institutional or discursive. As Heinich explores holistically the 'ripples' created in society by visual art, she reminds us powerfully and persistently that neither the work nor our reaction to it can be considered *sui generis* and places our response within a wider context. In short, she highlights the contingent nature of the cultural practices in which our responses to the visual are enmeshed.

A key phenomenon studied by Heinich is the social construction of the 'artist'. While the sociology of art frequently seeks to downplay this figure, Heinich remains fascinated by our investment in it and by the tacit rules that govern evolving understandings of what an 'artist' is. Here she shifts the conceptual terrain away from art historical or creative autobiography approaches to look instead at the business of framing artists within specific value regimes. *Être artiste* (1996b) thus analyses the material situation and status of the artist from the Middle Ages to the present; from artisan to *peintre maudit* to the highly valorised elite figures who constitute a new aristocracy in what she refers to as a 'regime of singularity' (2005). Heinich is especially interested in artists who disrupt established categories of visual expression, test conceptual boundaries and tacit definitions of 'art', and invent new ways of being an artist. She readily returns to salient 'grands singuliers' (1996b: 69), including Van Gogh (whom she sees as pivotal in evolving conceptions of the artist), Duchamp, Dali, Beuys, Picasso and others. Through selected case studies she analyses in detail the politics and power structures of both admiration and rejection; rather than showing us whom she admires or rejects and why, she scrutinises admiration and rejection themselves, pointing out that even admiration is, paradoxically, a negative construction affirmed through violence, 'a struggle of admirers against non admirers, a struggle between good and bad admirers, a struggle over what is to be admired and what is the proper way to do so' (1996a: 122). Clearly, then, Heinich seeks to determine not the meaning of art, but how we *give* it meaning.

We find in Heinich a subtle and intricate *mise en dialogue* of the various 'actors' in the field of the visual: artists, institutions, museums, curators, critics, specialist admirers and the general public. Her distinctiveness is also that she looks not into but out from the work itself, approaching it not as a self-contained world of meaning but as another 'actor' studying its effects. Further, Heinich draws our attention powerfully to the apparatus which commissions, displays and valorises visual art, making important contributions to museology through, for instance, her 1989 study of the Pompidou Centre in Paris (she focuses on the paradox that the Centre's utopian, open architecture cuts across the democratising ambition that inspired it), or her emphasis in *The*

Triple Game on how contemporary art challenges the physical and conceptual structures of museums. In addition, Heinich has produced interesting studies on the idea of the 'event' in the art world (Heinich and Schaeffer 2004a: 105–30) and the way in which events fabricate, or facilitate the expression of, values.

What of Heinich's methods and thinking tools? Those interested in the sociology of art often quote Pierre Bourdieu's observation that sociology and art make 'an odd couple' (1993: 139). The antinomies to which this observation alludes are usefully spelled out by one sociologist as follows: 'art tends to rebel against scientific images of the world, while sociology tends to thrive on demystifying the enchanting in social life. Art tends to revolt against materialistic explanations of life, while sociology tends to exult in exposing the singular and unique as socially constructed and socially reproduced' (Harrington 2004: 9). The sociologist is thus 'an intruder in the world of belief that is the world of art' (Tanner 2003: 105). Heinich finds here a stimulating thinking tool, since it is precisely this disjuncture, this sense of incompatibility that can tease both art and sociology into more refined awareness of themselves as they put each other's assumptions to the test. Not only is the visual art world thrown into sharper (if not always welcome)[1] relief when sociology takes art as its object, but Heinich discovers new routes through sociology. For instance, a disciplinary epiphany experienced in the course of her research on the admiration of Van Gogh permits her to progress from what she refers to as a 'critical sociology' (a Bourdieusian model seeking to denounce the inequities of domination and *distinction*) to a 'comprehensive sociology' with a mediating role, seeking 'l'intercompréhension plutôt que la dénonciation' [intercomprehension rather than denunciation][2] (1998c: 81).

Distinguishing features of Heinich's writing on the visual are, then, its scientific control, its alertness to the epistemological implications of method and its principle of detachment. Such affective flattening is unusual in writings which engage with art, but it is precisely this feature that clears the terrain for Heinich's general study of the competing values at work in the field. The remit of the sociologist is not to decide whether the actors are right, but to set out and follow through their reasons: 'suivre les acteurs' [follow the actors] (1998a: 335) is Heinich's watchword. A priori theory thus gives way to empirico-inductive reasoning and Heinich confines herself rigorously to asking only those questions that emerge from the data and that are particular to the sociology of art (as distinct, for example, from those asked in art history). She thus makes us alert to the meaning of method in a way that writings on art from other discipline areas, less intent on setting out their approach to knowledge, seldom do.

Heinich's habits of working and thinking include a phenomenological approach to social and cultural practices and the strategic de-familiarisation and fine-grained, 'thick' description that are key techniques in ethnography. She gathers data *in situ* from participants involved in the rituals we create around art, visiting Auvers-sur-Oise for the centenary commemoration of Van Gogh's death (1996a: 123–39), observing and talking to visitors wandering in the Pompidou Centre (1989) and drawing upon the *livres d'or* [visitors' books] placed in exhibitions to garner and examine public responses (for example, 1998a: 321; 346). Her thinking often proceeds by negation (teasing out the specificity of a thing by working out what it is not) and by exposing the paradoxes at work in our relationship with the visual, which she enjoys for their illuminating potential.

At the start of my introduction I asked how Heinich mediates the visual for us. The answer is by focusing on what customarily remains unarticulated and by inviting us to reposition ourselves in a resolutely empirical space. We can look to Heinich for ways of standing back from the often fervent affective or intellectual involvement we have with the visual and sharpening our curiosity about precisely what it is that we do when we engage with art. Nowhere is the paradoxical contrast between such a position and the emotional involvement that many of us sustain with art and artists more pronounced than in her highly original study of Van Gogh.

Van Gogh: the trace and the touch

It is not a personal reaction to Van Gogh's vibrant palette or distinctively powerful rhythms that motivates Heinich's major study, but a sudden recognition as she forages through library catalogues of the astonishing momentum in studies of the painter. From there her interest in 'the making of' Van Gogh and in how our (often competing) practices of admiration are structured around the visual traces he has left. Heinich adopts a constructivist notion of genius as not intrinsic to the artist but resulting from successive efforts 'to aggrandise and universalise him' (1996a: 99) and explores the exponential logic inherent in the collective construction of greatness by way of celebration, wherein 'admiration feeds off its own impact on the admired object' (*ibid.*: 112). We have made Van Gogh 'very present in words, actions and things' (*ibid.*: xiii). Mechanical means of reproduction have ensured our overwhelming familiarity with his images and with images of him: his iconic sunflowers, starry nights and self-portraits punctuate our visual landscape while legends of his life and severed ear abound. It is true that the visual universe of other major artists has also seeped into our everyday, but what is it that has distinguished our admiration, or 'love', of Van Gogh from our admiration of them? How might we account for what is, in the case of the collective relationship with Van Gogh, such a passionate desire to *see*?

To explore this question Heinich dissolves the hierarchies inherent in art appreciation, focusing even-handedly on the 'vulgar' question of hagiography as well as on scholarly questions of hermeneutics. Her 'anthropology of admiration' involves an exhaustive trawl through critical, biographical and fictional works on the artist and draws productively upon art history, biographical and hagiographical traditions, psychiatry and psychology, economics and the sociology of religion, with its interest in pilgrimages, atonement and the status of relics. The first two parts of Heinich's study delineate stages in the making of Van Gogh: for instance, from silence to hermeneutics; from biography to hagiography; and from the incomprehension to the aestheticisation of madness. The final part develops the idea of a mass psychodrama lived out with regard to the painter, and sees the popularity of his work through the prism of atonement. We will limit ourselves here to examination of two interwoven aspects of Heinich's study: the intense symbiosis of work and man that underpins collective admiration; and the concept of atonement.

The personalisation of artistic value

The collective imaginary has made Van Gogh a key figure in the evolving notion of the 'artist'. A number of conceptual shifts coalesce through our involvement with him, including displacements of interest from the art to the artist, from the normal to the abnormal, from conformity to rarity, from success to incomprehension, from the present to posterity and from the regime of community to the regime of singularity, which is of particular interest to Heinich (*ibid.*: 68). Van Gogh is thus an essential stepping stone towards the dynamic of the contemporary art world wherein initial incomprehension is, paradoxically, almost a prerequisite of excellence. Critically, the personal bond connecting audience to artist also emerges with Van Gogh and includes a strong ethical dimension: those for whom this genius/saint/hero painted are deemed *guilty* for refusing to recognise his visionary capacity, while his severed ear is equated with the blinded eye of Oedipus as 'one of the great self-sacrificial acts of Western culture' (*ibid.*: 72). The tenacity of the paradigm of sacrifice in the case of Van Gogh is all the more remarkable since, as Heinich points out, far from being misunderstood he was praised almost unanimously by specialists from the beginning doubtless because they had been prepared by the Impressionists to see value in deviance from the canon. His work was recognised a mere ten years after his death by numerous publications and a retrospective in a prestigious Paris gallery, and if he sold only one painting and saw just one article published on his work during his lifetime, this was simply because his career was so short.

Heinich's study of reception attends to specific features of Van Gogh's visual idiom which are insisted upon in both critical writings and popular responses. She is interested in how, progressively, his work is ritually seized upon as a visual indicator of the man and a vehicle for proximity to him. What is prized are those features that seem porous and raw; that appear to resonate with the artist's 'madness'; that invite a personalised response and that call, intensively, to communion, rendering his painting iconic in a quasi-religious sense. Such features include the artist's signature, the excessive and deranged quality of his touch, and his intensive recourse to self-portraiture. The aesthetic shock each of these elements is capable of creating in the spectator is commensurate with their ability to evoke the exceptional person of Van Gogh. 'Vincent', the artist's familiarly intimate signature, originated in his knowledge that his name was often ill-pronounced and in his desire 'that those who see me understand that I am saying "thou" to them' (*ibid.*: 70). It is interpreted as an invitation to proximity with the hero-martyr-saint (Vincent) rather than an invitation to critically assess the work of the genius of modern art (Van Gogh). The extreme particularisation of his brush strokes, always easily identifiable, provides graphic reminders of his tormented psychic state as he 'touched' the canvas, touching spectators in turn with a frenzied directness of gesture that re-enacts and enlivens our sense of what it was to paint and to paint in madness. The madness of gesture that severed the painter's own ear is the same madness that governs the unorthodox intensity of the movements he traced in paint. Painting here is both process and product, evoking the man as much as the subjects represented (*ibid.*:

69). Through the art-critical writing on Van Gogh which she studies, Heinich traces the evolution of terminology concerning the 'living flesh' of the paintings or their 'biological matter' (*ibid.*: 115). Such metonymic vision, wherein a brush stroke evokes a man, achieves a special intensity in Van Gogh's many self-portraits. Disregarding the painter's insistence that he painted himself because he could not pay others to sit for him, critics seize on the implied introspection of the self-portrait as further confirmation of the inextricable oneness of work and life. There emerges, then, an ethic of the trace in responses to Van Gogh, which situates the viewer not just before a painting, but before a 'material object [which is] part of a human being' (*ibid.*: 107).

'Our works are relics and small bones':[3] atonement through gaze, presence and money

In order to understand the relationships we bear to Van Gogh(s), Heinich draws on anthropological theories of social exchange and depicts activities around art that are linked to gift-giving. More particularly, she develops the thesis that we are indebted to the artist and that we persistently seek atonement for his martyrdom through three media: the gaze, presence and money. We will first explore her theorising of the gaze and of presence as practices of atonement. These are peculiarly consistent with current emphases on haptic contact and on emotion in response to the visual: if emotion in art is being theorised anew,[4] in adoration of Van Gogh it has remained a constant. Heinich insists here on proxemics, on affect, on how we are 'touched', and draws on the theology of presence applied to relics.

If the value and power of Van Gogh paintings lie in the mediated access they provide to Vincent, then beholding such paintings is both mysterious and sacred (see Plate 5). Heinich draws a sustained analogy between the cultural practices involved in making a pilgrimage to venerate the relics of a saint and making a journey to admire the painter's works in a gallery. All such 'pilgrims' are, she argues, in an emotionally charged and culturally prescribed 'quest for presence'; all commune with the relics or 'relic-works' of the dead; all are intent on achieving proximity to authenticated real objects; all display their admiration and return 'enriched with small objects sold to commemorate the moment' (1996a: 113–14). This model emphasises a transcendence of the aesthetic towards the spiritual or sacred as the gaze aims to look less at the work than through it to its author. Further, Heinich posits that an exchange of offerings takes place through the gaze: the spectator is provided with a 'highly emotionally charged experience', 'an aesthetic shock', 'a feeling of love' (*ibid.*: 116) and in return offers to Van Gogh tribute, reparation and atonement. The gaze is 'dutiful', 'admiring' and 'active' (*ibid.*: 119) in the sense that strong involvement is called for in this intimate encounter with the painting/person. All the rhetoric surrounding exhibitions primes this kind of gaze, as Heinich amply illustrates. Gazers also expect satisfaction at having done their duty and are thus 'caught up in [a] community web of commitments, promises, and exchanges' (*ibid.*: 120). If an exhibition *has to* be seen, this is because seeing it counters the indifference suffered by the living painter. Finally aesthetic pleasure and guilt feed on each other: the guilt cannot be extinguished and is renewed and heightened by contact with the paintings.

Participant observation in galleries allows Heinich to confirm how strong an imperative motivates the demonstration of looking, and of looking in certain ways. She posits that morality is harboured in the gaze, so that one courts shame if one does *not* look. Indeed, 'to abstain publicly from looking at admirable objects may be experienced as just as much of a transgression as looking privately at reprehensible objects' (*ibid.*: 121). The museum has thus become a moral space – a space for 'the public exercise of admiration, where looking is an obligation, where seeing becomes a duty' (*ibid.*). An extension of such duty, and one which is especially marked by what Durkheim terms the 'contagiousness of the sacred' (*ibid.*: 205), is outlined in Heinich's final chapter on atonement through presence. Here the focus shifts from a 'virtual pilgrimage' to gaze on the visual traces left by Van Gogh to a literal pilgrimage to his body in Auvers-sur-Oise – a village which has itself become a relic – in order to give the gift of presence 'to one who experienced the martyrdom of isolation' (*ibid.*: 133). Heinich's rich ethnographic description of her visit to the village in July 1990 for the centenary of Van Gogh's death studies the organisation of remembrance around 'the cult of the martyr' (*ibid.*: 124). She describes a multitude of ritual celebrations, the culmination of which is a procession to the painter's graveside to atone for collective indifference at the time of his suicide. Such rituals are linked more to cults than to visual culture and as such we will not linger on them except to observe the peculiarly post-modern saturation of images that characterises Auvers-sur-Oise, for key sites and motifs in the village – the Ravoux Inn where Van Gogh lived and died, the Daubigny Museum, the Notre-Dame-d'Auvers church – are surrounded by paintings of themselves. Thus, as Heinich comments, 'the world is reconstituted as an imitation of the images that have depicted it' (*ibid.*: 125).

Let us glance too at money as a medium of atonement, for the investment in Van Gogh is not solely emotional: painted 'relics and bones' are at the centre of a lucrative industry and the purchasing of Van Gogh's work is 'the commodity form in which the injustice committed against Van Gogh the man can be redeemed' (*ibid.*: 110) (here Heinich neatly links the terms 'achat' [purchase] and 'rachat' [redemption]). The regular increase in his market value, frequently characterised as irrational, is in fact a further manifestation of collective guilt at deferred recognition. Further, it is bound up in the complex inflationary logic that we have already described wherein the marks of admiration (excessive prices in this instance) serve to reinforce the artist's greatness, 'which then appears as the cause rather than the effect of monetary inflation' (*ibid.*: 111). Thus we are bound with Van Gogh into 'a debt that deepens in being paid back' (*ibid.*: 110) and one that compares well with the theory of *potlatch* dear to anthropologists of the gift. Auctions, as Heinich points out, are equally risky, agonistic systems of expenditure, involving public, ostentatious and sometimes ruinous acts of giving and receiving (*ibid.*: 102).

Our active construction of the painter/hero is further sustained by another cycle: that constituted by the often bitter rivalry between camps whose modes of appreciation differ and whose condemnation of each other is integral to their admiration. An important aspect of Heinich's study is precisely to 'grasp the system of positions involved in celebration' (*ibid.*: 63), including the various modes of disapproval that structure it. The principal division is between 'elite' admiration (scholarly, aesthetic, relatively private and engaged primarily with the work) and 'ordinary' admiration (un-learned, affective, relatively collective and engaged primarily with the man), although these forms are not symmetrical in their denunciation of each other since the ordinary has less need to denounce the elite (*ibid.*: 136–7). Nor are these 'pure' positions: they mesh in certain manifestations, and ordinary admiration is dependent on elite institutions in its quest for 'the grace of pure presence' (*ibid.*: 119). Other forms of disapproval include the parodic, Bakhtinesque fringe events that Heinich observes in Auvers-sur-Oise (*ibid.*: 130), and the condemnation, by admirers of all stripes, of an art market which encourages fakes, removes works from the public sphere and does violence to the memory of an impoverished man by its indecent prices. Whatever the denunciation, its intensity shows that the stakes involved in the psychodrama we live out with Van Gogh and in the beliefs and practices we thus nourish are high.

Heinich, then, provides a fine-grained analysis of collective investments in Van Gogh and illustrates the way, through the *doxa* that coalesces around him, a boundary is definitively established between the traditional concept of the artist (as craftsman) and the modern concept of the artist (as misunderstood genius). Thanks to Van Gogh, new readings of artists past and present become possible 'through the prism of the motif of incomprehension' (*ibid.*: 141); bohemia, madness and poverty are validated; the unfinished work becomes open to celebration; and the motif of moral indebtedness 'spread[s] to the totality of artistic production' (*ibid.*: 110). Some of the features that have come into play in our appreciation of him remain of great relevance to contemporary art, including the personalisation of the artist; an emphasis on emotion; an interest in madness and the visual; and a fascination for the trace, and for what might be disclosed by touch. One may dispute certain aspects of this study of Van Gogh. Not all readers will recognise the logic of atonement as outlined by Heinich or readily concede that their interaction with visual art may be understood as 'pilgrimage'. Nevertheless, Heinich's clinical defamiliarising of the rituals that we construct around the visual is a spur that enables us to consider afresh the way our aesthetic tastes and emotional responses may be bound up in the virtuous exponential circle of her 'anthropology of admiration'.

Transgression and assimilation: contemporary art's 'triple game'

A further centre of interest for Heinich lies in contemporary art and the *avant-gardes*. In *The Triple Game* she sets out to circumscribe the contemporary, an aesthetic paradigm whose 'mental framework' she sees as more distinct from the modern than the modern is from the classical (1998a: 328). Focusing upon the ways in which art proceeds through disruption, transgression and the testing of limits, she organises her study by examining the way the boundaries that structure the field are repeatedly challenged. These include the conceptual boundaries around what constitutes art; the physical boundaries of the museum; and the boundaries of authenticity, morality, and legality. Contemporary art is seen as a series of visual provocations which elude established formats, which need recuperating *as* art (by the textual apparatus on which they depend for their integration within the museum) and the assessment of which necessarily involves a range of factors beyond the visual. Heinich's terminology reflects the unstable definition of 'art' by referring to those creations that are available for inclusion in art history and institutions as 'artistic propositions'. Each successive proposition is a test case for the question of what art is. This neutralising vocabulary is characteristic of Heinich and consistent with other shifts in contemporary terminology, such as the replacing of *artiste* with *plasticien(ne)*.

The Triple Game provides a richly referenced panorama, exploring the more or less scandalous modes of disruption associated with specific creators, exhibitions and events since the early twentieth century. Heinich is interested in unclassifiable propositions or 'objets-frontières' (2006: 35) [boundary objects] (land art; performance art; conceptual installation pieces; works using the artist's body as field) which challenge gallery spaces and curators by the complexity of their installation or preservation. She spreads before us the heterogeneous range of materials involved and selects examples which work on the spectator's emotions, producing shock, amazement, pleasure, displeasure or disgust. Among the numerous examples she explores are Christo's (1985) packaging of the Pont-Neuf; the self-mutilations of Gina Pane and Orlan; Joseph Beuys's interactive 'social sculptures' and his performances combining felt, fat, wire and wood; and Piero Manzoni's *Merde d'artiste* (1961) consisting of ninety 30-gramme tin cans filled with his own excrement. Clearly, it is not only the definition of contemporary works *as* art that is unstable, but their very permanence: deliberately ephemeral, often incorporating fragile or perishable matter, they are frequently impossible to reproduce or to conserve. They are, in addition, especially dependent on the philosophy and theory which have become integral to our understanding of what and how contemporary art means. As in Heinich's work on Van Gogh, this study sees her teasing out a detailed spectrum of reception, including analyses by a range of major thinkers on art.[5] But where Van Gogh allows her to study expressions of admiration, contemporary art involves exploring the spectrum of rejections, both 'profane' (1998a: 204–25) and 'learned' (*ibid.*: 226–46), that routinely accompany art and artistic events.

The museum as physical reality and as conceptual entity also receives detailed consideration in this study. Heinich shows how it extends its remit of 'housing' what specialists agree is art to become instead the co-author or co-originator of visual propositions (*ibid.*: 331; 334). She thus argues that the locus of production of artistic values is not the artist and the work, but the institution itself. To consider the latter as merely mediating is a mistake (*ibid.*: 336), and therein lies one of the many paradoxes that Heinich enjoys revealing. There emerges from her study a clear picture of the contradiction between the logic of subversion which defines contemporary art and the logic of institutionalisation. The institutions of art 'commission', or have a hand in determining the nature of the transgressions which the artists produce and which are then absorbed into the establishment. Thereafter it is not just the object itself that is exhibited: in a self-referential gesture, the museum exhibits itself exhibiting the exhibited object (*ibid.*: 343).

As Heinich's title makes clear, it is the metaphor of the game that structures her view of contemporary art; more specifically the Victorian parlour game of 'Hot Cockles' [*le jeu de la main chaude*], a variant of the children's game 'Blind Man's Bluff' characterised by escalating provocation, collusion, bluff and double bluff. The art world functions through ever-intensifying cyclical play between transgression (effected by the work), rejection (by the public) and integration and assimilation (by specialists and by the institution, which is the hidden game-master). The extremity of transgression accelerates exponentially: artist's gestures are more and more shocking; spectators are more and more shocked; specialists work harder and harder to mediate and constantly demonstrate their power to restructure the meaning of art (*ibid.*: 341). Heinich singles out one particular project, Paraponaris's 1996 installation *Tout ce que je vous ai volé* [*Everything I Stole From You*], exhibited in the Musée d'Art Contemporain in Marseille, as particularly exemplary of the 'triple game' dynamic (*ibid.*: 329–35). In exhibiting forty-two everyday items which he had stolen from individuals, institutions or companies, the artist at once highlighted and threatened a number of aesthetic and ethical boundaries, not to mention legal ones (both he and the museum's curator were taken away in handcuffs and duly charged). As happened in the case of Manzoni's conserved faeces, a can of which was opened in public twenty-eight years later by artist Bernard Bazile (*ibid.*: 92), further 'works' were subsequently generated: artists whose belongings had been purloined and exhibited contacted the police and turned the recuperation of their goods into a performance, of which a video film was made; Paraponaris created *Further Replica* (2007), described by the gallery as 'an act of memory permitting renewal of both the act and the object' and incorporating three elements: a second collection of stolen objects; painted or photographed reproductions of these objects; and *L'Affaire est dans le sac* [*The Affair Is in the Bag*], a series of empty white plastic bags each bearing the definition of a stolen object which was confiscated by the police and each for sale at €14.18.[6] The meaning of these 'propositions' and their validation as art depend entirely on the narrative of controversy surrounding them and on the museum's proactive desire to embrace theft as an artistic act.

Case studies in rejection

In her sustained examination of the multiple incidents of defiance and rejection which shape contemporary art, Heinich persistently asks who says 'no', to what and how. Her treatment of individual works eschews interpretation, pursuing instead a 'pragmatic' approach (2001: 96–9), by which she understands analysis, conducted through empirical fieldwork observation, not of what an art work means or is worth, but of what it *does.* How does it impact upon emotions, cognitive categories, value systems, and frameworks of perception defined by sensory experience and models of evaluation (1998a: 96)? How does it recompose our familiar world? What happens when we come up against it? In *L'Art contemporain exposé aux rejets* (1998) and *The Triple Game*, she analyses public reaction to selected works which have aroused incredulity, indignation or anger, such as Daniel Buren's controversial *Les Deux Plateaux* (1986) (see Plate 6), a series of columns installed in the *cour d'honneur* of the Palais-Royal (1998a: 41–2). In the range of methods used to criticise this project (petitions; letters to newspapers or ministers; graffiti; vandalism) and in the spectrum of arguments employed, it is possible to see not only the opposition between partisans and adversaries, but also the diverse register of values – civic, aesthetic, ethical, pragmatic/functional, legal, etc. – in the name of which indignation was expressed. Heinich's holistic presentation of this *cause célèbre* provides a useful, emotionally voided space wherein interested parties may consider dispassionately the stakes at play in Buren's installation (see Plate 6).

One case in particular illustrates especially sharply Heinich's concerns. The proposition in question is produced by Christian Boltanski, an artist to whom Heinich frequently returns since his installations and projects exemplify some of the ways in which contemporary art perpetually courts rejection by destabilising understandings of 'art', 'the artist' and the museum. His work erodes art–non-art boundaries in several ways, including the powerful bridging it effects between art and ethnology (*ibid.*: 89) and its reliance on mundane materials (family photographs; used clothes; biscuit boxes; light bulbs) which distance it from the 'singularity' associated with artists and art, thus affirming the enduring power to disturb of the ready-made. While he explores in various ways the idea of the fetish, Boltanski rejects the fetishising of artworks themselves, of the pedestals on which they stand and of the idea explored in Heinich's work on Van Gogh that they are 'sainte[s], parce que touchée[s] par un grand saint' (*ibid.*: 116) [holy, because touched by a great saint]. He dismisses the reverence for permanent incarnations of art upon which exhibiting institutions and markets depend and shifts the emphasis towards performances, reinterpretations or reconstitutions of propositions which use new materials each time (*ibid.*: 325).

Following in the traces of the Bauhaus, Boltanski increasingly explores the possibilities of working outside the limits of the museum and 'deterritorialising' the work of art (*ibid.*: 100). To him, museum space produces a levelling effect where one artwork is equated to the next and the 'active gaze' which engages with art is severed from everyday life. Boltanski's attempts to free himself from the museum network and challenge the museum's physical limits include experiments with the idea of 'mail art' (*ibid.*: 102); an installation of used clothes (*Dispersion* (1994)) which dissolved the frontier of the museum by inviting visitors to take the exhibits away (*ibid.*: 121); and an archive piece installed in the museum's basement which could be seen through a glass slab in the floor but not visited.[7] Such projects clearly undermine the museum, although Heinich does not fail to point out the paradoxes at work here since *plasticiens* such as Boltanski certainly do still depend on the museum network: their motto might be, she remarks, 'en être sans y être' [be of it but not in it] (*ibid.*: 98).

To study the reactions of rejection provoked by Boltanski, Heinich focuses on a characteristically troubling installation that was part of his *Dernières années* exhibition at the Musée d'Art Moderne de Paris (1998). This consisted of piles of used clothing stuffed on to shelves in the museum's storerooms (*ibid.*: 80; 2001: 98). By focusing in particular on the work's 'repulsion effect' and by noting the range of reactions elicited in this register, she is able to highlight the conflict that takes place at the fraying edges of some common-sense categories which are habitually operative in assessing art. These include beauty, durability, transparency of meaning, the value attached to the material used and evidence of specific competence in the artist's work. Of course, one may strongly admire Boltanski's work precisely because of his transgressions, but the intense charge transmitted by his installations cannot be described just in terms of admiration or rejection: the interesting question is where such reactions come from. Heinich shows that what disturbs and provokes is the composite status of the objects used, their confusing closeness to us and the difficulty we experience in relating them to a given category. These clothes, humanised by being visibly used, fit nowhere. They exemplify contemporary art's penchant for de-functionalising functional objects and absorbing the everyday. They are carefully folded and piled so cannot be seen as rubbish; they are not merchandise to be sold for they are displayed in a museum; they are not detached from those who wore them and whose imprint and odour they still bear, yet they are de-personalised and not (quite) relics; they call us to identification, yet defy such identification by their sheer number. Their logic is that of another universe built on negation: that of the concentration camp. The unsettling indeterminacy of this installation and its implied, yet unarticulated, ethical dimension provide a clear instance of contemporary art's propensity to challenge categories as well as of its need for accompanying narratives. One might also observe (although Heinich herself does not) that her work on the reception of art, whether it concerns Van Gogh or a contemporary artist such as Boltanski, is of a piece in that it is marked by the intense fascination with traces which runs throughout postmodernity.

Concluding thoughts: Heinich and Baudrillard

We have seen, then, a sample of what ensues when, through Heinich, the 'odd couple' of art and sociology come together. We have seen that her studies valorise works – especially 'objets-frontières' – because they express the broader society, culture or Zeitgeist and reveal the construction of values. Clearly, to follow Heinich in her exploration of visual art means to remain alert to methodology and epistemology and to find a neutral space of analysis at a remove from affective/aesthetic investment in art/the artist. A characteristic of art, however, is precisely that it calls into question the a-critical impartiality of the sociologist (1998a: 337; 343). In her work on Van Gogh, Heinich anticipates the difficulty of persuading the painter's admirers that to study the phenomenon of admiration is not to negate it. In the case of contemporary art, she is similarly conscious that merely to describe the interdependency in the 'triple game' of actors that proclaim their autonomy reads like a criticism of the art world's apparatus. Description and denunciation are in fact inseparable in this instance, since to describe is indeed to expose the fictions around which 'le pacte muséologique' [the museological pact] (*ibid.*: 344) is organised: for instance, that artistic transgression repeatedly comes up against the conservatism of institutions. Uncharacteristically, Heinich follows through the logic of denunciation to conclude *The Triple Game* with a trenchant value judgement. The final part of her study criticises the universe of contemporary art for deepening the fracture between elite and 'ordinary' culture (*ibid.*: 346); for sustaining and concealing the paradox of institutionalised transgression; and for having become 'le lieu par excellence de la mauvaise foi' [the locus, par excellence, of bad faith] (*ibid.*: 344). Most radically, she describes the vicious cycle of the triple game as a pathology that blights the social body of contemporary art (*ibid.*: 337). This (fleeting) polemical attack on the closed system of the art world suggests affinities with sociologist Jean Baudrillard whom Heinich mentions as a formative influence – an 'auteur de prédilection' [a preferred author] (2006: 13) – in her early career. In the interest of plotting connections between the theorists in this volume, it is with observations on the interfaces between these two major figures that this chapter will conclude.

Notable commonalities include attentiveness to everyday phenomena and an emphasis on structures and systems at the expense of specific art objects. What fascinated Heinich in Baudrillard's *Le Système des objets* (1968), as indeed in the work of Bourdieu and Roland Barthes, was its 'concrétude' [concreteness] (*ibid.*), and she allies herself to the creative, disruptive shift which forced an opening for serious analysis of 'les pratiques ordinaires que dédaigne la pensée académique' [ordinary practices disdained by academic thought] (2007b: 130).

Heinich and Baudrillard both sharpened their positions in what became known as the 'querelle de l'art contemporain' [the contemporary art quarrel], which crystallised a sense of crisis in the French art world of the 1990s, taking centre stage both in specialist reviews (notably *Esprit*) and in articles in the national press, including Baudrillard's 'Le Complot de l'art' [The Art Plot] which was published in *Libération* (20 May 1996). Baudrillard, to whose article Heinich refers (2006: 57; 1998a: 232–3), was among those intellectuals who castigated contemporary (as opposed to modern) art as institutional, elitist, posturing and empty. This diagnosis is, as we have seen, precisely the motivation underpinning Heinich's own concurrent research towards *Le Triple Jeu* on the institutionalisation (therefore the impossibility) of transgression in art and the frustration of the uninitiated at art's mystifying depthlessness.

Other shared preoccupations can be traced: both thinkers interrogate the spaces of art, especially where projects of spectacular scale are involved – both wrote, for instance, on the dysfunction of the Pompidou Centre;[8] both highlight the commercial frenzy of the art world; both comment on the Bauhaus (2006: 9) and on reality television (2002b: 213–44); both are interested in elitism and democracy in the world of visual culture; both are intent on laying bare this world's systemic mechanisms, whose pervasive logic all too easily blinds us to their operations.

There are contrasts too: where Baudrillard has theory (of sign systems and simulation), Heinich has method; where Baudrillard participates *in* art's controversies, Heinich presents data *about* them; where the implications of Baudrillard's analyses of the power of the visual image in modern industrial societies are bleak, data presented by Heinich on vigorous acts of rejection to art can be energising. To conclude our brief plotting of interfaces, we might usefully note that Heinich's ongoing, self-reflexive commentary on her contemporaries is undertaken not to elucidate their approach but energetically to stress the stand-alone distinctiveness of her own (her career-long engagement with Bourdieu remains the major example). In this way she seeks to remain above the fray, above the seduction of controversy, gathering data and presenting detailed evidence from a position of 'neutralité engagée' [engaged neutrality] (2002a) in what she determinedly (if not always entirely successfully) presents as an opinion-free zone. Heinich's virtue is that she keeps us so coolly alert to one overriding and consistently rewarding question: in precisely what processes and structures is our looking enmeshed?

References

Bourdieu, P. (1993), *Sociology in Question*, London: Sage.

—— and Darbel, A. (1966) *L'Amour de l'art. Les Musées d'art européens et leur public*, Paris: Éditions de Minuit.

Gielen, P. (2005) 'Art and social value regimes', *Current Sociology* 53(5), 789–806.

Grenfell, M. and Hardy, C. (2007) *Art Rules: Pierre Bourdieu and the Visual Arts*, London: Berg.

Harrington, A. (2004) *Art and Social Theory*, Cambridge: Polity.

Heinich, N. (1989) 'The Pompidou Centre and Its Public: The Limits of a Utopian Site'; trans. Chris Turner, in Robert Lumley (ed.), *The Museum Time Machine* London: Comedia/Routledge, 119–212.

—— (1991) *La Gloire de Van Gogh. Essai d'anthropologie de l'admiration*, Paris, Éditions de Minuit; trans. P. L. Browne (1996a), *The Glory of Van Gogh. An Anthropology of Admiration*, Princeton, NJ: Princeton University Press, 1996.

—— (1993) *Du peintre à l'artiste. Artisans et académiciens à l'âge classique*, Paris, Éditions de Minuit.

—— (1996a) *The Glory of Van Gogh: An Anthropology of Admiration*, trans. P. L. Browne, Princeton, NJ: Princeton University Press.

—— (1996b) *Être artiste: Les Transformations du statut des peintres et des sculpteurs*, Paris: Klincksieck.

—— (1998a) *Le Triple Jeu de l'art contemporain: Sociologie des arts plastiques*, Paris: Éditions de Minuit.

—— (1998b) *L'Art contemporain exposé aux rejets: Études de cas*, Nîmes: Jacqueline Chambon.

—— (1998c) *Ce que l'art fait à la sociologie*, Paris: Éditions de Minuit.

—— (1999a) *Pour en finir avec la querelle de l'art contemporain*, Paris: L'Échoppe.

—— (1999b) 'La Sociologie et les publics de l'art', in Raymonde Moulin (ed.), *Sociologie de l'art*, Paris: L'Harmattan, 267–78.

—— (2000) 'From rejection of contemporary art to culture war', in Michèle Lamont and Laurent Thévenot (eds), *Rethinking Comparative Sociology. Repertoires of Evaluation in France and the United States*, Cambridge: Cambridge University Press, 2000, 170–212.

—— (2001) *La Sociologie de l'art*, Paris: La Découverte.

—— (2002a) 'Pour une neutralité engagée', *Questions de communication*, 2, 117–27.

—— and Edelman, B. (2002b), *L'Art en conflits: L'œuvre de l'esprit entre droit et sociologie*, Paris: La Découverte.

—— (2003a) *Face à l'art contemporain: Lettre à un commissaire*, suivie de *Retour sur les retours*, Paris: L'Echoppe.

—— (2003b) 'The Van Gogh effect', in Jeremy Tanner (ed.), *The Sociology of Art, A Reader*, London: Routledge, 122–31.

—— and Schaeffer, J.-M. (2004a) *Art, création, fiction. Entre sociologie et philosophie*, Paris, Jacqueline Chambon.

—— (2004b) 'Factuel, fictionnel, fictif: retour sur le cas Van Gogh', in Thierry Lenain (ed.), *Mensonge, mauvaise foi, mystification: Les mésaventures du pacte fictionnel*, Paris, Vrin, 29–37.

—— (2005) *L'Élite artiste. Excellence et singularité en régime démocratique*, Paris: Gallimard.

—— (2006) *La Sociologie à l'épreuve de l'art. Entretiens avec Julien Ténédos*, vol. 1, Paris: Aux lieux d'être.

—— (2007a) *La Sociologie à l'épreuve de l'art. Entretiens avec Julien Ténédos*, vol. 2, Paris: Aux lieux d'être.

—— (2007b) *Pourquoi Bourdieu*, Paris: Gallimard.

—— (2007c) *Comptes rendus à ... Benjamin, Bourdieu, Elias, Goffman, Héritier, Latour, Panofsky, Pollak*, Paris: Les Impressions Nouvelles.

—— (2008) 'Entre éthique et esthétique: art et animalité', in Yolaine Escande and Johanna Liu (eds), *Frontières de l'art, frontières de l'ésthétique*, Paris: You Feng.

Laermans, R. (2000) 'Nathalie Heinich, Sociologist of the arts: a critical appraisal', *Boekmancahier*, 12(46), 389–402.

Tanner, J. (ed.) (2003) *The Sociology of Art, A Reader*, London: Routledge.

Notes

1 For the art establishment's cold-shouldering of Heinich following publication of *The Triple Game* see Heinich (2003a).

2 Bourdieu was a mentor from whom Heinich rapidly differentiated herself and with whose shadow she vigorously boxes. His emphases on the social conditions of cultural practice and particularly on the less educated general public's responses to art (for example, Bourdieu and Darbel 1966) provide an important predecessor to her own studies. For an introduction to Bourdieu's sociology of art see Grenfell and Hardy (2007).

3 Christian Boltanski interviewed in *Journal of Contemporary Art* 2(2) (1989), 22–3.

4 For example: Grenier, C. (2008), *La Revanche des émotions*, Paris: Seuil.

5 Her chapter on the function of specialist writings (305–26) explores contributions from Alechinsky, Paz, Krauss, Didi-Huberman, Bourdieu, De Duve, Goodman and Baudrillard.

6 The gallery's supporting text and an entertaining inventory of the objects stolen are available on www.bureaudescompetences.org

7 For the 1993 Lyon Biennale of Contemporary Art.

8 For references to these themes in Baudrillard, see Chapter 12 in this volume.

Part IV
Memory, body, image

9

Seeing and touching: Jean-Luc Nancy and the ground of the image

Ian James

Introduction

Jean-Luc Nancy is perhaps best known to date for his thinking on community in texts such as *La Communauté désœuvrée* (Nancy 1986), his reworking of Heideggerian ontology, and of phenomenological accounts of world disclosure in key texts of the late 1980s and 1990s such as *L'Expérience de la liberté* (Nancy 1988), *Une Pensée finie* (Nancy 1990), *Le Sens du monde* (Nancy 1993) and *L'Être singulier pluriel* (Nancy 1996). These major works of Nancy's philosophy explore a complex legacy of phenomenological thought, principally that of Husserl, Heidegger and Merleau-Ponty. There is little in these works to suggest a sustained engagement with, or interest in, the visual. This sense of a marginalisation of the visual in favour of another register might perhaps be confirmed by Derrida's important work *Le Toucher, Jean-Luc Nancy* (Derrida 2000) where it is the figure of touch, which according to Derrida forms a constant and central point of reference in Nancy's philosophical writing.

Yet, from the mid-1990s onwards Nancy's work begins to engage in a sustained manner with questions of art, aesthetic experience and of artistic presentation, in which the problem of the visual, of the gaze, and of the image, takes on a central importance. Nancy's two major volumes of collected essays on art, *Les Muses* (Nancy 1994) and *Multiple Arts* (Nancy 2006), both engage extensively with the visual arts, most notably with painting and sculpture, but also with photography. He is the author of an important essay on film, *L'Évidence du film* (Nancy 2001b), and has written extensively on painting, both secular and religious, in works such as *Le Regard du portrait* (Nancy 2000a), *Visitation (de la peinture chrétienne)* (Nancy 2001c) and *Noli me tangere* (Nancy 2003b). In 2003 he also published an important philosophical work on the nature of the image and the faculty of the imagination, *Au fond des images* (Nancy 2003a). Taken together these works represent a sustained engagement with a wide range of visual art forms but also with the question of the visual per se, the visual in the artistic image or aesthetic form, but also in representation, presentation, image formation and perception more generally.

Across this body of work it is arguable that Nancy develops, in a sustained if not entirely systematic manner, an innovative rethinking of the question of realism and representation in the artwork. It might be worth recalling at this point the extent to which thinking about literature and art in the wake of much French literary theory of the 1960s and 1970s has emphasised the impossibility of realism, mimesis and the representational function of the work of art. This kind of theory, of course, stressed the way in which literary meaning and signification is produced through the organisation and arrangement of linguistic signifiers and culturally signifying codes (a good example of this would be Roland Barthes's seminal text *S/Z* (1970)). What follows will argue that Nancy's philosophical engagement with the question of the visual and with the status of the image allows the question of realism, and of the relation of the artwork to worldly existence to be rethought in an original and innovative manner.

In *Le Toucher* Derrida referred to Nancy as developing an 'absolute post-deconstructive realism', yet, he adds, this is an absolute realism which is 'irreducible to all traditional forms of realism'. If we take this comment by Derrida as a guiding thread, it might be argued, Nancy can be seen as a major contender for a thinking that moves through, and in decisive ways beyond, theoretical and critical work associated with post-structuralism and the postmodern, and, in particular, poststructuralist critiques of representation.

There have, of course, been a number of critical responses to Nancy's thinking and, more specifically, to what one might call his philosophy of finitude. Foremost among these is the response of the French philosopher Alain Badiou. Badiou is critical of Nancy for the way in which his philosophical writing turns around the questioning and affirmation of finitude. This questioning and affirmation leaves its mark on Nancy's work, most explicitly in the works on community but also in his quasi-ontology of sense, his thinking of being in the singular plural and in works such as *Une pensée finie.*[1] In an essay dedicated to Nancy's thought, Badiou writes: '"Finitude" est le signifiant-maître du discours philosophique de Jean-Luc Nancy' ['finitude' is the master signifier of Jean-Luc Nancy's philosophical discourse] (2004: 17). This for Badiou is an inescapably Heideggerian gesture and readers of his major work of ontology, *L'Être et l'événement* (1988), will know that his own thought affirms uncompromisingly that contemporary philosophy needs to be plotted from Cantor onwards. For Badiou the only possible ontology which could avoid falling back into a traditional metaphysics would be an ontology articulated through post-Cantorian set theory. It is only the mathematics of set theory, Badiou contends, that allows for, 'le discernement de la pluralité des infinis, et de sa conséquence pour les orientations fondamentales de la pensée' [the discernment of the plurality of infinites, and the consequences of this plurality for the fundamental orientations of thought] (Badiou 2004: 21).[2] The task here is to think the multiplicity of being, as infinite multiplicity and outside of any totalising horizon, outside of any finitely bounded whole. 'Je ne crois pas' he writes, 'que l'injonction est celle de la fin, du fini et de la finitude. Ma conviction est que c'est l'infini qui fait défaut' [I do not believe that the injunction we are to follow is that of the end, of the finite and of finitude. My conviction is that it is the infinite which is lacking] (*ibid.*: 15). For Badiou, then, 'ce avec quoi il faut en finir, c'est la finitude' [that which we should be done with, is finitude] (*ibid.*). On this basis he rejects Nancy's thinking as still enmeshed in the very metaphysical and totalising horizons of thought from which it is trying to extricate thought more generally.

Derrida offers a more nuanced, less polemical yet not entirely dissimilar critique of Nancy's thinking of the finitude of sense. As has been indicated, he focuses, in particular, on the lexicon of touch in Nancy's thought and the relation of this to what he calls the 'haptocentrism' of European philosophy, the legacy of which is intimately bound up with the metaphysics of presence. More than any other text, Derrida's *Le Toucher* has shown the extent to which Nancy's use of the term touch sets his thought in a relation to a broader European philosophical tradition. According to Derrida the figure of touch organises a manifold tradition of thinking which would incorporate, among others, such diverse names as Maine de Biran, Ravaisson, Kant, Husserl, Merleau-Ponty and Deleuze. This tradition, Derrida argues, has given rise to what he calls 'une affaire, une sorte de complot, une intrigue philosophique du toucher' [an affair, a plot, a sort of conspiracy, a philosophical intrigue of touch] which has been played out along the cultural boundaries which separate France, Germany and England (2000: 159). Derrida also poses the hypothesis that this tradition is continued, complicated and interrupted in twentieth-century thought, most prominently in the development of phenomenology from Husserl onwards and then, specifically, in the work of Nancy such as it develops from the 1970s to the 1990s. The figure of touch, then, becomes the privileged motif of a '"tactilist" or "haptocentric" tradition'. Or put another way, it is posed as a key organising concept in an interlocking history of European 'métaphysique haptocentrique'. What is at stake here, as elsewhere in Derrida's work, is the question of an ontology of presence, and all its attendant philosophical baggage: 'partout avec le toucher, il va s'agir de « l'être », bien sûr, de l'étant, du présent, de sa présence et de sa présentation, de sa présentation de soi' [everywhere with touch it is going to be a question of 'being', of course, of the beings, of the present, of its presence and of its presentation, the presentation of itself] (*ibid.*: 17). Nancy's thought therefore potentially falls back into a metaphysics of presence – or at least that is the risk that has to be constantly negotiated when one tampers with the lexicon of touch and persists with this lexicon in such a sustained manner.

By way of a preliminary response to both Badiou and Derrida it might be worth noting that language of finitude and touch in Nancy needs to be read very carefully, and needs, in particular, to take account of the style of Nancy's philosophical writing. In relation to his thinking of the visual, and specifically of the image, it will be argued here that finitude in Nancy is thought in a way to which Badiou does not really do justice in his arguments. Nancy emerges in this context as being far less evidently or orthodoxly Heideggerian than Badiou appears to believe. Derrida, of course, maintains an ambivalence in relation to Nancy's thinking of touch throughout the pages of *Le Toucher* and he never suggests that Nancy's thought is entirely or unequivocally recuperated into the orbit of the tradition and into a metaphysics of presence.

Nancy's recent thinking around the question of the visual, and more specifically his thinking of the image, makes far more explicit the figure of touch operates in his writing only as the touching of an untouchable; the proximity it implies is only ever a distance, and the presentation that touch enables is, for Nancy, only ever, and also, a withdrawal. Indeed, his thinking resists the kind of recuperation into a metaphysics of presence that Derrida suggests might be the risk of his lexicon of touch. It certainly has to be conceded that, from the 1970s through to the mid-1990s in particular, Nancy's philosophy is dominated by the question of finitude (of finite embodiment, sense, thought, existence, etc.). Yet

Nancy's finitude is one which is always thought within an economy of excess, his ontology is always an ontology of excess, that is to say, he consistently seeks to affirm or think that which, within finite existence or being, infinitely *exceeds* finite existence or any horizon of ontology.

The image

In *Au fond des images* (2003a) Nancy's thinking of the visual and the image can be understood against the backdrop of the account of image offered by gestalt psychology. The distinction made within gestalt psychology between figure and ground, is of key importance when it comes to understanding the way Nancy unfolds his thinking in *Au fond des images.* If Nancy does follow Heidegger, in this context, he does so to the extent that he engages with, and draws out, the implications of Kant's problematic description of the schematising work of the imagination as 'an art concealed in the depths of the human soul' (Kant 1998: 273) and he follows Heidegger also in so far as his engagement with the question of the image is an attempt to think: 'comment la production de la possibilité d'une prise-en-vue en général renvoie, en amont de toute espèce d'image mimétique, à la valeur originelle du Bild en tant qu'aspect qui se fait voir' [how the production of the possibility of a taking-sight in general refers, prior to any kind of mimetic image, to the original value of a 'Bild' [picture], understood as an appearance which lets itself be seen] (Nancy 2003a: 156). *Au fond des images*, therefore, represents not just a narrow focused thinking of the status of particular kinds of image, artistic or poetic images for example (although this is of key importance). What is at stake in this work is the visual in general insofar as its condition of possibility is thought in relation to a fundamental dimension of the image as sensible–intelligible form.

Gestalt psychology – figure and ground

In gestalt theory the perception of a figure which emerges as distinct from the ground is a consequence of an internal choice that, although quasi-instantaneous, involves a complex of internal processes. The meaning connected with a figure is a critical aspect of its relation to the ground in the instant that the distinction between figure and ground is made.[3] If we look at this example we see a classical image drawn from the canon of gestalt psychology where there is a possible confusion between figure and ground (see Plate 7). One can see either a kind of vase or two faces opposed to each other; indeed, it is easy to perceive an oscillation between the two.

What one might perceive instantaneously, automatically or pre-reflectively, however, is, for the gestalt psychologist at least, related meaningfully to what might be called 'ground' of the viewer's experience. This 'ground' would be a rich mix of all of past experiences of the self, of world, and their myriad interactions plus the feelings, beliefs, values and the needs that are embedded in the internal world. In this context the ground defines the figure and gives it meaning. It is, if you like, the force which allows the figure to distinguish itself from the ground, to create the unity of an image from a diversity of sensible appearance. It should be noted that gestalt psychology is not mentioned explicitly in *Au fond des images* (despite its insistent and implicit presence in the reference to ground within the title itself).[4] However, the distinction between figure and ground in gestalt theory allows for a clarification of some of Nancy's apparently obscure formulations in this work.

The distinct

Central though the motifs of 'finitude' and 'touch' in Nancy's discourse are, it may be suggested that both Badiou and Derrida do not fully take into account the sustained way in which this discourse also deploys the motifs of 'infinity' and of the 'untouchable'. These motifs have taken on a greater prominence in Nancy's philosophical writing since the mid-1990s and have, in particular, played a key role in his writing on art, aesthetic experience and sense perception more generally. The opening essay of *Au fond des images*, 'L'Image–Le distinct', focuses on the notion of the 'distinct' and of the distinct as a key element of image formation. The 'distinct' in this essay is articulated, and decisively so, around the figure of the 'untouchable', and around figures of distance, separation and setting apart. It also organises itself around the key signifier of the 'infinite', rather than that of the finite or of finitude.

Nancy begins the essay with a meditation on the sacred as a setting apart from the profane. This, in turn, leads to the identification of the concept of the distinct as that which is set apart, distanced or distinguished, yet one which is removed from the difficult relation to religion etc. that the notion of the sacred will always have. Nancy begins to unfold this concept of the distinct in the following terms:

> Le distinct, selon l'étymologie, c'est cela qui est séparé par des marques [...] cela qu'un trait retire et tient à l'écart, en le marquant aussi de ce retrait. On ne peut l'y toucher [...] c'est que le trait distinctif sépare ce qui n'est plus l'ordre du toucher, pas exactement, donc un intouchable, mais plutôt un impalpable. (*ibid.*: 12)[5]

> [The distinct, according to its etymology, is what is separated by marks [...] what is withdrawn or set apart by a line or trait, by being marked also as withdrawn. One cannot touch it [...] because the distinctive line or trait separates something that is no longer of the order of touch; not exactly the untouchable then, but rather an impalpable.]

A key emphasis is given to the term 'trait' in French, which, as in English, can signify line, stroke, dash, characteristic, or feature. The 'distinct', then, is that which does not allow itself to be confused with something which is analogous or neighbouring; it is demarcated, other, different, independent, or separated. With reference to the gestalt image (Plate 7) it is easy to see how the white area can be seen as distinct from the black in the tracing of a line which demarcates one colouring from another. Just as Nancy emphasises the line or 'trait' of the image, so too he places an emphasis on withdrawal, and notes also that what is withdrawn here, is, not of the order of 'touch'. What is withdrawn is most obviously the background (which for the time being can be distinguished from the 'ground' of the image proper; 'background' would here be either the white or the black depending on whether one sees faces or a vase). The background is withdrawn in the sense that what can be perceptually, sensibly and intelligibly grasped is the figure only, either faces or vase. The background cannot exactly be identified, for if one tries to grasp the background as such it becomes the alternative figure and the other colour recedes into and as the background (in trying to grasp the background as such one will perceive only an oscillation between the two figures). The ability of the image to figure an intelligible form resides, for Nancy, entirely upon this power of distinction, of the distinct, that is to say, the detachment of figure from background, and the process of separation and withdrawal this implies. Nancy specifies this process further:

> Le distinct est au loin, il est à l'opposé du proche. Ce qui n'est pas proche peut être écarté du contact ou bien de l'identité. Le distinct est distinct selon deux manières. Il ne touche pas, et il est dissemblable. Telle est l'image: il faut être détachée, mise dehors et devant les yeux. (*ibid.*)

> [The distinct is at a distance, it is the opposite of what is near. What is not near can be set apart in two ways: separated from contact or from identity. The distinct is distinct according to these two modes: it does not touch, and it is dissimilar. Such is the image: it must be detached, placed outside and before one's eyes.]

This could easily be read as a more or less direct riposte to Derrida who in *Le Toucher* emphasised that with touch, the dominant motif of

Nancy's thought, it is always proximity, nearness and presence which is at stake, therefore also sameness, and a recuperation of difference within the logic of the same and the identity of the concept. The distinction of the image is, Nancy argues, a detachment, separation or distancing – distancing from a background, certainly, but also distancing from the perceiver and therefore a distancing or separation of the perceiver from that which is figured or imaged. In figure 1 the distinctness of the vase, if vase I see, emerges from the withdrawal of the background, a tracing of a line which detaches the image, separates it from the background and places the image before the eye *at a distance*. Yet the figuration or imaging of the vase is not, at a fundamental level, Nancy maintains, grounded in the identity of a concept, a signified or represented empirical vase. Rather the distancing, detachment and separation that the 'distinctive trait' of the image traces, is a fundamental order of dissimilarity and difference:

> L'image est une chose qui n'est pas la chose: essentiellement elle s'en distingue [...] Ce qui est à saisir, c'est comment la force et l'image appartient l'une à l'autre dans la même distinction. Comment l'image se donne par un trait distinctif [...] et comment ce qu'elle donne ainsi est d'abord une force, une intensité, la force même de sa distinction.
>
> [The image is a thing that is not the thing: it distinguishes itself from it, essentially [...] What remains to be grasped is how the force and the image belong to one another in the same distinction. How the image gives itself through a distinctive trait [...] and how what it thus gives is first a force, an intensity, the very force of its distinction.] (*ibid.*: 13)

The image, then, is a thing which is not the thing that it images. In this context Nancy aligns the 'distinct' with the term 'force' insofar as he speaks of the image in terms of 'the very force of its distinction' and insists that: 'force and the image belong to one another in the same distinction'. Earlier in relation to the distinction made by gestalt psychology between figure and ground, the ground was described in terms of a 'force which allows the figure to distinguish itself from the ground, to create the unity of an image from a diversity of sensible appearance'. The 'ground' of the image, as distinct from the background, is the mix of past experiences of self, world, feelings, beliefs, values etc. It is in this context that Nancy comes to understand the 'ground' as a diffuse horizon of sense (in excess of any symbolic order of signification) which exerts a force which allows the image to emerge as a sensible–intelligible appearance, but does so only on the basis of its withdrawal (the ground is withdrawn from the distinct image just as the background is necessarily withdrawn).[6]

In the 'becoming distinct' of the image Nancy is trying to think the separation or emergence of figure from (back)ground as resulting from the imposition of a force which gives form, which detaches, separates, distances in the tracing of the distinct line of the image. In this the image is a distinct form, it is the thing but not the thing, it is held to the seeing eye but only in distance, it is detached from the ground, but only in the withdrawal of the ground from the visibility of the finite image. Nancy deploys a difficult figural language here in his attempt to think the emergence of the image, that of force, but also that of 'ciel', that is to say of heaven or sky.

Nancy resorts continually in the opening essay of *Au fond des images* to the language of force and speaks of 'the intimate force of the image'. At the same time this language of 'intimate force' is closely linked to the notion of sky or heaven. Nancy speaks of sky as celestial force. Such figural language, initially rather obscure to the reader perhaps, poses a particular difficulty for interpretation. Most immediately Nancy would appear to be mobilising a theological or even religious vocabulary derived from Christianity. This Christian inheritance is perhaps unavoidable yet Nancy does take some care to distinguish between the overtly theological connotation of 'celestial' and 'heaven' by indicating that he derives his use of the term 'ciel' here from painting. He is trying to find a means of articulating the way in which an image achieves distinction, or a clear and distinct figuration, only insofar as it is the bearer, within that very distinction, of a source of illumination, or the casting of light, as if it were a silhouette (one need only think of the celestial lighting cascading from above in Christian painting, or the more diffuse ambient light passing through windows in the painting of Dutch masters such as Vermeer):

> Toute image a son ciel, fût-il représenté comme au dehors de l'image ou ne fût-il pas représenté: il lui donne sa lumière, mais la lumière d'une image vient de l'image elle-même. L'image est ainsi son propre ciel. (*ibid.*: 20)

> [Every image has its sky, even if it is represented as outside the image or is not represented at all: the sky gives the image its light, but the light of an image comes from the image itself. The image is thus its own sky.]

Ground, in its withdrawal, allows the tracing of the figure as a separation of shadow and light. The image detaches itself from the ground, and emerges as a distinct form in the withdrawal of ground, and this emergence of figure can only be thought in terms of a separation of shadow and light in the realm of the visible (that is, of the image); the ground therefore is of the realm of the invisible, the withdrawn. Nancy's language here is itself densely figural but density serves to articulate a complex relation of figure and ground which enables the emergence of a sensible–intelligible image. It is only in the context of this complex relation that Nancy's rather enigmatic formulations regarding the ground of the image can be understood. In this context, then, the ground, for Nancy, is:

> la force de l'image, son ciel et son ombre. Cette force se presse « au fond » de l'image ou plutôt elle est la pression que le fond exerce sur la surface – c'est-à-dire sous elle, en cet impalpable non-lieu qui n'est pas simplement le « support » mais le revers de l'image. Celui-ci n'est pas un « revers de la médaille » [...] mais le sens insensible (intelligible) comme tel senti à même l'image. (*ibid.*: 23)

> [the force of the image, its sky and its shadow. This force is pressed 'in the ground' of the image or rather it is the pressure that the ground exerts on the surface – that is to say beneath the surface, in that impalpable non-place which is not simply the 'support' but the reverse side of the image. This is not a 'reverse side of the coin' [...] but insensible (intelligible) sense as such sensed directly on the image.]

In this short passage gestalt theory's language of the ground, a post-Nietzschean language of force, and Nancy's understanding of the term 'sense' all come together. Indeed his thinking of the image, of perception and the intelligible-sensible visibility of worldly appearances hangs on this conjunction of terms. The ground of the image is for Nancy: 'insensible (intelligible) sense as such sensed directly on the image'. There is a paradox here: intelligible sense is 'insensible' insofar as it is withdrawn with the presentation of sensory form of the image and yet sensed 'directly on' that visible form insofar as it is a force which, in its withdrawal, articulates the presentation of the image as such. The force is the force with which the figure is detached from the ground in the emergence of a form which makes sense in its sensible appearance.

This emphasis upon affective force resonates to a certain degree with Jean-Louis Schefer's account of the image as discussed by Patrick ffrench in Chapter 11 in this volume. For both Schefer and Nancy the form of the image bears an emotion or force which can be related to a certain materiality or bodily affect. The difference between the two is that where, for Schefer, the force of the image appears to solicit singular affects related to the pre-symbolic drives of an individual body (and therefore related also to more personal memories, biographical experience etc), for Nancy the affective force of the image, in its embodied materiality, solicits a sense which is collective, shared, or spaced in the touching and distance of a multiplicity of bodies who share a world and share the sense of a world. Nancy does not invoke a Lacanian model whereby a symbolic order of signification represses a pre-symbolic body of infantile drives at the moment that the subject is constituted as lack and divided from itself in that very symbolic order. Unlike Schefer, the impersonality of affective force in Nancy already articulates a shared order of sense and world.

Nancy's overall account of the image in *Au fond des images* suggests that the unity of the image, its ability to assemble a figure from a potentially amorphous diversity or heterogeneity of sensory appearance, derives not from the systematic unity of reason – but from an exertion of force, the force of the ground itself as it withdraws in the emergence of figure and delineates or traces a separation shadow from light. This force is the affective, imposing force of shared sense itself. Sense in Nancy is that horizon of referential implications or inscription, which prior to language or any order of the symbolic, imposes itself, as the force of the image, it is the ground of the image, withdrawn in the very detachment of the image from ground.[7] The unity, assemblage, or reassemblage of the image is not one of concept (Hegel), reason (Kant), intentional directedness or logical essence (Husserl), it is the intimate force of sense itself as it absents itself in the presentation of a sensible–intelligible image; a visible, clear, distinct form.

One might revisit more explicitly now the critiques of Nancy offered by Derrida and Badiou. It has already been clearly shown that Nancy's thinking of the image is organised around figures of the untouchable, of distance, separation, withdrawal – a lexicon which opposes itself to that of proximity, nearness and presence that Derrida associates with touch and the 'métaphysique haptocentrique' he identifies in *Le Toucher*. The dominant motif of Nancy's account of the image, and by extension his account of the visual, perception, originary intuition, and the disclosure of worldly appearances, is one of presentation in withdrawal; if sense is ontologised in Nancy, if it is posed as the very being of the world, it is so only to the extent that it is always withdrawn from presence or presentation, it is only insofar as it is an excess; sense, for Nancy, is that which 'in the phenomenon exceeds the phenomenon itself'.

Sense, as the diffuse withdrawn ground of the image, is always in excess of the finite tracing of the visible form of the image itself; sense in Nancy is only ever characterised as in excess of the world, over language and the symbolic, it is an excess over all limits of the visible and the finite. In this context the image is doubly removed and distinct from finite existence: as image it is distinct from the worldly thing it images, yet it is distinct also from the excess of sense, from that 'insensible (intelligible) sense', withdrawn from the image yet 'sensed directly on the image'. Nancy expresses this in the following manner:

> L'image est hors du monde, étant en soi l'intensité d'une concentration de monde. Elle est aussi hors du langage, étant en soi le rassemblement d'un sens sans signification. L'image suspend le cours du monde et du sens [...] mais elle affirme d'autant plus un sens (donc un « insensible ») à même ce qu'elle fait sentir [...] Il y a dans l'image, qui pourtant est sans « dedans », un sens non signifiant mais pas insignifiant, aussi sûr que sa force (sa forme). (*ibid.*: 27)

> [The image is outside of the world, being in itself an intensity of a concentration of world. It is also outside of language, being in itself the gathering of a sense without signification. The image suspends the course of the world and of sense [...] but it affirms all the more a sense (therefore an 'insensible') directly on that which it is sensed [...] There is in the image, which, however, is without an 'inside', a non-signifying but not insignificant sense, just as sure as its force (its form).]

It is in this context that, for Nancy, the image *in art* is always a relation, albeit one of non-relation, to the world (as his elliptical formulation 'une concentration de monde' implies). The artistic image, here, is not a re-presentation of the thing, or something which is of the order of symbolic signification. The artistic image is not mimetic, but rather participates in that primordial faculty of imaging which constitutes sensible–intelligible appearances per se. The entirety of Nancy's discourse on art and realism, on the realism of the artistic image, is at stake here. Within the text of *Au fond des images* Nancy's thinking shifts in a rather unstable manner between the discussion of individual images within specific works of art and art-forms on the one hand (*ibid.*: 17, 22, 33) and a fundamental order of imaging on the other. This fundamental order of imaging, on the basis of which sensible–intelligible experience of any kind *makes sense*, is always engaged in and by the aesthetic form of the artwork. Such a fundamental order of imaging is simultaneously the condition of possibility of worldly sensible–intelligible–visual perception, of 'taking sight' in any meaningful manner, and at the same time the condition of possibility of the intelligible presentation of distinct aesthetic forms in art.

In 'L'Image–Le Distinct' Nancy draws on a number of different examples and different genres: an extract from Edith Wharton's *Summer*, Hans von Aachen's painting, *Young Couple*, and a 'musical image' form Verdi's *La Traviata.* Citing and analysing Wharton's image of an open door, the emergence of a young girl and an expanse of city and sky, Nancy specifically focuses on the visual nature of the image but at the same time takes pains to resist any strictly mimetic interpretation, according to which the reader, assimilating a string of images, would visualise a scene which could then be said to re-present a recognisable pre-existing external reality. 'Il s'agit moins ici' [It is less a question], he suggests:

> de l'image que nous ne manquons pas d'imaginer (celle que le lecteur forme ou forge de sa façon et selon ses modèles): il s'agit d'une fonction d'image, lumière et juste rapport d'ombre, encadrement et détachement, sortie et touche d'une intensité. (*ibid.*: 17)

> [of an image which we cannot fail to imagine (one which each reader forms or forges in their own way and according to their own models) than it is a question of an image function, light and precise relation of shadow, framing and detachment, opening and touch of an intensity].

What interests Nancy is the manner in which the image traces or figures a form which has no pre-existing model or 'reality' (for the image to work as it does it is not necessary that Wharton actually witness and reproduce the open door, emergent girl, city, etc., or that they ever really existed). What is of interest here is what Nancy terms the line of the image [*le trait de l'image*]. The French word 'trait', translated here as 'line', serves the double function of suggesting a tracing or figuration (such as one might associate with the term 'line-drawing') but also a separation or differentiation: a line is that which separates or divides two volumes or planes of space. Nancy suggests that with the appearance of the young girl through the open door, a world also appears. Yet he also suggests that this world, like the girl, stops at the threshold, stops, and stops us the readers at the threshold of the novel, at the line or figure traced by its writing, such that we enter a world, but are held before or at a distance from it. In the image the reader does not simply visualise an environment but, through a certain intensity of the image, s/he is exposed to 'une totalité indéfinie de sens' [an indefinite totality of sense] or world (*ibid.*: 18). This is an exposure in which the tracing or figuration of form in the line of the image also marks the infinite separation and distance of that which is traced. The reader is held on the threshold of the line which divides/shares [partage] inside and outside, light and shade, life and art (*ibid.*). If, Nancy adds, it is possible that the same line [*trait*] can both separate and communicate:

> C'est que le trait de l'image [...] est lui-même [...] sa force intime: car cette force intime, l'image ne la 'représente' pas, mais elle l'est, elle l'active, elle la tire et elle la retire, elle l'extrait tout en le retenant, c'est avec elle qu'elle nous touche. (*ibid.*)
>
> [It is because the line of the image [...] is itself its intimate force: because the image does not 'represent' this intimate force, but it is that force, it activates it, it draws and withdraws it, it extracts just as it withholds it, and it is with that force that it touches us.]

Here, then, Nancy returns his analysis once more to the motif of touch: the image touches us but not in a way which suggests emotion or sentiment and not in a way which implies a continuity or homogeneity of that which touches and that which is touched. What touches here, in the very instant of a proximity-in-distance, is the force of sense, the tracing of a line which both presents and withdraws, brings into contact and separates. The language of touch is doubled with a language of force, intensity or affect.

The manner in which the images of art engage a fundamental order of the image lies at the basis of Nancy's assertion that: 'l'art touche au réel' [art touches the real] (Nancy 2003a: 54). It should be clear by now, however, that, this affirmation of touch here, an affirmation that so worries Derrida in *Le Toucher*, can and must only be read in the context of Nancy's primary emphasis on the untouchable, the distinct, the distancing of withdrawal, etc.

This is true also for Nancy's emphasis on the finite and finitude. His account of the image in *Au fond des images* highlights the extent to which, for him, the finite space of the visual, of vision, or of the visible, is always exposed as visible, but is so *only* in its relation to the withdrawn invisible of sense. The finite in Nancy is, we might say, only articulated in and on the basis of, a certain thinking of the infinite. This is illustrated in the following two citations which, between them, gather together all the thinking about the image that has been unfolded so far: 'L'image est l'évidence de l'invisible' [The image is the evidence of the invisible] (*ibid.*: 30), it is an index:

> D'un seul coup, qui est son coup, l'image livre une totalité de sens ou une vérité (comme on voudra dire). Chaque image est une variation singulière sur la totalité du sens distinct: du sens que n'enchaîne pas l'ordre des signi-

> fications. Ce sens est infini, et chaque variation est elle-même singulièrement infini. Chaque image est un détournage fini du sens infini, lequel n'est avéré infini que par ce détournage, par le trait de la distinction. (*ibid.*)
>
> [At a stroke, which is its stroke, the image delivers a totality of sense or a truth [...] Each image is a singular variation on the totality of distinct sense: of sense which does not enchain the order of significations. This sense is infinite, and each variation is itself singularly infinite. Each image is a finite detour of infinite sense, which is only recognised as infinite by this detour, via the trait of distinction.]

The image, in its evidence, its absolute givenness to perception, is a space of visibility which is rendered visibly distinct only in the 'trait', tracing or demarcation of lines which articulate the limits, finite boundaries, or finitude of the visible itself. Yet at the same time, as 'the evidence of the invisible', the image opens out in excess of the visible, it troubles the totality or self-enclosure of the finite insofar as sense, the ground of the image, is withdrawn, distinct from all visible form. It is infinitely in excess of the finite. Nancy's thinking of the image, and of the finitude of visible appearances or sense perception, emerges only on the basis of a thinking of the *infinitisation* of finitude. The image, here, and the space of visible form that it makes possible, are always, and infinitely, in excess of all determinate or finite signification, yet they always nevertheless make sense, a sense presented in the form of the image yet at the very same time infinitely withdrawn as an invisible excess.

In his major philosophical work *L'Être et l'événement* Alain Badiou writes: 'La thèse de l'infinité de l'être est nécessairement post-chrétienne' [The thesis of the infinity of being is necessarily post-Christian] (Badiou 1988: 162). Thinking being not as finitude but rather as infinity is the only way, Badiou consistently affirms, for contemporary thought to extract itself from a metaphysics of presence, and engage philosophically with the real of the world. This affirmation was the explicit centre of Badiou's rejection of Nancy's thought seen as unfolding within the orbit of the master signifier of finitude. And yet if we look at Nancy's account of the image it is clear that both Badiou and Nancy see the inscription of infinity within being, or the thought of infinity *as* being, as central to a thought which might begin to extricate itself from its entanglement within the metaphysics of presence. Both, of course, think the infinity of being in very different ways: for Badiou infinity can only be thought mathematically according to post-Cantorian set theory, and according to a rigorous set of protocols which he begins to enumerate within the text of *L'Être et l'événement* itself. For Nancy, as has been shown, infinity is the infinite excess of sense itself, sense as the diffuse ungraspable ground of the image which infinitely withdraws in the presentation or emergence of the distinct line, figure or form of the image itself. Badiou would no doubt view Nancy's infinity as inescapably 'bad' given the way in which he develops his thinking in figural terms, eschews the formalisations of mathematics in favour of a working through in philosophical–figural language of Kant, Husserl, Heidegger, Merleau-Ponty and others. Ultimately though what Nancy offers us in his account of the intimate force that renders the image distinct is a thinking of affection. Affections, or affection, need to be understood here as the affective allure or force which is the condition of the visual and of intelligible sense perception and awareness of both self and world. More specifically Nancy's account of the image tells us that: every affection is an affection of the finite through the infinite and that this is what constitutes the finite: finite existence. Or, put another way, affection is affection by and through exteriority, 'le dehors', in French: there is no affection if not through exteriority.

This brings Nancy close to both Derrida and Badiou. Derrida, it might be recalled, said of difference that: 'finite difference is infinite and vice versa'. Arguably then the differences between Nancy and Derrida or Nancy and Badiou should be addressed, not in terms of the risks Nancy runs in his language of touch, nor in terms of his inexcusable persistence with the language of finitude. Nancy's thinking of the infinite shares the aim of Badiou's philosophy. The question posed by the difference between these thinkers may ultimately be the question of how contemporary philosophical thought can best 'cure' itself of 'bad' infinity through a rigorous thinking of being as 'actual' infinity. In this context Nancy's thinking of the visual and his account of the image stands, alongside the rival mathematical ontology of Badiou, as one of the most important contributions to recent French philosophy.

References

Ash, M. G. (1995) *Gestalt Psychology in German Culture, 1890–1967*, Cambridge: Cambridge University Press.

Badiou, A. (1988) *L'Être et l'événement*, Paris: Seuil.

—— (2004) 'L'Offrande réservée', in François Guibal and Jean-Clet Martin (eds), *Sens en tous sens*, Paris: Galilée, 2004, 13–24.

Barthes, R. (1970) *S/Z*, Paris: Seuil.

Derrida, J. (2000) *Le Toucher, Jean-Luc Nancy*, Paris: Galilée.

Husserl, E. (1982) *Ideas Pertaining to a Pure Phenomenology and to a Phenomenological Philosophy*, trans. F. Kersten, The Hague: Nijhoff.

Gombrich, E. H. (2001) *Art and Illusion*, Princeton, NJ: Princeton University Press.

James, I. (2006) *The Fragmentary Demand: An Introduction to the Philosophy of Jean-Luc Nancy*, Stanford, CA: Stanford University Press.

Kant, E (1998) *Critique of Pure Reason*, trans. Paul Guyer and Alan W. Wood, Cambridge: Cambridge University Press.

Nancy, J.-L. (1986) *La Communauté désœuvrée*, Paris: Christian Bourgois.

—— (1988) *L'Expérience de la liberté*, Paris: Galilée.

—— (1990) *Une Pensée finie*, Paris: Galilée.

—— (1993) *Le Sens du monde*, Paris: Galilée.

—— (1994) *Les Muses*, Paris: Galilée.

—— (1996) *Être singulier pluriel*, Paris: Galilée.

—— (1997) *Hegel: L'Inquiétude du négatif*, Paris: Hachette.

—— (2000a) *Le Regard du portrait*, Paris: Galilée.

—— (2001b) *L'Évidence du film Abbas Kiarostami*, Bruxelles: Yves Gevaert.

—— (2001c) *Visitation (de la peinture chrétienne)*, Paris: Galilée.

—— (2003a) *Au fond des images*, Paris: Galilée.

—— (2003b) *Noli me tangere*, Paris: Bayard.

—— (2006) *Multiple Arts*, Stanford, CA: Stanford University Press.

Notes

1 For an overview of Nancy's philosophy, see James (2006).

2 Set theory is the branch of mathematics which studies sets, thought as grouped multiplicities of objects (most usually objects that are important for mathematics). Badiou's insistence that being be understood as 'pure multiplicity' (rather than as univocal, or in any (onto-)theological figure of the One) leads him to identify set theory as the sole means to think being, or to articulate an ontology that does not return thought to metaphysics. As pure or infinite multiplicity, being can *only* be properly thought in the mathematics of number and sets. Any other way of approaching the infinite multiplicity of being would impose a totalising horizon that would reduce it to a figure of the one.

3 For a broad historical account of the development of gestalt theory, see Ash (1995).

4 Gestalt theory, of course, is much more explicitly referenced in Ernst

Gombrich's classic art-history work on image-making *Art and Illusion*. Gombrich is more critical of certain aspects of gestalt theory, however: see Gombrich (2001: 222–7).

5 Nancy does not in fact elucidate further upon the etymology of 'distinct'; it derives from the Latin 'stinguo' which in turn derives from the Greek 'stígo', meaning to 'prick'. Beyond that the Greek term has an Indo-European root 'stig-' meaning to prick or mark by pricking. The basic idea, then, is to mark things off from one another.

6 The term force, however, such as Nancy uses it, almost certainly needs to be understood in terms of its resonance with a Nietzschean theory of force.

7 On 'sense' in Nancy, see James (2006: 89–97, 105–13).

10

Georges Didi-Huberman: images, critique and time

Nigel Saint

Introduction

Since the early 1980s, and in some thirty books, Georges Didi-Huberman has forged a rebellious form of art history that renews the interpretation of visual images by working with Freud, Warburg, Benjamin and Bataille, and by drawing on phenomenology and post-structuralism. By displacing Vasari, Kant and Panofsky in the process, this overhaul of interpretative practice revalorises images through a sustained reflection on their disruptive power and complex temporality. This reflection has led to a body of work organised around a number of positions relating to time, history, art theory and the body, and deploying a particular visual sensibility that sees writing as an integral part of the enquiry, whether in the analysis of art history in *Devant l'Image* (1990a), or the reinvestigation of modernity and time in *Devant le Temps* (2000a), or the controversial polemic of *Images malgré tout* (2003), through to the hybrid essayistic approach adopted in the studies of contemporary art and dance (Didi-Huberman 1998, 2000b, 2001b, 2001d, 2006a; Convert 1999). This chapter will consider Didi-Huberman's visual sensibility, his style, his development of Benjamin's dialectical image, his interest in Warburg and his approach to the relationship between history and images.

Opening and interpreting images

There are several fruitful entry points into Didi-Huberman's work: the essay 'Question de détail, question de pan' [On the detail and the patch], which is the appendix to *Devant l'Image* (1990a: 273–318); 'Ouverture' [Opening], in *Devant le Temps* (2000a: 9–55); the intellectual self-portrait, again entitled 'Ouverture', in *L'Image ouverte* (2007c: 25–62); and the essay 'L'Image brûle' ['The Image Burns'] in a volume devoted to his work, *Penser par les images* (2006b: 11–52). For Didi-Huberman, works of art are not simply objects hanging on the walls or presented in the space of a gallery, facing their spectators (2006a: 13). The experience of the work is also a situation, where space is opened up and transformed (Demorand 2001: 44). 'Opening' is a key term and organising principle, with the first sentences summoning us to open ourselves to the image and the imaginary, to new spatial and mental dimensions: 'Pour savoir il faut s'imaginer' [In order to know you have to imagine] (2003: 11); 'La peinture souvent déconcerte' [Paintings are often troubling] (1990b: 9); 'Toujours, devant l'image, nous sommes devant du temps' [When we confront images we always confront time] (2000a: 9); and 'La *Vénus* de Botticelli est aussi belle qu'elle est nue. Mais elle est aussi reclose, aussi impénétrable qu'elle est belle' [Botticelli's *Venus* is as beautiful as she is naked. But she is as sealed and impenetrable as she is beautiful] (1999b: 11).

This last statement comes from what could be called Didi-Huberman's version of Kenneth Clark's *The Nude* (1956), *Ouvrir Vénus* (1999b), whose front cover shows a woman's viscera being cut out, from the second of Botticelli's paintings of the *Story of Nastagio degli Onesti* (1482–83), in contrast to the images adorning editions of Clark's study (Clark 1956, 1960, 1972): Botticelli's *Birth of Venus* (1484–86), the torso of Michelangelo's *David* (1504) or the 'profane' woman from Titian's *Sacred and Profane Love* (1514). Didi-Huberman's approach, drawing on his reading of Freud and Warburg, underlines the negative side of beauty, beauty's excessive power, its ability to wound spectators and to defy linguistic expression (1990a: 231–47). Our journeys to museums and galleries involve risk, since for Didi-Huberman the image is associated with our potential loss and our disempowerment: 'L'image impose[r] sa visualité comme une ouverture, une perte – fût-elle momentanée – pratiquée dans l'espace de notre certitude visible à son égard' [The image imposes its visuality like an opening, a loss – even if only momentary – affecting the space of our visible certainty about the image] (1992: 76).

In *Devant l'Image* Didi-Huberman analyses '*main stream*' art history (1990a: 117 n. 22), which in his view can be traced back from Panofsky's humanistic iconology via Kant's theory of knowledge to Vasari's discourse of artistic originality and immortality. In the wake of the new histories of art being produced from the 1970s on both sides of the channel and the Atlantic, Norman Bryson argued that this premise no longer seemed innovative (Bryson 1993: 337). However, Didi-Huberman, like Arasse and Damisch (see Chapters 3 and 4 in this volume), was addressing Panofsky's reception and his enduring legacy in France (and beyond), and the specific emphasis of his critique was also distinctive.

The arrival in French in 1967 of *Gothic Architecture and Scholasticism* (1957), with an afterword by Pierre Bourdieu (where he introduced his concept of the 'habitus' (1967)), and *Studies in Iconology* (1939, 1962), introduced by Bernard Teyssèdre (1967), was followed by *Meaning in the Visual Arts* (1955) in 1969, again introduced by Teyssèdre. The latter's commentaries are very detailed and offer multiple links with art history, philosophy and sociology, urging readers to adopt international rather than German approaches to art history and culture, and to aim for a historical critique of symbols, which in October 1967 Michel Foucault, declaring himself a 'Panofskian neophyte', calls 'a sort of cultural symptomatology' (Foucault 1994: 621–2). Teyssèdre sees Warburg's history and Cassirer's philosophy combined successfully in Panofsky (Teyssèdre 1967: 9). It was the need to reconsider Warburg and Cassirer that led Didi-Huberman to question this happy reception of Panofsky, wondering if there were aspects of all these thinkers that had precisely not been received. In Didi-Huberman's view, unlike some of the critics debating the intellectual trajectory of Panofsky from 1920s Hamburg to 1950s Princeton (Recht and Douar 2008), it is the earlier, German and conceptually adventurous Panofsky that is sacrificed when the American Panofsky sets out to establish iconology in his new homeland from the mid-1930s.

The principal question posed by Didi-Huberman in *Devant l'Image* concerns the way signs are read in Panofsky's iconological scheme. The twin poles of the visible (analysed via the theory of mimesis) and the readable (dealt with by iconology) should cover everything in a painting but Didi-Huberman suggests that they can instead obscure our investigation into the visual and the figurative (1990a: 212–23). The interpretation of significant details is a crucial part of the approach, since they provide the key to determining which figures and which stories are being represented: first the figure or object is recognised ('pre-iconographical description'), then its significance is explained according to symbolic associations of the figure or object within a mythological, religious or historical framework ('iconographical analysis'), and finally the overall meaning of a painting may be determined from how its combined associations can be understood ('iconological interpretation') (Panofsky 1970: 51–81).

In the essay 'Question de détail, question de pan' (1990a: 273–318), Didi-Huberman is interested in how a section of a painting can defy explanation and integration into a coherent whole. In his view the idea of the detail makes painting too dependent on its referent in reality, since it relies too much on the mimetic transparency of the iconic sign (*ibid.*: 296–302). Some sections of a painting or painted surface may be more accurately called patches – *pans* – whose visual force disrupts the initial reading. Inspired by Proust's 'petit pan de mur jaune' [little patch of yellow wall], which refers to a section of Vermeer's *View of Delft* (1656) that greatly affects the novelist Bergotte in *La Prisonnière* (Proust 1983: 222–3), the *pan* restores attention to the parts of a painting where the referent is not dominant and where the material of paint and its visual intensity are equally important, so that in fact they disrupt mimetic coherence.

In the case of Fra Angelico, discussed in *Devant l'Image* and explored at length in *Fra Angelico: Dissemblance et figuration* (1990b), Didi-Huberman finds justification for his approach in the abstract use of paint dripping and other non-mimetic patches of colour in the frescoes at St Mark's convent in Florence. By including these *pans* in his interpretation, he saves his analysis from an all-encompassing religious context that would function as a guarantor of the invisible, metaphysical dimension to the narrative image. Instead the painted blood, milk and sperm are material visual signs of incarnation that 'make a sign towards' the divine 'according to an economy of the figure', rather than 'signify iconographically', and are in this way not dependent visually on an invisible deity (*ibid.*: 111). In Didi-Huberman's view the *pan* not only spills over onto the whole of which it is a part but also indicates a different structure at work, which he investigates by combining Freud's ideas about the surface–depth relationship in symptoms and the convergence of figures in a dream. The instability of the *pan* may therefore be explained by its temporal and spatial fluidity. Images can be read as symbols but in Didi-Huberman's view they are also symptoms, so that they contain both ideas and phantasms, what he calls elsewhere 'le double régime de l'image' (1995: 9–12; 2003: 103).

As well as the parallels explored in this book with the work of Arasse and Damisch, also discussed by Bernard Vouilloux (2011: 281), Didi-Huberman's work on opening up interpretation reflects the influence of Louis Marin (1931–92), his former supervisor and mentor. Where

Marin studied narrative, semiotics and the power and limits of textual and visual representation, Didi-Huberman's critique of visual representation set out to examine how figures displace their referents (Marin 1981 and 1994). Then where Marin's later work sought to explore the limits of representation through the figure of the sublime, Didi-Huberman concentrated on the displacement brought about by the opening caused by images (Marin 1995b; Didi-Huberman 1990a). There is probably more of a dialogue possible between the two thinkers than has existed up to now, especially where the later Marin is concerned, notably in his thinking around the figure in his work on Philippe de Champaigne, Port-Royal biography and portraiture, and representations of political power and theological truth in *Des Pouvoirs de l'image* (Marin 1993, 1995a, 1997). *Des Pouvoirs de l'image*, published the year after Marin's death, pointed to a dual enquiry into the aesthetics and anthropology of the image, which would have led to further connections with Didi-Huberman's work.

Writing the image

The examples given above of the language of opening and loss indicate Didi-Huberman's debt to psychoanalysis, but they also oblige us to consider Didi-Huberman as a writer. In his review, Norman Bryson made writing the key to appreciating the purpose of *Devant l'Image*. Such is the force of his rhetoric that the transformation in interpretation Didi-Huberman encourages 'happens before your eyes': the mode of ekphrasis takes you beyond the categories of the legible and the visible (Bryson 1993: 337). For Bryson, Didi-Huberman's *approximations* (the tear/rip, the symptom, incarnation and death; 1990a: 171–269) are sometimes 'too portable'; however, Didi-Huberman is seeking to develop an alternative dictionary of philosophical concepts, drawing on a variety of disciplines, in order to look differently at works of art, to include as well gesture, solitude, night and depth (2006a: 78).

The book on Simon Hantaï, *L'Étoilement: Conversation avec Hantaï* (1998), is based on conversations and written exchanges between the two men over a number of years. Didi-Huberman's interest in a new dictionary of concepts, or metaphors, strikes gold with Hantaï. A chain of nouns stretches across the 120-page text from *bâillon* [gag], through *camisole* [camisole], *duite* [conduit], *filet* [netting], *maille* [mail], *tablier* [tablecloth], *envers* [verso], *poche* [pocket], *charpie* [shred], *treillis* [trellis], *onde* [wave], *étoile* [star], *faille* [fault], *serpillière* [floorcloth], *corporal* [altar cloth], ending with *linceul* [shroud]. Each keyword is defined in 4–24 lines, first the literal meaning, sometimes backed up or nuanced with reference to Littré's *Dictionnaire de la langue française.* The translations given here in brackets for the chain of nouns linked to Hantaï are limited to one word for reasons of space; in Didi-Huberman's text figurative and specialised meanings follow the initial definition; then artistic usages and finally uses in or links to painting end the entry. The cultural resonance of the word is emphasised: we are given a source of ideas for reading the folded paintings.

The *treillis*, which cannot in fact just be translated as trellis or lattice, is a large piece of canvas used for bags and clothes; a wooden and iron enclosure; a grid placed against windows; in the fourteenth century a decorative adornment to certain letters of the alphabet; a meshing used for helmet visors and in stained-glass windows; and lastly in painting the device used to check proportions. *Treillis* is distinguished from *grille* [grid], since the lattice-work of the Hantaï canvas is made of the parts of the folded canvas that are not reached when it is dipped into paint, prior to its reopening when it is unfolded (*ibid.*: 68–83). Didi-Huberman discusses the way variations in the folding work out materially and visually, beyond the artist's control: 'We could call it a *requirement of the wave*: never establish the framework, always leave the choice of technique open to variation and heighten the potential of the formal structure of the works by encouraging indeterminacy' (*ibid.*: 82).[1] Nuance and reprise structure the chapters of Didi-Huberman's own text, from the keyword definitions to the open-ended conclusions.

L'Étoilement is the first in a series of texts by Didi-Huberman called 'Fables du lieu', devoted to contemporary artists (Hantaï is accompanied by Convert, Penone, Parmiggiani and Turrell). All five featured in an exhibition curated by Didi-Huberman at Le Fresnoy, Tourcoing, in 2001. In the catalogue he considers the way the notion of place is being explored and suggests that our expectations are resisted. The artist is the catalyst in the conversion of the visible space of the gallery into the visual experience of the place, which is itself a reprise of the contrast made between the visible and the visual in the context of the *pan* and Fra Angelico. In *L'Homme qui marchait dans la couleur*, Didi-Huberman, writing about the light installations and viewing chambers of the American artist James Turrell, cites the fable of creation in Plato's *Timaeus*, because space is described there as a hybrid entity that is perceived as if in a dream (Plato 1971: 70–1; Didi-Huberman 2001d: 36–7). Indeed, at the beginning of the Turrell text, before any question of art is addressed, Didi-Huberman embarks on a fable about a man walking in a desert-like space (2001d: 9–10). The experience of a place is written about, an extreme place or absolute landscape – suggesting another link with Marin, this time his work on the landscapes of Champaigne featuring Desert Fathers (Marin 1995a: 29–75). Moses's forty years of wandering in the desert are implied in Didi-Huberman's opening passage, but the text emphasises the originary experience of wandering, the collapse of time, the lack of direction and knowledge, the vagueness of the limits and edges to experience and the power of the colours perceived.

'On peut décrire un espace, on ne peut qu'*écrire* un lieu' [You can describe a space, but you can only *write* a place], Didi-Huberman wrote in the catalogue (2001a: 13). In his view Turrell's *Skyspaces* avoid symbolism and any predetermined programme: 'Is it a "mystical art"? Absolutely not, if it limits itself to emptying spaces to produce places without names, without symbols, without slogans, without laws, without any function other than visual. Places which ought to invoke nothing other than the absence in which all desire to see places us' (Noever 1999: 54).[2] In his Turrell study he combines historical, theological and philosophical contexts on the one hand and an attempt to write about the visual experience of the *Skyspace*, on the other, wishing to emulate the Hopi balance between 'human intervention' and 'immemorial limitlessness' (*ibid.*: 52; Didi-Huberman 2001d: 76). Didi-Huberman also draws on Merleau-Ponty in his exploration of the experience of the edges and limits of Turrell's spaces (2001d: 79–80; Merleau-Ponty 1945: 320–1). The Hopi context and the emphasis on the complexity of our experience of vision, with reference again to Merleau-Ponty, suggest to the reader that for Didi-Huberman neither the spaces of Turrell's work nor Merleau-Ponty's phenomenology tries to guarantee the foundational unified spectator-subject that Lyotard had criticised Merleau-Ponty for privileging (2001d: 61; Lyotard 1971: 20–3).

The dialectical image

In the 'Fables du lieu' series, artworks and literary or philosophical commentaries are set to work dialectically, stretching the resources of invention and theoretical exploration. Time is also a major preoccupation. In a dialogue with Pascal Convert Didi-Huberman had underlined its importance: 'Le temps est notre doute et nous ne pouvons détruire ce qui nous fonde, sauf à nous détruire nous-mêmes' [Time is what we are unsure of and we cannot destroy what constitutes us, except by destroying ourselves] (Convert 1999: 46). Didi-Huberman's work on the image required an adequate model of time. The model he has worked with and adapted is dialectics, a way of thinking and reasoning with an ancient lineage that, when applied to visual images, enables him to think about the production of images and their interconnections (Williams 1988: 106–8).

In *Devant l'Image*, the term dialectic is used to refer to how to think beyond the positivist approach to interpretation that implies that through knowledge all will be clear and decipherable. 'L'étape dialectique' [the dialectical stage] is a consideration of the opposite, meaning that we relinquish our grasp of the image in order to allow the image to lead us: '*se laisser dessaisir de son savoir sur elle* [l'image] ... Nous accepterions de nous livrer aux aléas d'une phénoménologie du regard' [*let ourselves be released from our knowledge about it* [the image] ... We would be ready to give ourselves up to the unpredictable course of a phenomenology of the look] (1990a: 25). This can be contrasted with Ernst Gombrich's mantra of 'refrain[ing] from polluting the intellectual atmosphere by pretending to know more than we do' (Gombrich 1996: 8): Gombrich and Didi-Huberman have different conceptions of knowledge. Didi-Huberman devotes most of *Ce que nous voyons, ce qui nous regarde* (1992) to a theorisation and demonstration of the 'dialectical image', as outlined by Benjamin in his *Arcades Project*. Benjamin's friend and correspondent Adorno was fascinated but unsure as he witnessed this concept develop and in November 1934 he made the following demand: 'the concept of the "dialectical image" should also be expounded with the greatest possible clarity' (Adorno and Benjamin 1999: 54). Seven months later, Benjamin writes from Paris that he aims to make the world of dialectical images 'immune to all objections that can be raised by metaphysics' (*ibid.*: 89), showing his confidence in his revision of historical and cultural concepts.

Put briefly, Benjamin's dialectical image revitalises the relationship between contemporary society and the past, allowing the spectator to see the past and the present in dynamic conjunction. Didi-Huberman locates three important influences on Benjamin's thinking: Marx for providing a way to think beyond a fixation on the archaic in the image, Proust for summoning up images again in a new form, Freud for offering a model of interpretation (1992: 146). In Didi-Huberman's view, Benjamin's modernist montage enhances the visuality of the Marxist materialist method. The dialectical image is considered by

Benjamin to be a crystal of time with the past meeting the present with crucial impact, as in this famous passage:

> It is not that what is past casts its light on what is present, or what is present its light on what is past; rather, image is that wherein what has been comes together in a flash with the now to form a constellation. In other words: image is dialectics at a standstill. For while the relation of the present to the past is purely temporal, the relation of what-has-been to the now is dialectical: not temporal in nature but figural <*bildich*>. Only dialectical images are genuinely historical – that is, not archaic – images. The image that is read – which is to say, the image in its now of recognis-ability – bears to the highest degree the imprint of the perilous critical moment on which all reading is founded. (1999a: 463)

When it comes to the critical function of the dialectical image, Didi-Huberman emphasises its reflexive action: 'In fact, the *dialectical image* provided Benjamin with the concept of an image able to *remember* without recourse to imitation, able to bring back into play and to *critique* what it has been able to bring back into play' (1992: 82).[3] This ability lends a '*parameter of ambiguity*' to the structure of the dialectical image (2000a: 241). This may be linked with what Benjamin contends in his essay on the collector Eduard Fuchs, namely that the dialectical alliance of past and present in our reenergised consciousness disrupts 'the continuum of history' (Benjamin 1999b: 352). The legacy is not a positivist one.

This rereading of dialectics as a cultural force and a working method leads Didi-Huberman to explore the dialectics of montage in the photos by Boiffard in the review *Documents*, in the films of Eisenstein, and in the work of Brecht and Godard (1995, 2009b and 2003), and to discuss the dialectics of temporality in the work of Warburg (2002) and the sculptures of Pascal Convert (2007a). I will consider his analysis of Brecht and Godard briefly, before turning in the rest of this chapter to Convert, Warburg and further questions of history.

Godard's project in *Histoire(s) du cinéma* (Godard 1998) appeals to Didi-Huberman's image dialectic because it creates through montage previously unseen images of film-makers, artists, events and characters out of combinations of images and supplements of text: 'The dialectic should be understood as a multiplied collision between words and images: images collide with each other so that words appear suddenly, words collide with each other so that images appear suddenly, images and words collide so that thought can happen visually' (2003: 173).[4] Rather than the creation of images directly, the imagination understood dialectically sets up the exchange between images. This exchange is also addressed by Didi-Huberman in his study of Brecht, *Quand les images prennent position: L'Œil de l'histoire 1* (2009b), where he emphasises the critical function of the image dialectic, notably in Brecht's *Work Journal* and *ABC of War*. The montage of war photos and text disrupts conventional historical interpretation and politicises aesthetic considerations, avoiding the subordination of images to textual evidence. The political function of montage is noted too by Max Silverman who has detected a move on Didi-Huberman's part to 'reflect on the primary function of the image … to reach out to the world and resist the ever-increasing atomisation of our senses and our knowledge' (Silverman 2010: 61).

Didi-Huberman has also explored temporality and dialectics in the case of Pascal Convert's *Souches* (1995–98), sections of tree stumps retrieved from the battlefields of Verdun and from Hiroshima, which are then covered in Indian ink in the first case and black lacquer in the second (1999a: 151–64; see Plates 8 and 9). In 'La Souche', Didi-Huberman attempts to let the form of the treated tree stump determine the outcome of the essay, with a dialectical approach used to follow up each stage. The roots also act as branches, the energy of these structures is contrasted with their immobility, their organic function with their present stricken state. A characteristic move is to align the organic volume of time contained in this form with the domination of the surrounding space. It seems that these 'formes hérissées' [bristled forms] will resist words and remain as distant and silent as the chestnut tree encountered by the narrator in Sartre's *La Nausée* (1999a: 157).

Didi-Huberman emphasises that the form of the stump is the key to its singularity and familiarity. The tree stumps have been displaced and now tell a particular story or fable: 'The extraction tells the story of at least three time periods which come together in the same object: the *immemorial time* of genealogies, of tree rings, of the transmission of forms; the *sudden time* of burning and bloodletting, of the destruction of history; and the *time of the artwork*, anachronic and meticulous, with the transformation into an image (moving the object, inking, lacquering, exhibition, links with other images, etc.)' (*ibid.*: 163–4).[5] In that way, the work of art has converted these three dimensions of time: dialectical immemorial time, looking forwards and backwards (2000a: 91–2); the fragility and power of the time of the object that has survived near-destruction; and the sculpting of time. Derived from Benjamin, therefore, Didi-Huberman's image is anachronic because of the collision of past times with the present and because of previous images resurfacing in present ones; 'anachronic' is preferable to the pejorative 'anachronistic' here and also takes up the term being used by Alexander Nagel and Christopher Wood in their work, albeit with different emphases from Didi-Huberman, on the 'plural temporality' of Renaissance artworks (Nagel and Wood 2005 and 2010: 7–19). The anachronic state of Convert's *Souches* is dialectical because the collision and reappearance occur non-mimetically and critically. This is what Didi-Huberman had in mind when he spoke of seeking an untrivial model of time; his gloss or advance on Benjamin's dialectical image is to consider the way images resurface and to explore the experience of desire and loss before the image. Didi-Huberman's dialectic reignites the relationship between the visual and temporal.

Warburg's time

Didi-Huberman subscribes to a counter-tradition of philosophy and critical thinking from different epochs, which has reinterpreted the notion of aesthetic form, displacing ideal form in favour of an investigation of the formation of visual objects, the presentation of artworks and the creation of critical thinking (1992: 161). Aby Warburg is Didi-Huberman's hero in the domain of art history. In *L'Image survivante* (2002), Didi-Huberman is first interested in the complex time of images understood through Warburg's concept of *Nachleben*, translated into French as *survivance* and English as *afterlife. Nachleben* defies chronology and refers to the process whereby images incorporate cultural memory, comprising elements which tenaciously return in different places and under different guises. Hand in hand with *Nachleben* goes the term *Pathosformel*, since it is the 'pathos' of images, the convergence of feeling and gesture in art and ritual, which Warburg sees being channelled by their anachronic time and symptomatic structure. Griselda Pollock has commended Warburg's pathos formula for jointly attending to 'form and meanings, rationality and irrationality', and for avoiding the anterior narrative obsession, 'for which the artwork is reduced to belated illustration, rather than a creative intervention both in and outside of [its] time' (2007: 18, 45). Time, structure and pathos would all be set to work in the experimental final project of Warburg, the *Mnemosyne Atlas* (1927–29), which spurns synthesis and seeks to mobilise images, enabling us to follow the unconscious element of time across and between images.

Our conventional understanding of anachronism is subverted by the concept of *Nachleben*. Peter Burke has posited the standard view of anachronism – the lack of any sense of historical perspective and change – as the primary weakness of historians prior to the Renaissance. The past can only be judged properly if anachronism is avoided and if evidence and causation are considered (Burke 1969: 1). Didi-Huberman is not in fact overturning this view, but is instead arguing that it provides an inadequate model of time, indeed that history guided by perspective risks simplifying time. In his view, art historians need to take note of the fact that history is not the same as time. The complexity of time is a better model for thinking about memory and the afterlives of images: 'On ne peut pas accepter la dimension mémorative de l'histoire sans accepter, du même coup, son ancrage dans l'inconscient et sa dimension anachronique' [You cannot acknowledge the memorial dimension of history without accepting at the same time both its anchoring in the unconscious and its anachronic dimension] (2000a: 37). Didi-Huberman's model of history crucially draws on the complex relationship between history and time asserted by Michel de Certeau (2003: 125–30). There are risks for spectators in galleries and risks for historians in the archives.

Working on Warburg has led Didi-Huberman to adopt a broader cultural approach to images, taking up and developing Warburg's interest in anthropology (Warburg 1995; Didi-Huberman 2002: 354–62). Certainly there is a move from the study of 'art' to the study of 'images' (see the interview with Vouilloux in Chapter 14 in the present volume). The *Mnemosyne* project is a montage of black-and-white photographs arranged by topic or motif on forty screens. Almost devoid of text, these montages assemble images (including 'details') of sculptures and bas-reliefs from Greece and Rome, as well as sculptures and paintings from Renaissance Florence, juxtaposed with Babylonian terracotta reliefs, Etruscan bronzes, Ptolemaic miniatures, Egyptian reliefs, photographs of Native American sacred dances and of contemporary subjects. Although Gombrich felt that the project was undermined by lacking a formula to 'subsume' Warburg's interest in Greek mythology and the gestures of human passion (Gombrich 1970: 291), in Didi-Huberman's view the agile spectator can find links between the images, according to the 'rules' of *Nachleben* and *Pathosformel*, enabling him or her to see the temporality and creativity of the montage.

Some eighty years after Warburg, three bas-relief wax sculptures by Pascal Convert (*Pietà du Kosovo, Madone de Bentalha, Mohammed Al Dura*) feature in the sculptor's book *Lamento 1998–2005*, which is part collaborative volume and catalogue, part Warburgian Atlas '*in progress*' (2007b: 201), a montage of images assembled by Didi-Huberman in relation to Convert's three works of lamentation, which were all themselves based on photographic or film images. The first double page of Didi-Huberman's 'Esquisse d'atlas' [Sketch for an Atlas] is taken from Warburg's own *Mnemosyne* as a starting point (*ibid.*: 204–5), followed by filmic, plastic, pictorial and photographic (including documentary) images: among them Niccolò dell'Arca's *Lamentation over the Dead Christ*, Goya's *Disasters of War*, Eisenstein, *Guernica* (Picasso's painting and aerial and reportage photographs), Robert Capa, Eugene Smith, Don McCullin, Donatello, Caravaggio and Michelangelo (see Plates 10–12: dell'Arca's *Lamentation*; Arca reworked; and cries from various sources, including dell'Arca, Franz Xavier Messerschmidt and the *Laocoon*). The sources are numerous and the connections established draw on a wide range of periods and media linked to the main focus of each sequence (usually one particular artist's work).

The relationship between Convert's sculptures and the photographs relating to conflicts by Mérillon and Zaouar, and the film still of the death of Mohammed al Dura, can be expanded and enriched in Didi-Huberman's view by means of this Warburgian montage of previous images of lamentation. A further reference may be made here to Griselda Pollock's 'counter-archive' project, the 'Virtual Feminist Museum', since both thinkers seek to displace establish academic and museum demarcations according to period, nation and style. Pollock's distinctive contribution has a feminist and explicitly political agenda, directed at change and drawing on Kristeva's diagnosis of the social and symbolic sickness afflicting dominant notions of time (Pollock 2007: 10, 47, 60; Kristeva 1993: 329). Didi-Huberman's reinvestment in Warburg's *Mnemosyne* project, meanwhile, creates a montage in relation to Convert's *Pietà* that connects with the forms and memorial charge in culture of these rituals, so that through the montage of images it is possible to release the singular power in these gestures of lamentation – 'to sustain the weight of the time, or of *the times*, that such a gesture brings into being' (2007b: 201) – and to amplify the political charge of both Convert's works and the images with which they coexist.

Conclusion: further questions of history

Cultural history has been of greater concern to Didi-Huberman since working on Warburg, while history is central to the analysis of four

Auschwitz photographs included in the 2001 exhibition 'La mémoire des camps' (2001c), *Images malgré tout* (2003), which reprints and then develops the exhibition catalogue essay, and, more recently, studies of Samuel Fuller's film *Falkenau* (2006c) and Brecht's *Work Journal* and *ABC of War* (2009b). Didi-Huberman's reading of the four Auschwitz photographs, taken by members of the Sonderkommando and then smuggled out in defiance of Nazi attempts to hide or destroy evidence of the camps, certainly proved controversial. Fully aware that the idea of the unrepresentability of the Holocaust had dominated studies for two decades, Didi-Huberman pointed to these four small and fragile photographs as indications of the way the understanding of the subject had allowed itself to become iconophobic and dogmatically obsessed with the impossibility of witnessing what had taken place (2003: 37–41, 79–85). In the context of the tension between aesthetics and history, the obsessive approach to unrepresentability involved a sublimation of the difficulty of representation: aestheticised history and historicised commentary on the images were asking either too little or too much of them (*ibid.*: 48–50). Also overlooked were the way the danger and necessary haste involved in taking the photos is reflected in their blurred state, their unorthodox framing and the 'lack' of a subject in the last case. There is a documentary value to the images, but there is also the event of their creation.

In seeking an alternative reaction to silence in the face of the unrepresentable, Didi-Huberman points to the attempt by the members of the Sonderkommando to achieve a representation of their situation in spite of the danger and in spite of the horrors of the camp: 'Tout acte d'image s'arrache à l'impossible description d'un réel' [Every image act saves itself from the impossibility of describing the real] (*ibid.*: 156). As Didi-Huberman puts it, they can scarcely be accused of wanting to fetichise these images, of trying to replace the exterminated prisoners with an image. Those problems are acknowledged in other cases but simply irrelevant in this one. Because the 2001 catalogue essay 'Images malgré tout' was the subject of two attacks in *Les Temps modernes*, Didi-Huberman responds point by point (*ibid.*: 69–113), but he does not confuse polemic with an analysis of the aesthetic at work in Lanzmann's *Shoah* or Godard's *Histoire(s) du cinéma* (*ibid.*: 151–87).

At the same time, in view of his desire to 'open up' the image, his style combines the language of drama, tension and horror relating to the taking of the photos and their content, while also seeking the tone appropriate to the desperate artistic modesty of these photographic images. Libby Saxton has commented on the repetition of 'malgré tout' in Didi-Huberman's text, suggesting a 'potential crisis of figurability and testimony' before these images (Saxton 2008: 59). They cannot represent the whole of Auschwitz and yet they cannot avoid the many associations of the place, the 'tout' that seems inescapable. For Didi-Huberman the use of 'tout' is deliberate, affirming the need to object to the totalising discourse of the absolutely unimaginable: 'Il faut désormais entendre dans ce *malgré tout* une objection au *tout*, un faisceau d'arguments et de faits donnés *malgré le tout* de l'inimaginable érigé en dogme' [From now on we have to hear in this *in spite of all* an objection to the *all*, an array of arguments and facts presented *in spite of the all* of the dogma of the unimaginable] (2003: 83).

How Didi-Huberman's thinking has evolved from the opening up of the visual in Fra Angelico in *Devant l'Image* and *Fra Angelico: dissemblance et figuration* to the reopening of our eyes before the Sonderkommando photographs suggests both a persistent investment in the critical force of images and a desire to intervene where contemporary debates risk reducing images to adjuncts of ideological arguments. Hence we have the paradox that where considering an image 'readable' in the context of a visible symbolic scheme (its iconography) had been criticised for underestimating the visual, by the time of the debate surrounding images of the death camps the question of 'readability' was invoked as an urgent political issue needing salvaging from the discourse of the unrepresentable. With the media of photography and film, in the case of the Sonderkommando photographs and the films of the liberation or rather opening of the camps in 1944–45, the readable is a quality that has to be revived in order to keep thinking, in spite of the visual horror, about how the experience of the camps and their opening is represented.

'Ouvrir les camps, fermer les yeux' addresses these questions directly, leading to a commentary on Fuller's *Falkenau* (2006c). In Didi-Huberman's view, as set out in *Images malgré tout* and his discussion of *Falkenau*, an ethics of looking cannot transcend history nor can it isolate singularly powerful images. The dialectical energy of Didi-Huberman's thinking, influenced by Pierre Fédida, has been directed consistently – and in the last decade more explicitly – at the crucial combination of text (readability) and image (visibility) (Fédida 1995). Opening up the image, acknowledging the power of the visual, recognising the dialectical temporality of images and promoting their survival are all part of Didi-Huberman's approach to the image, which may be summed up as follows: 'we must always keep our childlike eyes wide open before the image (accepting the ordeal, the not-knowing and the peril of the image, and the weakness of language) and as adults we must always keep constructing the "knowability" of the image (involving knowledge, point of view, the act of writing and ethical reflection)' (2006c: 1047).[6] Didi-Huberman's critique of the beauty, history and politics of images, and of our reactions to them, continues to be expressed in groundbreaking critical interventions, accompanied by ongoing collaborations with artists and diverse essays on topics such as flamenco (2006a) or film extras (2009a), reflecting the persistent vitality and experimentation in his thinking.[7]

References

Adorno, T. W. and Benjamin, W. (1999) *The Complete Correspondence 1928–1940*, ed. H. Lonitz and trans. N. Walker, Cambridge, MA and London: Harvard University Press.

Benjamin, W. (1999a) *The Arcades Project*, trans. H. Eiland and K. McLaughlin, Cambridge, MA and London: Belknap Press of Harvard University Press.

—— (1999b) 'Eduard Fuchs, Collector and Historian', *One-Way Street and Other Writings*, trans. E. Jephcott and K. Shorter, London and New York: Verso.

Bourdieu, P. (1967) 'Postface', in E. Panofsky, *Architecture gothique et pensée scholastique*, Paris: Minuit, 135–67.

Bryson, N. (1993) 'Georges Didi-Huberman, *Devant l'Image*', *Art Bulletin* 75(2) (June), 336–7.

Burke, P. (1969) *The Renaissance Sense of the Past*, London: Edward Arnold.

Clark, K. (1956) *The Nude: A Study in Ideal Form*, London: John Murray [later editions: Harmondsworth: Penguin, 1960; Princeton, NJ: Princeton University Press, 1972].

Convert, P. (1999) 'Dialogue sur l'inestimable, entretien avec Georges Didi-Huberman', *artpress* 248 (July–Aug.), 43–7.

—— (2007) *Lamento 1998–2005*, Luxemburg: Musée d'Art Moderne Grand-Duc Jean.

Demorand, N. (2001) 'Entretien. Georges Didi-Huberman: Le philosophe de la maison hantée', *Beaux-Arts Magazine* 202 (Mar.), 42–5.

Didi-Huberman, G. (1990a) *Devant l'Image: Question posée aux fins d'une histoire de l'art*, Paris: Minuit; *Conflicting Images: Questioning*

the Ends of a Certain History of Art, trans. J. Goodman, University Park, PA: Pennsylvania State University Press, 2004.
—— (1990b) *Fra Angelico: Dissemblance et figuration*, Paris: Flammarion; *Fra Angelico: Dissemblance and figuration*, trans. J. M. Todd, Chicago, IL and London: University of Chicago Press, 1995.
—— (1992) *Ce que nous voyons, ce qui nous regarde*, Paris: Minuit.
—— (1995) *La Ressemblance informe, ou le gai savoir visuel selon Georges Bataille*, Paris: Macula.
—— (1998) *L'Étoilement: Conversation avec Hantaï*, Paris: Minuit.
—— (1999a) *La Demeure, la souche: Apparentements de l'artiste*, Paris: Minuit.
—— (1999b) *Ouvrir Vénus: Nudité, rêve, cruauté (L'Image ouvrante, 1)*, Paris: Gallimard.
—— (2000a) *Devant le Temps: Histoire de l'art et anachronisme des images*, Paris: Minuit.
—— (2000b) *Être Crâne: Lieu, contact, pensée, sculpture*, Paris: Minuit.
—— (2001a) 'Fables du Lieu', *Fables du Lieu: Pascal Convert, Simon Hantaï, Claudio Parmiggiani, Giuseppe Penone, James Turrell*, exhibition curated by G. Didi-Huberman (Le Fresnoy, Studio national des arts contemporains), 11–16.
—— (2001b) *Génie du non-lieu: Air, poussière, empreinte, hantise*, Paris: Minuit.
—— (2001c) 'Images malgré tout', in Clément Chéroux (ed.), *Mémoire des camps: Photographies des camps de concentration et d'extermination nazies (1933–1999)*, Paris: Marval, 219–41.
—— (2001d) *L'Homme qui marchait dans la couleur*, Paris: Minuit. [see 'The Fable of the Place', in Noever, *James Turrell*, 45–56]
—— (2002) *L'Image survivante: Histoire de l'art et temps des fantômes selon Aby Warburg*, Paris: Minuit.
—— (2003) *Images malgré tout*, Paris: Minuit; *Images in Spite of All: Four Photographs from Auschwitz*, trans. S. B. Lillis, Chicago, IL: University of Chicago Press, 2008.
—— (2006a) *Le Danseur des solitudes*, Paris: Minuit.
—— (2006b) 'L'Image brûle', in Laurent Zimmermann (ed.), *Penser par les images: Autour des travaux de Georges Didi-Huberman*, Nantes: Éditions Cécile Defaut, 11–52.
—— (2006c) 'Ouvrir les camps, fermer les yeux', *Annales: Histoire, Sciences sociales* 61(5) (Sept.–Oct.), 1011–49.
—— (2007a) 'Construire la durée', in Convert, *Lamento 1998–2005*, 25–35.

—— (2007b) 'Esquisse d'atlas', in Convert, *Lamento 1998–2005*, 199–261.

—— (2007c) *L'Image ouverte: Motifs de l'incarnation dans les arts visuels*, Paris: Gallimard.

—— (2009a) 'People Exposed, People as Extras', *Radical Philosophy* 156 (July/Aug.), 16–22.

—— (2009b) *Quand les images prennent position: L'Œil de l'histoire, I*, Paris: Minuit.

Fédida, P. (1995) 'Le souffle indistinct de l'image', *Le Site de l'étranger*, Paris: Presses universitaires de France, 187–220.

Foucault, M. (1994) 'Les mots et les images', *Dits et écrits, I: 1954–1969*, ed. D. Defert and F. Ewald, Paris: Gallimard, 620–3.

Godard, J.-L. (1998) *Histoire(s) du cinéma*, Paris: Gallimard.

Gombrich, E. H. (1970) *Aby Warburg: An Intellectual Biography*, London: Warburg Institute.

—— (1996) *The Essential Gombrich: Selected Writings on Art and Culture*, ed. R. Woodfield, Oxford: Phaidon.

Kristeva, J. (1993) 'Le Temps des femmes', *Les Nouvelles Maladies de l'âme*, Paris: Fayard, 297–331.

Lyotard, J.-F. (1971) *Discours, figure*, Paris: Klincksieck.

Marin, L. (1981) *Le Portrait du roi*, Paris: Minuit.

—— (1993) *Des Pouvoirs de l'image: Gloses*, Paris: Seuil.

—— (1994) *De la Représentation*, ed. Daniel Arasse *et al.*, Paris: Seuil/Gallimard.

—— (1995a) *Philippe de Champaigne ou la présence cachée*, Paris: Hazan.

—— (1995b) *Sublime Poussin*, Paris: Seuil.

—— (1997) *Pascal et Port-Royal*, ed. Alain Cantillon, Paris: Presses universitaires de France.

Merleau-Ponty, M. (1945) *Phénoménologie de la perception*, Paris: Gallimard.

Nagel, A. and Wood, C. S. (2005) 'Interventions: Toward a New Model of Renaissance Anachronism', *Art Bulletin* 87(3) (Sept. 2005), 403–15.

—— (2010) *Anachronic Renaissance*, New York: Zone Books.

Noever, P. (ed.) (1999) *James Turrell: The Other Horizon*, Ostfildern-Ruit: Hatje Cantz.

Panofsky, E. (1970) *Meaning in the Visual Arts* (1955), Harmondsworth: Penguin.

Plato (1971) *Timaeus* and *Critias*, trans. H. D. P. Lee, Harmondsworth: Penguin.

Pollock, G. (2007) *Encounters in the Virtual Feminist Museum: Time, Space and the Archive*, London: Routledge.

Proust, M. (1983) *La Prisonnière*, Paris: Gallimard, Collection Folio.

Recht, R. and Douar, F. (eds) (2008) *Relire Panofsky*, Paris: Musée du Louvre/Éditions Beaux-arts de Paris.

Saxton, L. (2008) *Haunted Images: Film, Ethics, Testimony and the Holocaust*, London and New York: Wallflower.

Silverman, M. (2010) 'The Violence of the Cut: Michael Haneke's *Caché* and Cultural Memory', *French Cultural Studies* 21(1) (Feb.), 57–65.

Teyssèdre, B. (1967) 'Présentation', in Erwin Panofsky, *Essais d'iconologie*, Paris: Gallimard.

—— (1969) 'Présentation', in Erwin Panofsky, *L'Œuvre d'art et ses significations: Essais sur les arts visuels*, Paris: Gallimard.

Vouilloux, B. (2011) 'Saint Georges à la croisée des chemins: Question posée aux fins d'une anthropologie des images', in *Devant les images: Penser l'art et l'histoire avec Georges Didi-Huberman*, sous la direction de Thierry Davila et Pierre Sauvanet, Dijon: Les Presses du Réel, coll. Perceptions, 271–343.

Warburg, A. (1995) *Images from the Region of the Pueblo Indians of North America*, trans. with an interpretive essay by M. P. Steinberg, Ithaca, NY and London: Cornell University Press.

Williams, R. (1988) 'Dialectic', *Keywords*, London: Fontana, 106–8.

Notes

1 'Appelons cela une *exigence de l'onde*: ne jamais fixer la trame, nuancer toujours les choix de procédures par une marge d'indécidable, « soulever » toujours les structures formelles par un appel à l'indétermination' (1998: 82).

2 'Est-ce une œuvre « mystique »? Absolument non, si elle accepte d'en rester à ceci: évider des espaces pour produire des lieux sans noms, sans symboles, sans mots d'ordre, sans loi, sans fonction autre que visuelle. Des lieux qui ne devraient invoquer rien d'autre que l'absence où tout désir de voir nous place' (2001d: 83–4).

3 'En fait, l'*image dialectique* donnait à Benjamin le concept d'une image capable de *se souvenir* sans imiter, capable de remettre en jeu et de *critiquer* ce qu'elle avait été capable de remettre en jeu' (1992: 82).

4 'La dialectique doit se comprendre dans le sens d'une collision démultipliée des mots et des images: les images s'entrechoquent entre elles pour que surgissent des mots, les mots s'entrechoquent entre eux pour que surgissent des images, les images et les mots entrent en collision pour que la pensée ait lieu visuellement' (2003: 173).

5 'L'extraction raconte au moins trois temps qui se mêlent dans le même objet: *temps immémorial* des généalogies, des anneaux de croissance, des transmissions de formes ; *temps fulgurant* des mises à feu et à sang, des destructions de l'histoire; *temps œuvré*, anachronique et méticuleux, de la transformation en image (déplacement de l'objet, encrage, laquage, exposition, mise en relation avec d'autres images, etc.)' (1999a: 163–4).

6 'ne pas cesser d'écarquiller nos yeux d'enfants devant l'image (accepter l'épreuve, le non-savoir, le péril de l'image, le défaut du langage) et ne pas cesser de construire, en adultes, la « connaissabilité » de l'image (ce qui suppose le savoir, le point de vue, l'acte d'écriture, la réflexion éthique)' (2006c: 1047).

7 I would like to thank the British Academy for two small research grants in support of this chapter.

11

Jean-Louis Schefer: the body of the image

Patrick ffrench

The inclusion of Jean-Louis Schefer in this volume devoted to modern French visual *theorists* is problematic; Schefer's œuvre does not offer an immediate image of coherence. He does not propose a systematic theory of the visual field ('Je ne propose donc pas une méthode ni un programme d'études' [I propose therefore no method nor programme of study] (1995b: 10); 'je [ne] soutiens aucun propos de philosophie ou de théorie, ni un engagement pour une forme d'art' [I do not support any philosophical angle nor any commitment to a specific form of art] (1998a: 13)), his work does not focus uniquely on any specific period, neither are the objects of his analyses of equivalent type or scale. The objects on which Schefer writes are heterogeneous in the extreme: Uccello, Chardin, El Greco, Roman law, Marie Antoinette's shoe, Walter Benjamin, Cy Twombly, Dracula, Todd Browning, Carl Dreyer, Fatty Arbuckle, Hitchcock, Chris Marker, the colour red, David Lynch, Francis Bacon, Tim Burton. This heterogeneity is highlighted by the titles of the books he has published; while some are devoted to a single object, their title signalling a privileged motif (*Lumière du Corrège*, *Sommeil du Greco*), the majority are collections. The collection per se interests Schefer in so far as it is the binding together of varied objects within a single volume which suggests, retrospectively or as if in secret, the affective, emotional response which had always provided their consistency. Consistency, therefore, is *affective*, and *transversal*. The subtitles of the collections propose non-intuitive transversal motifs which bind the objects together: *Choses écrites: Essais de littérature et à peu près*; *Images mobiles: Récits, visages, flocons*; *Cinématographies: Objets périphériques et mouvements annexes*. The second or *sub*title, which indicates the underlying continuity, is often either a formal or imaginary motif; with *Images* *mobiles*, for example, the subtitle 'récits, visages, flocons' [tales, faces, flakes], focuses on the elements which fascinate the author – fragmentary narratives or fictions, faces, the decomposition of the image into the 'grain of the image' (to echo Barthes). Fascination is a crucial motif; what fascinates is what holds the gaze, what calls for sense to be made (even while it resists this sense-making) what fascinates is what calls for writing to be done in relation to it. There is a specific kind of consistency to Schefer's work, which addresses the notion of constancy when it comes to the critical, textual consideration of visual objects. Let us immediately attempt to circumscribe this coherence.

In his short essay or review of Schefer's first book *Scénographie d'un tableau* Roland Barthes focuses on the fundamental tenet of Schefer's work, which intimately links the visual object and the written text which considers it; the relation between the painting and the language used to analyse it, to read it, to write about it, *is the painting itself*; 'Un tableau n'est jamais que sa propre description plurielle' [A painting is never anything but its own plural description] (Barthes [1969] 1982: 140). This has significant consequences: the painting *is* the story I tell about it; there is no 'neutral' or 'objective' state of the object. Neither, however, is the painting the object of a 'purely mythical elaboration', susceptible to a purely subjective account: 'un lieu infiniment disponible d'investissements subjectifs' [an infinitely free place of subjective investments] (*ibid.*: 140). Barthes does not make the point himself, but the parallel with his own *S/Z*, a 'textual analysis' of Balzac's novella *Sarrasine* (Barthes 1970), would suggest that the reading of a single painting is constrained or determined by the multiple texts, the systems of representation, the historically situated layers of meaning that the painting generates, and by which it is supported. Just as in *S/Z* Barthes codifies the associations of the fragmented lexical units which his own dissection of the text has spotlighted, and relates them to the cultural codes of the epoch (Balzac's nineteenth century), Schefer reads Paris Bordone's *Une partie d'échecs* [The Chess Players] according to the cultural codes and epistemologies of the period. As in *S/Z*, reading is a potentially infinite analysis, endlessly deferring an (impossible) ultimate signified. There is no single code which determines the painting in a more or less linear fashion; reading activates or performs the plurality of connotations which the painting can generate.

While Barthes identifies the productive nature of Schefer's writing on painting, the way in which, according to this theory, the painting *is* the writing it produces, he stops short of a freer, more ludic account of the relation between painting and writing. He notes that Schefer's analysis of *Une partie d'échecs* is characterised by 'un bonheur d'écriture qui fait enfin passer le critique du côté de l'écrivain' [a joy in writing which finally allows the critic to pass onto the side of the writer] (Barthes [1969] 1982: 141), but he does not perhaps fully acknowledge the subjective engagement of the subject in the writing. This hesitancy is no doubt to do with the scientific or pseudo-scientific ambitions of the moment (1969), and reflects a generalised tendency towards scientificity in French intellectual discourse on the aesthetic, at this moment. But one can see the logic of the development of the greater presence of the subject in Schefer's later work (and, incidentally, that of Barthes). In so far as the painting 'n'existe que dans le récit que j'en donne' [exists only in the story I tell about it] (*ibid.*: 140) it is necessarily a site of subjective investment. The painting is not only what is written about it within the limits of the historical 'contexts' that define it (and both Barthes and Schefer would no doubt question this notion of context). It is also what is written from the place of the subject, what the painting induces me to write, or causes to be written in me, in a relation of seduction or desire which would be theorised not very much later by Barthes in *Le Plaisir du texte* (1973).

Arguably Schefer's methodology throughout his extensive work is more far-reaching and subtle than that of Barthes in *S/Z*, in that the object of study is the site of tension, conflict, the overlapping of chronologically different systems of representation, and different critical methodologies. In the brief essay 'L'Objet de figuration' (1978: 17–25) Schefer postulates that the system of representation inherited by Europe is determined by a tension between the pagan practices and epistemologies of ancient Rome, which are essentially juridical and polytheistic, and the system of representation implied by Christianity, which is monotheistic (or monotheistic as mediated via the Trinity). A symptomatic and determinative text in this regard is Augustine's *City of God*. Schefer argues that Augustine is obliged to construct a methodology and an epistemology which postulates what he calls the anthropological subject. This, and the shift from a polytheistic to a monotheistic religiosity, entails the repression of a quotient of libido. Schefer employs a further Freudian motif in proposing that this process also involves a displacement of the body as the referent of the image. The practice of scriptural commentary from which, he argues, the European system of representation derives, implies and produces a double or split subject, the schism being between the writing subject, or the one who writes (cf.

Schefer's account of this in the essay 'Celui qui écrit' (*ibid.*: 245–51)), and the subjectivity implied by the interpretation, the 'moral subject' demanded by the Scriptures. This split instigates and coalesces with the mediation of the representation of the body via the whole epistemological panoply of Christianity, such that the body – by which Schefer intends in Barthesian manner the body of *jouissance* – is occluded from the scene of representation. Schefer's work as a whole is focused on the tension that this occlusion creates. Our lived body is absent from the 'official' systems of knowledge which our culture supports. Paul Smith elegantly highlights this with the title of his excellent translation into English of key texts of Schefer's œuvre, *The Enigmatic Body*, and with the proposition that Schefer's disparate work is held together by the 'fantasy of an enigmatic body' (1995a: ix).

This is what Schefer proposes in perhaps his most significant work on a single painting, *Paolo Uccello, Le Déluge* (1999a). Uccello's fresco *The Universal Deluge* is emblematic of the kind of effects with which Schefer is concerned. The barely discernible fresco is the site, according to Schefer, of a resistance to the rules of 'classical' painting. It is the body in particular which functions as the symptom of this conflict between the orthodox or 'doxical' system of representation, linked to the systems of knowledge supported by and supporting Christianity, and the pagan body, the 'prefigural' body repressed by Christianity (*ibid.*: 95). In particular, Schefer finds the tensions and conflicts inherent in the painting in the strange figure of the *mazzocchio*, usually represented as a form of headdress, but here worn around the neck of the figure in the foreground holding a club. The *mazzocchio* is a geometric figure formed through the drawing of a circular disc or torus in perspective ('un tore projeté', *ibid.*: 161). In the context of Uccello's painting Schefer reads it as the embodiment of a system of knowledge heterogeneous to the order of the painting, and, as a geometric or logical figure, outside the referential domain. It is thus a 'corps étranger' [foreign body] (*ibid.*: 163) or a 'corps nouveau' [new body] (*ibid.*: 8). It is of a different order from the other bodies featured in the painting; the painting thus dramatises the temporal disjunction of its different bodies: 'Cette fresque met en scène, en jeu et en mouvement des corps qui ne sont pas contemporains les uns des autres' [This fresco puts on stage, in play and in motion bodies which are not contemporary with each other] (*ibid.*). If the *mazzocchio* is the embodiment of the science of geometry, it is in tension with the knowledge implied by the other bodies of the fresco. This other knowledge is corporeal, infantile. Paul Smith points out that from the book on Uccello onwards, Schefer's work stages the conflict between orthodox knowledge, and the 'primitive or childish knowledge' put into play by the paradoxical bodies figured in paintings such as *Le Déluge* (1995a: 68). This conflict and these tensions bear many parallels to the schema of anamorphosis analysed by Lacan in his remarks on Holbein's *The Ambassadors* (Plate 2) in *Les Quatre Concepts fondamentaux de la psychanalyse* (1973: 92–104). While in Schefer's work this meditation will not support a full-fledged psychoanalytic system of references, it will, as Smith notes, accompany an 'increasingly autobiographical' writing (1995a: 68).

The book on Uccello thus inaugurates a continued focus on the body in Schefer's work; the body becomes its central and perpetual point of reference. The 'paradoxical' bodies 'washed up' in Uccello's flood come back to haunt the Christian doxa like its murdered child: 'son archaisme, sa mémoire, sa raison païenne' [its archaism, its memory, its pagan reason] (1999a: 90). Memory plays an important role here in Schefer's thinking, as Paul Smith justly underlines (1995a: 68). It is as if the painting calls upon a primitive memory, linked to primal fears, to prehistory and to childhood (an image that recurs in the book is of a child leading the author to a dark corridor to indicate that this is the place of her fear (1999a: 79)). This produces a writing of impressive and startling aggressivity, the often elliptical sentences list the affects of the painting and its bodies: 'Pisse, cadavre, éponge, chiure de lait, étrave de la tête palpant les yeux fermés sur la nuit. Mémoire traversée de corps fabuleux' [Piss, corpse, sponge, flyspecks of milk, the stem of the head groping in the dark with eyes closed. Memory traversed by fabulous bodies] (*ibid.*: 59); 'Pluie de corps. Catafalque de viandes blanchies' [Rain of bodies. Catafalque of whitened meat] (*ibid.*: 58). The violence of the writing is unleashed by the bodies that the painting reveals, as if the waters of the flood, receding, were to offer up the bloated corpses seeking out their voice, the writing which was their due. Schefer writes that the bodies of the painting, of painting solicit our bodies and our voices to live again; they are spectres whose function it is to haunt:

> Rien m'ôtera de l'idée que ces corps-là font un suspens énigmatique: ils attendent le nôtre afin qu'un battement de notre cœur ou la nuée vague de notre savoir perdu donne écho à leur voix faible ou que l'affect expérimental né d'une sympathie pour l'expression de leurs passions leur donne, tour à tour et de temps en temps, notre voix. (*ibid.*: 13)

> [Nothing will take from me the idea that these bodies are enigmatically in suspense: they await ours, so that a beat of our heart or the vague cloud of our lost knowledge will give an echo to their weakened voices, or so that the experimental affect born from a sympathy for the expression of their passions will give them our voice, turn by turn and from time to time.]

Uccello, Schefer writes, is an obsessional system (*ibid.*: 53). Unlike in orthodox art history, the painting is not symptomatic of its time, representative of the ideology of its time; it is a site of conflict, and of the violence produced by the foreclosure of the affective body from the rules of representation. This violence is visited upon the reader. The writing in this book leads the reader into a space of threatening proximity to the affective force of the image, to the obscenity or madness, perhaps, of the body's resistance to knowledge. Schefer writes that the aim of his book was to:

> laisser venir l'interprétation dans un imaginaire onirique ou moral par lequel 'le corps' a été un objet singulier, isole et réduit à des effets d'expression, dans notre culture. (*ibid.*: 7)

> [allow interpretation to move into an oneiric or moral imaginary space through which 'the body' has been a singular and isolated object, reduced to a few effects of expression, in our culture.]

Criticism, in Schefer's view, must construct the imaginary world of the painting, and allow the reader to inhabit it:

> Ce livre tente une sorte de précipité physique des effets ou des inductions imaginaires de la peinture dans le monde subjectif de celui qui regarde. Ces inductions, passagèrement, donnent forme ou configuration à un monde vague. C'est à peu près cela qui s'appelle la critique ... (*ibid.*: 11)

> [This book attempts a sort of physical precipitation of the effects or imaginary inductions of painting in the subjective world of the one who looks. These inductions, intermittently, give form or configuration to a vague world. This is more or less what is called criticism ...]

Let us return now to the questions of consistency: given the absence of 'ready made' motifs of consistency – scientific, philosophical or historical – what is at stake in Schefer's work, as the book on Uccello bears out for the first time, is the proposal of different *fictions*. These fictions bear an intimate relation to the body; they are produced to try to account for the strange experience of the body and for the disjunction between experience and representation. Schefer considers images of different kinds as offering varied manifestations of a deformed or reformed body.

The history of painting and of cinema is a history of the phantasmatic projections of the body to which humankind has been prey, since the first images on the walls of caves and since the first images by the child to represent or form those bodies that inhabit his/her world. These fictions are as if 'visited' upon the spectator, who is: '[le] lieu d'expérimentation ou de vérification, des hypothèses ou des fictions touchant la forme humaine' [place of experimentation or verification of the hypotheses or fictions concerning the human form] (1998a: 12). Schefer writes of the kinds of affective, emotional and moral relations we may entertain with the monstrous or experimental bodies we see. The consistency of his work thus lies in this affectivity, or more simply put the consistency of his work is affective. This is to say that it is both fictional and writerly. Schefer refers to himself as 'un auteur sans romans' [author without novels], for whom 'tout est fiction' [everything is fiction] (1995b: 9). His work bears many parallels with that of Roland Barthes, for whom many things were pretexts for writing, and for whom writing was the utopia which catalysed desire, the space of seduction in which desire and other affective energies could be played out.

Visual figures, then, are 'des énigmes avec lesquelles nous dialoguons' [enigmas with which we are in dialogue] (1998a: 8). But the writing produced by such images is not necessarily of the order of interpretation. The relation is one of seduction: 'nous ne parlons pas d'un objet mais commentons une relation de séduction aisée ou difficile' [we are not speaking of objects but comment on a relation of seduction, which can be easy or difficult] (*ibid.*). Schefer writes: 'je suis incapable de parler de ce que je n'aime pas' [I am incapable of speaking of what I don't like] (*ibid.*: 8); to this extent Schefer's work, like that of Barthes, is coherent in offering an account of all of the objects with which, at one moment or another, he has loved. We can recall Freud's hypothesis that the subject may be constituted by the residual traces of all of the objects which he/she has loved and lost ([1923] 1961: 29). To this extent Schefer writes a continuous autobiography, and it is not coincidental that alongside the regular publication (and republication) of writings on art, cinema and literature, Schefer publishes a regular 'journal', *Main courante*, now in four volumes, the title of which points us to the activity which forms the continuity of his work – the hand moving across the page in the act of writing. In an interview on *Paolo Uccello*, Schefer writes in effect that the only connection that the objects he considers have is that they are 'de l'ordre du scriptible' [of the order of the writerly] (1978: 48). We can recall that Barthes's notion of the 'scriptible' is that which installs or instigates a desire to write; writing is a space of seduction (Barthes 1970: 10). Schefer's work may thus be characterised as novelistic (*romanesque*), if this word is taken to refer to the form that an affectivity, a sensibility or a morality may take in writing, without ever taking on the dogmatic shape of a single fiction or a novel. Schefer continually writes the novel that the images he considers suppose, and postulates what he calls 'un fantôme romanesque' [a novelistic phantom] (1998a: 8). Echoing the title of Barthes's final course at the Collège de France, Schefer's writing is the continuous preparation of a novel: 'Sans doute y-a-t-il dans ces textes (referring to the articles and essays collected in *Figures peintes*) 'un roman qui, peu à peu, fait sa toilette ou dont l'idée du moins cherche les corps dans lesquels elle pourrait vivre' [Perhaps in these texts there is a novel adorning itself little by little, or a novel whose idea, at least, is searching for those bodies in which it can live] (*ibid.*).

Schefer is thus an irresponsible art historian, or aesthetician. His work does not obey the demands of system, nor does it obey a strict sense of scale, its motif (like that which governs the later work and perhaps the entire œuvre of Barthes) is pleasure and seduction, or affectivity in general. He considers this sense of irresponsibility, and justifies it, in *Questions de style*: 'Quelques amis d'historiens d'art m'ont dit d'avoir regretté la liberté de main de certains livres (Uccello, Le Corrège, le Greco). Je ne peux rien y changer, telle est ma manière' [Some art-historian friends have said to me that they were disappointed by the freehand nature of certain books (Uccello, Correggio, El Greco). I can't change; this is my way] (1995b: 10). Method, Schefer suggests, is the convenient motif that allows heterogeneous objects to be linked together, objects whose presence in the same context (the context of a book, for example) is often one determined by affective motives. The finality, Schefer proposes, of writing on art, is not scientific (*ibid.*: 13); culture and writers are nomadic. Schefer cites Baudelaire as one of the first 'modern' writer in so far as 'il a compris et expérimenté ceci: la culture et l'écrivain sont nomades' [he understood and experimented with this fact: culture and the writer are nomadic] (*ibid.*: 12). This nomadism affords the writer an extraordinary freedom; in so far as the responsibility of the writer is to his/her affective engagements, objects deriving from wildly differing historical periodisations can become contemporary. Schefer's books are thus of a different type than most books of art history or theory, ask to be read as texts, in other words, as exercises in writing themselves. They do not serve their objects; the latter, rather, provide the occasion for the writing itself. Analysis and interpretation are not the description of the code which will enable the reader to discover the meaning of the painting. Interpretations are the fictions that the painting has induced in those who consider it. Interpretation is a 'fiction d'interprétation' (*ibid.*: 9).

Let us look at two texts in more detail. *Questions de style*, published by L'Harmattan in 1995, announces, in its 'Avant-propos', that it consists only in 'le développement d'une diagonale d'interprétation: son premier objet est la couleur rouge' [the development of an interpretative diagonal: its first object is the colour red] (*ibid.*). Across this book and through other essays by Schefer the colour red functions as what Adrian Rifkin has called an 'anachronistic thing' or 'anamorphic object' generating different figures through different chronological zones (2005: 371). The 'second objects' are also the 'corps d'appui' [supporting bodies] of the first, the textual or visual bodies which support the primary object; a passage from Aristotle, an altar piece by Uccello, and a painting from the Rhenish School entitled *La Vierge au jardinet*; his consideration of this last object takes up most of this relatively short book, and Schefer reveals here the particular affective force that this painting holds for him. It relates to the question of origins: the text by Aristotle that is commented on relates to the origin of colour, 'l'engendrement des couleurs' (1995b: 25); on the altarpiece by Uccello Schefer writes that 'L'invention d'Uccello est la libération et comme l'invention de la couleur rouge dès le moment où l'hostie est profanée, c'est à dire au moment même où la pertinence du signe est interrogée' [Uccello's discovery is the liberation and in some sense the invention of the colour red from the moment of the profanation of the host, that is to say from the very moment when the pertinence of the sign is interrogated] (*ibid.*: 33). The *Vierge au jardinet*, Schefer writes, concerns another myth of origins: 'cette fois tout personnel. Un autre rouge y traduit, maintient, varie, *plisse* exactement un léger affect' [completely personal this time. Here a different red translates, maintains, varies and *folds*, precisely, a light affect] (*ibid.*: 39). The painting relates to a moment in Schefer's own affective life, and pertains to the writing, rewriting and analysis, of an affective fiction. 'Cette jeune fille du Moyen Âge finissant ne m'explique rien du tableau; celui-ci est un miroir tendu de très loin dans mon histoire et qui fait le portrait, méconnaissable en détail, d'une durée amoureuse seulement préservée par ce portrait' [This young girl from the late Middle Ages explains nothing of the painting to me; this is a very distant mirror held upon my past and which presents the picture, unrecognisable in detail, of an amorous moment preserved only by this portrait] (*ibid.*). The writing 'of' the image is in some sense generated by the desire to animate it, to give life to the novel that it supposes. Thus Schefer writes of the virgin in question: 'elle n'est jusqu'ici que le personnage silencieux d'un roman que l'on écrit dans la seule idée de la tutoyer un jour, c'est à dire de l'animer, de rendre à la vie l'illusion de cette âme silencieuse ou tue à jamais' [she is nothing more here than the silent character of a novel being written with the sole idea of speaking intimately to her one day, that is of animating her, giving back to life the illusion of this silent or forever silenced soul] (*ibid.*: 41). The bodies of pictures are characters in a novel which it is the task of the writer-critic to produce.

The image has a special resonance for Schefer, and it seems that the memory attached to it is rising, with difficulty, as in Proust's description of the *madeleine*, from murky depths. There is a Proustian note to this confession: 'De combien de joies, d'effusions silencieuses cette petite image a-t-elle été la gardienne, la lointaine maîtresse, pendant toute ma vie d'enfant, puis d'homme jusqu'à ce que je la retrouve . . .' [How many joys, silent effusions has this little image kept hidden, like a distant mistress, during my entire childhood life, and then my adult life, until I found her . . .] (*ibid.*: 43). As if the image holds a part of Schefer's affective life within it, and the writing *of* or *on* this image – produced by the image – could unlock, as the narrator's effort to focus seeks to do in *Du côté de chez Swann* – the key to part of the affective life of the writer. According to this logic, images are the secret and silent guardians of our life stories – of the fictions of our souls and the text of our affects. After some time, and through a writing the rhythm of whose syntax seems to accord with the logic of the heart rather than that of the mind, Schefer gives us the biographical key to the image: 'Comme par un tour de passe-passe, ou la manipulation d'un magicien, ce portrait laisse venir en filigrane l'image changeante, inassurée dans ses traits d'une jeune fille qui m'en donna, à la fin de notre enfance commune, la photographie' [Like a juggling trick or a magician's sleight of hand, this portrait lets the changing image tentatively emerge, features yet trembling, of a young girl who, at the end of both of our childhoods, gave me a photograph of it] (*ibid.*: 45). Thus we see that the interpretation that Schefer gives to the image is overdetermined by the emotional associations it holds for the writer, associations which relate to seduction and to childhood, or more specifically, to the threshold between childhood and adult life, around which desire and seduction are woven, the moment at which the body becomes a sexual, libidinal body. The 'tour de passe-passe' Schefer considers is in fact the oscillation between the reasons of the heart – reasons related to childhood love, to seduction and to emotion, and the reasons of the mind, the work of analysis, history and criticism. There are two art histories in Schefer's work – the broader sweep of the history of images of the body of *jouissance*, and the fiction of the writer, where this is the story of seduction and of love. Schefer suggests that the second is there to hide the first, but, paradoxically, to lead back to it. The image of the Virgin in the garden is, Schefer continues, 'une allégorie mystérieuse ou indéchiffree d'un moment de ma vie' [a mysterious or undeciphered allegory of a moment of my life] (*ibid.*: 49) – the colour red, the primary object of analysis – relates to an origin in so far as it signals the end of childhood, the first and the last moment of love, Schefer tells us. It is also 'ce qui revient' [what returns] – in so far as the memory of the childhood love Schefer recalls seems to emerge out of the colour red. Schefer imagines that the opulent and ample red dress that falls around the knees of the virgin hides him, and hides him from himself: 'Est-ce cependant moi que les plis de sa robe rouge dissimulent comme un donateur minuscule, ou un orant aux mains jointes, agenouillé et perdu dans les plis d'étoffe qui le cachent, même à mes yeux' [Is it me that the folds of her red dress hide like a miniature supplicant, someone praying with hands joined, kneeling and lost in the folds of cloth which hide him, even from my eyes] (*ibid.*: 50).

Whoever writes on painting, then, is confronted with an enigma which (in true Proustian fashion) is not 'out there' but 'within myself'. Schefer writes of the critic that 'Ce qu'il lui reste à expliciter n'est pas "le sens" du tableau, c'est l'usage qui constitue dans cette œuvre une énigme dont il a responsabilité de déchiffrement et de construction, parce que cette énigme est la sienne; qu'elle mobilise de façon transitoire et purement fictive *une chose inconnue* qui est en lui et à laquelle il cherche avidement, ardemment, des formes de résolution et de transition' [What it remains for him to explicate is not the 'meaning' of the painting, but the usage which in this painting constitutes an enigma, for the construction and deciphering of which he is responsible, because this enigma is his own; it mobilises, in transitory and purely fictive fashion, an *unknown thing* which is in him, and whose forms of resolution and transition he avidly and lovingly seeks] (*ibid.*: 55; my italic). The painting is thus, in some sense, an external object which plays an interpretative role in a practice of confession, auto-analysis and auto-biography. Schefer does nothing but write his own biography, the history or the fictions which the enigmas of varied images have produced within him, and which have invited him to express and explore his own enigmas. Schefer refers to an expression taken from Sade, which also gave the title to the earlier collection of essays *L'Espèce de chose mélancolie* (1978), to explain what he intends here: 'J'essaie de leur faire éprouver l'espèce de chose qui trouble et bouleverse ainsi [si cruellement] mon existence' [I am trying to make them feel the species of thing which thus so cruelly troubles and upsets my existence] (*ibid.*). What is at stake is an account of subjectivity which holds it to be secretly determined by 'something' or 'some species of thing', some thing without orthodox form which determines one's existence, which is hidden from oneself, or which is the enigma of one's own biography 'l'inconnue de moi-même' [the unknown of myself] (*ibid.*). If we recall Freud's description of the melancholic as someone for whom 'the shadow of the object has fallen on the ego' ([1917] 2005: 209), we can see how it would make sense to see the 'espèce de chose' which Schefer imagines as determinative of the writing on or of art, as the return of a lost self, but one experienced precisely as a foreign body, 'un corps étranger'. The activity of interpretation is a process which – in a manner reminiscent as much of Proust as of Freud – risks the reanimation of this 'other' body, which can be experienced as monstrous: 'Comment interpréter sans que s'interpose quelque moi, quelque chose, ou corps étranger. Car, avant cet acte le moi inconnu n'était pas une chose et pas non plus une masse invisible déformant le champ visuel, c'est la chose inconnue qui vient d'un monde habité de fictions et qui va tuer le narrateur' [How can one interpret without there coming between some ego, some thing, or foreign body. For before this act the unknown self was not a thing and nor was it an invisible mass deforming the visual field, it is the unknown thing which comes from a world inhabited by fictions, and which will kill the narrator] (*ibid.*: 56). The world of painting (and *a fortiori* of cinema, perhaps) is a world of hybrid forms, hybrid in so far as they appear as precipitates of the process on the one hand of the deformation and reformation of visual bodies in the history of art, and on the other of the deformation and reformation of the ego through the incorporation and expulsion of its objects of cathexis. Thus writing on painting appears as a dialogue with figures which have taken on the form of the phantasmatic objects with which in the course of a life one has entertained relations of seduction. In Schefer's writing, this knowledge is bound up with subjectivity: 'Nous ne sommes pas sûrs de ce que nous mettons dans la littérature; nous sommes à peu près certains que notre subjectivité (qui s'est appelée esprit, sensibilité) y a droit de mélange avec notre savoir' [We are not sure of what we put into literature; we are almost certain that our subjectivity (which has been called intelligence, sensibility) is side by side there with our knowledge] (*ibid.*: 57). Schefer postulates this as a 'science nouvelle ou romantique; qui distribue des objets historiques et fait place à celui qui opère cette distribution' [a new or romantic science, which distributes historical objects and makes a place for the one who effects this distribution] (*ibid.*).

The distinction between the 'primary object' and the secondary objects or 'corps d'appui' [supporting objects], and the notion of the enigmatic body or the 'espèce de chose' [species of thing] whose interpretation generates the writing, allows us to consider Schefer's books as variations of different 'interpretative fictions', associations of motifs strung around historical objects. *Questions de style*, as we saw, is a meditation on the colour red which focuses on the question of origins or myths of origins, and seems to revolve around the confessional motif of the painting of the Virgin in the Garden. *Polyxène et la vierge à la robe rouge* offers a different interpretative fiction, strung between a different series of secondary objects, but featuring the same painting of the Virgin of the Garden, and the same essay from seven years earlier. Schefer asserts that the book is not a confession, but the 'development' of a 'confusion de sentiments' [confusion of feelings] (2002a: 7). Again the basis of the book is a fiction. What Schefer imagines here, he says, is 'un monde antérieur à celui de nos culpabilités historiques' [a world before that of our historical guilt] (*ibid.*), that is, a world earlier than that which is determined by the guilt of which we are conscious. Implicit here is the notion that the history of representation and of the sign relates to the Christian era, a proposition that is explored in the work of Louis Marin and Jean-Luc Nancy, among others (see Chapters 6 and 9 in this volume). Before Christ takes on the responsibility of sacrifice and the history of art becomes that of the representation of the crime of the crucifixion, the fault is unknown and the crime immemorial: 'C'est un jeu essayé des responsabilités sur une faute inconnue et la réalité d'un crime si ancien qu'il n'a plus de mémoire' [It is an experiment with the responsibilities for an unknown fault and a crime so ancient that it has no memory] (*ibid.*). Once more Schefer's work takes on a Freudian resonance, this time with reference to *Totem and Taboo*, and the proposition that the foundation of the social body depends on a crime committed in common – the murder of the father. Although the crime in question here is different, the motif of the original crime (we can recall the title of the book published by Clima in 1985; *Origine du crime*) resonates with that of the enigma, or the 'espèce de chose', which calls for interpretation. The archaism of the 'crime', here, is both historical and psychic: the Greek vase depicting the sacrifice of Polyxena comes from the prehistory of art, while Schefer also postulates a psychic archaism at work here: 'C'est l'obscurité du désir qui imagine sa propre antiquité' [The obscurity of desire which imagines its own antiquity] (*ibid.*: 8). Again the 'interpretative fiction' is referred to as a novel, as yet in fragments ('ce roman mis en miettes' [this novel in pieces] (*ibid.*: 11) and is woven around its 'secondary' objects, a vase in the British Museum, Giovanni Bellini's painting *The Drunkenness of Noah*, the image of a courtesan being forcibly penetrated with a wooden bird figure from Oshima's film *Ai no Corrida*, and the Virgin in the Garden from the Rhenish School already considered in *Questions de style*. The cohesion of these figures seems to relate to a sacrifice – to a moment of cruelty which is nevertheless indissociable from a moment of *jouissance* (recalling the tenor of the work of Georges Bataille): 'cette scène est donc sacrée, c'est une scène de dévotion, d'absolution du crime avant le crime' [this scene is thus sacred, it is a scene of devotion, of the absolution of the crime before the crime] (*ibid.*: 60). In the 'Journal' which acts as a kind of post-face to the texts on each of four objects Schefer again considers the importance that the image of the Virgin has for him: the work of the writer of/on painting, Schefer proposes, is driven by a search for those objects which will allow the 'unknown' to be written, which will allow 'le seul roman de ma vie' [the only novel of my life] to write itself (*ibid.*: 79). The concern is again for the myth of an origin, the 'chose inconnue' or the 'espèce de chose'. To this extent Schefer abdicates the position of 'author': 'dans tout cela je ne suis pas l'auteur mais le pantin ou la marionnette de sentiments, ou la plume enregistrant en un graphique inégal les courbes exagérées des incertitudes du cœur' [in all of this I am not the author but the puppet or the marionette of emotions, or the pen recording in an unequal script the exaggerated curves of the uncertainties of the heart] (*ibid.*: 11).

To consider now Schefer's *Chardin*, from 2002, we can see that the mode of attention of the writer to the image is affective, one of seduction; it is an erotic relation. Barthes commented on a photograph in *La Chambre claire* that it gave him the desire to live there (Barthes 1980: 66). Schefer engages the same kind of relation with the images of and on which he writes. Of Chardin, he comments that the images (reproduced at the beginning of the book) give him the desire or nostalgia for a kind of peace: 'aspiration à la familiarité d'une vie domestique, calme, chaleureuse que je ne connaissais pas' [an aspiration for the familiarity of a calm, warm domesticated life, which I never knew] (2002b: 19) The book is inspired then by 'une envie romanesque' [a novelistic desire] (*ibid.*: 17), to live in this world, or more precisely, to give substance to this world by providing it with its description, with its theatre (thus Schefer also considers the other 'novels' to which these images have given rise, in the writing of Diderot, the Goncourts and Proust). Here perhaps it is most clear that Schefer's writing does not offer us a theorisation of painting, nor a historicisation, but a writing of the *jouissance* of the painting, a writing that attempts to account for the relation of *jouissance*, seduction, pleasure and affection that we entertain with the image. A single paragraph from the end of the book can witness this Proustian and Barthesian aim: 'Élégant déhancement du corps de *la Pourvoyeuse*, étalant le beau bleu de Prusse de son tablier, fichu du même blanc de plomb travaillé d'ombres bleues, la saignée du coude serrée d'un ruban carmin, dont le tour du cou reprend comme un leitmotiv le même brouillage de blancs, rouges rosés, et bleu qui sont le motif le plus heureusement répété des portraits; les pains blonds foncés, poudrés de la même farine grisée que la Brioche' [The elegant curve of the hips of the *Servant Returning from Market*, displaying the beautiful Prussian blue of her apron, made of the same leaden white riven with blue shadows, the inside of her elbow pulled tight by a carmine ribbon, the turn of whose neck echoes as a leitmotif the same blurring of whites, reds, pinks and blues which is the most successful motif of the portraits; the dark blonde loaves, powdered with the same grey flour as the Brioche] (*ibid.*: 99–100). The play of colours, the absence of proposition, the dominance of the descriptive mode, of nominal and adjectival clauses, all of these qualities present a writing which bears a relation of love and of pleasure, to the object of its focus.

This contrasts dramatically with the fear which one encounters in Schefer's writing on cinema. One of the emphases of Schefer's writing on the cinema is the strangeness of this technology, the affective strangeness of the vision and the experience with which the cinema presents. The writing which this produces is the 'enseignement fantasmatique' [phantasmatic teaching] (to adopt an expression used by Barthes (1978: 43)) which the experience of cinema generates. Schefer imagines, for example, that in the cinema, rather than in Plato's cave, we are 'pour une inestimable éternité, suspendus entre un corps géant et l'objet de son regard' [for an inestimable eternity suspended between a giant body and the object of its gaze] (1980: 88). As in the writing on Uccello's *Déluge*, what Schefer shows us is the material and moral quality of the visual (and auditory) surface we see: 'cette poussière [...] cette lumière [...] ce corps gris' [this dust ... this light ... this grey body] (*ibid.*: 79), 'ce monde apparemment flottant, ce granit et ces flocons' [this apparently floating world, this granite and these flakes] (*ibid.*: 83), 'ce visage de mosaïque, fait de flocons, de points, de poussière' [this face of mosaic, made of flakes, points, of dust] (*ibid.*: 84), 'le tissu vocal' [the vocal tissue] (*ibid.*: 17). The film presents me with another, foreign world in which I am surprised to find I can also live: 'j'y apprends donc de m'étonner de pouvoir vivre simultanément dans plusieurs mondes' [I learn thus to be shocked to find myself able to live simultaneously in different worlds] (*ibid.*: 5). Schefer thus writes against a view of the cinema as representational, ideological, oneiric, its 'realism', or its illusory quality, is irrelevant, since we have already entered into this other space and are affected by it: 'il m'a déjà fait entrer dans la vérité et l'étrangété des affects entiers, nouveaux, et dominateurs, parce que leurs qualités sont inédites, parce que leurs rapports d'objet sont inédits' [it has already made me enter into the truth and the strangeness of whole, new and dominant affects, because their qualities are unknown, because the relations between objects they suppose are unknown] (*ibid.*: 16). Instead, there emerges a stress upon the affective quality of the individual's experience of this visual and auditory reality, in relation to which the spectator is something like a guinea pig, 'la conscience expérimentale' [experimental consciousness], 'un être expérimental' [an experimental being] (*ibid.*: 10). A recurrent image, in effect, is that of torture, subjugation: 'je reste en effet constamment non son lecteur mais son serviteur le plus soumis' [I remain in fact never its reader but always its most submissive servant] (*ibid.*: 5). This strange new world is a space of improbable births, and it appeals in the spectator to the memory of childhood, to the earliest experiences. The cinema solicits in us a depth of feeling and affect that is prior to meaning and which has to do with the early experience of vision: 'la toute première expérience de [la] vision' (*ibid.*: 7). It solicits the memory of our infantile, pre-symbolic bodies, 'une part de nous mêmes qui demeure sans expression: cette partie vouée au silence et à une aphasie relative' [a part of ourselves which remains without expression, that part destined for silence and a relative aphasia] (*ibid.*). The spectator looks something like the young Marcel in Proust's *À la recherche du temps perdu*, whose habitual somnolence is traumatically shattered by the intrusion of the images of the magic lantern. And this is also an autobiographical inflection: Schefer's insistence on fear, crime and guilt in the cinema relates very much to his own experience of watching silent films, as a child, while the war was raging elsewhere, in the other world: 'Au fond du cinéma (dans sa condition la plus ancienne pour nous et la plus brutale) subsiste la terreur ou la peur vague liée toute notre enfance à n'importe quel film' [In the depths of the cinema (in its oldest and most brutal state, for us) subsists the terror or the vague fear which throughout our childhood was linked to any film] (*ibid.*: 79); 'toute la peur de la guerre et quatre ans de terreur, et d'objets brisés et de visages disparus se fixèrent en un instant dans telle salle, sur l'image du premier film' [all the fear of the war and four years of terror, of broken objects and vanished faces were fixed in one moment in such and such a venue, on the image of the first film] (*ibid.*: 80). As such, Schefer does not write 'professionally' on cinema: 'je n'ai pas de qualité pour parler du cinéma' [I have no quality to write on cinema] (*ibid.*: 5), but as 'l'homme ordinaire'. The ordinary man that he is is nevertheless of a certain age, having lived through a certain history, which links the experience of cinema to the war, to a 'univers de chuchotement' [universe of whispering] (*ibid.*: 81). Schefer's first and most intriguing text on cinema, *L'Homme ordinaire du cinema*, thus resembles Barthes's *La Chambre claire* in many ways; it is written from the perspective of the 'amateur'. But the two books, published in the same year and by the same publisher (Cahiers du cinéma/ Gallimard), also resemble each other strangely: both feature commentaries on photograms (photographs, in Barthes's book, film stills in Schefer's), and both deviate from the doxical, 'studious' knowledge which the photogram produces to meditate on the subjective, affective element, the 'punctum', which pricks or wounds the subject emotively and morally. Schefer's book, however, extends the motif of the affective, subjective wound into a general principle, and makes fear into the dominant note; on a still from Terence Fisher's *Frankenstein Must Be Destroyed* (1969), Schefer writes: 'C'est un être jamais engendré dans le monde (ni dans l'histoire) qui vient ici, c'est un organisme intérieur au cinéma qui vient nous infecter de sa naissance impossible. Et comme spectateur je suis le lieu constant de cette naissance' [It is a being never before engendered in the world (nor in history) which now comes; it is an organism interior to cinema which comes to infect us with its impossible birth. And as a spectator I am constantly the place of this birth] (*ibid.*: 25). The monstrosity of the deformed body, automaton or vampire, becomes a theoretical principle applied to the cinema as a whole. More specifically, the cinema solicits in us, calls to life an aphasic, monstrous being, a puppet, 'ludion' (*ibid.*: 97) or automat (extremely resonant with Deleuze's 'spiritual automaton' in *Cinéma II*) which lives within us and is our double ('paradoxale addition d'un être à notre être' [paradoxal addition of a being to our being], 'existence fantomale' [phantom existence] (*ibid.*: 96).

Schefer's work as a whole thus offers an extremely rich, dense and intriguing series of meditations on the fictions supposed by images, and on the sensibilities and moralities implied by these suppositions. The recurrent comparison with Barthes in this essay perhaps suggests the kind of theoretician I consider Schefer to be, a factor which will undoubtedly frustrate those seeking a straightforward yield of theoretical knowledge, or an applicable methodology. The 'childish knowledge' which Schefer's writing supposes has the power, nevertheless, to unsettle the orthodox representations and legitimisations which we assume as history, and to reveal them as fictions.

References

Barthes, R. (1970) *S/Z*, Paris: Éditions du Seuil.

—— (1973) *Le Plaisir du texte*, Paris: Éditions du Seuil.

—— (1975) *Roland Barthes par Roland Barthes*, Paris: Éditions du Seuil.

—— (1978) *Leçon*, Paris: Éditions du Seuil.

—— (1980) *La Chambre claire: Note sur la photographie*, Paris: Cahiers du cinéma/Gallimard.

—— ([1969] 1982) 'La peinture est-elle un langage?', in *Essais critiques IV: L'obvie et l'obtus*, Paris: Éditions du Seuil.

Deleuze, G. (1985) *Cinéma 2: L'Image-temps*, Paris: Éditions de Minuit.

Freud, S. (2005 [1917]) 'Mourning and Melancholia', in *On Murder, Mourning and Melancholia*, trans. Shaun Whiteside, Harmondsworth: Penguin, 201 18.

—— ([1923] 1961) 'The Ego and the Id', in *Standard Edition of the Complete Psychological Works of Sigmund Freud, Vol. XIX: The Ego and the Id and Other Works*, ed. and trans. James Strachey, London: Hogarth Press, 1–68.

Rifkin, A. (2005) 'From Structure to Enigma and Back, Perhaps' *Journal of Visual Culture* 4, 365–81.

Schefer, J.-L. (1969) *Scénographie d'un tableau*, Paris: Seuil.

—— (1978) *L'Espèce de chose mélancholie*, Paris: Flammarion.

—— (1980) *L'Homme ordinaire du cinéma*, Paris: Cahiers du cinéma/Gallimard.
—— (1985) *Origine du crime*, Paris: Café Clima.
—— (1995a) *The Enigmatic Body*, ed. and trans. Paul Smith, Cambridge: Cambridge University Press.
—— (1995b) *Questions de style*, Paris: L'Harmattan.
—— (1997) *Du monde et du mouvement d'images*, Paris: Cahiers du cinéma.
—— (1998a) *Figures peintes: Essais sur la peinture*, Paris: POL.
—— (1998b) *Cinématographies: Objets périphériques et mouvements annexes*, Paris: POL.
—— (1998c) *Choses écrites: Essais de littérature et à peu près*, Paris: POL.
—— (1998d) *Main courante*, Paris: POL.
—— (1999a) *Paolo Uccello, Le Déluge, La Peste*, Paris: POL.
—— (1999b) *Images mobiles: Récits, visages, flocons*, Paris: POL.
—— (1999c) *Sommeil du Greco*, Paris: POL.
—— (1999d) *Lumière du Corrège*, Paris: POL.
—— (1999e) *Main courante 2*, Paris: POL.
—— (2001) *Main courante 3: Sommes-nous des moralistes?*, Paris: POL.
—— (2002a) *Polyxène et la vierge à la robe rouge*, Paris: POL.
—— (2002b) *Chardin*, Paris: POL.
—— (2005) *Figures de différents caractères*, Paris: POL.
—— (2008) *Main courante 4: Notre âme est une bête féroce*, Paris: POL.

Part V
The digital era

12

Jean Baudrillard

Paul Hegarty

From the 1968 book *Le Système des objets* to his late essays, books and pieces for the daily newspaper *Libération*, Jean Baudrillard's work addresses the visual culture that dominates the imaginary of the contemporary world. In that first book, he looks at the system of meanings that accrue to household objects, arrangements of furniture, cars, and technological objects (amongst others). It is the connotation (the sign value of an object) that provides the essential part of how objects work, with this idea a premonition of his gradual dismantling of the idea of a referent world that holds any actual reality. This critique of the belief in referentiality begins in earnest in *Pour une critique de l'économie politique du signe* (1972), where not only reality but also representation comes under attack. Baudrillard's world-view comes to be dominated by the concept of simulation, which is fully realised in *L'Échange symbolique et la mort* (1976) and the essay originally written in the same year, 'La précession des simulacres' ['The Precession of simulacra'] (in Baudrillard 1981: 9–68). This interest in what others would term representation, might suggest a simple view of visual culture where 'the visual' has somehow replaced a more concrete reality. Baudrillard's theory, appropriately enough, looks like this is what it does, but it is more subtle and more profound: in fact, the surface of things has replaced nothing, it is the status and import of 'the surface' that has changed so that it imbues all reality, to the detriment of the realness of that reality. Throughout his œuvre, simulation defines the other theorisations, which often derive, as does simulation, from visual phenomena (for example, his idea of transparency). At the same time, he constantly refers to art objects, architecture, media events, technological media, and cannot do otherwise as a thinker who attempts to write about the meaning of 'now' and the future (just as Marshall

McLuhan and Buckminster Fuller did in the 1960s). What Baudrillard does not often do, despite this promising combination of a visually derived philosophy, and interest in visual cultural objects, is analyse specific media or objects in great detail. Often, he gestures almost contemptuously towards analysis, and seems to be proposing a superficial, imagistic reading of his own (as in the five aphoristic *Cool Memories* books). This is both good and bad for the would-be user of Baudrillard to assess visual phenomena or objects: good in that it is necessary to apply his thought rather than cite his opinion on a given cultural product; and bad for the very same reason. Baudrillard's influence on artistic producers can often be tangential – it is not his direct statements on art that are of use, but, more tangentially, his thoughts about the status of reality, of politics or the media. Where there is influence, it is as if he and the artists are complicit with each other, or at least up to the same thing (that is, his praise for pop art, when his own writing could be seen as a theory equivalent of pop's approach to art and the world). Perhaps the best-known reference to Baudrillard in cultural production is in the Wachowski brothers' film *The Matrix* (1999), which creates a world where 'the real world' is a giant computer simulation, and humans are wired into the system while acting as batteries powering the very system that controls them. Arguably the film is a very literal interpretation of Baudrillard's theory of simulation, and one that still posits a real to be revealed when the simulation is removed, and overdoes its literalism by showing a copy of Baudrillard's *Simulacra and Simulation*.[1] But beyond the question of direct influence, cross-referencing of any Baudrillard writing from the mid-1970s (on reality TV, TV wars, cloning, simulation in general) or later work with developments in 'the media' or elsewhere, shows him to be highly prophetic, and if we mostly live in a world first defined by William Gibson and J. G. Ballard, we also live in more of a Baudrillardian world than even he expected, and such a world is visual to its (empty, burned-out) core.

Baudrillard's theory of simulation is the frame for all his thought and both product and driver of his views on visual culture. Simulation is the latest in a sequence of what initially seem to be historical, epistemological states. Culture is a sequence of simulacra, he claims (1976: 77). We move from 'the counterfeit', which relies on the belief that truth is contained in the original, an inherent part of it. The second 'order of simulacra' is that of representation, and this is where realists already start to part company with Baudrillard, for representation is just one, historically determined, process for defining the world, defining what reality is. It belongs to the industrial, capitalist period, and posits a world where truth is hidden, waiting 'deeper' than the level of appearances, to be revealed. This then gives way, gradually, to simulation, where there is no longer any reality: 'c'est aussi l'effondrement de la réalité dans l'hyperréalisme, dans la réduplication minutieuse du réel, de préférence à partir d'un autre médium reproductif – publicité, photo, etc' ['it is also the collapse of reality into hyperrealism, into a real duplicated right down to the smallest detail. This largely happens via an other reproductive medium – advertising, photographs, and so on'] (*ibid.*: 112). So, there is never unmediated access to a real world, and it seems not just that such a thing is hidden, in either Platonic or Kantian terms, away from our view, it just does not exist, except as a product of whichever simulacra dominate. Simulation arises through a combination of the collapsing economy in 1929 altering the functioning of capitalism, the decline of official communism, as shown in May 1968, and the spread of mass media.

This very visual 'theory of everything' actually emerges, in terms of Baudrillard's own development of the theory, through something even more specific: the Bauhaus, on which he writes in *Pour une critique*. The core of this book is Baudrillard's attempt to dismantle the representational truth apparently realised in the sign form (i.e. the combination of signifer and signified) and the identification of the parallel this has with the Marxist critique of capitalism. Other parts focus on art, with the theory of simulation emerging in the essay on the Bauhaus (Baudrillard 1970: 229–55), and the complex interplay of simulated value and aggressive destruction of value that can be seen in the art auction (127–43). This latter builds the key opposition in Baudrillard, of symbolic exchange on the one hand, and the spread of simulation on the other, but it is the highly privileged example of the Bauhaus that is of most note here.

The Bauhaus was part of the utopian modernism that sought to bring developments in the artistic avant-garde into social, built reality. Like Le Corbusier, Bauhaus artists envisaged a world built anew from new materials on principles that merged ultra-rationalistic planning of interiors and cities with the explosive creativity of modern art. The link happens in design, and for Baudrillard, the Bauhaus notion of designing everything, of making everything part of design, structures a new kind of environment, one that is above all semantic, even when apparently at its most functional (*ibid.*: 230).[2] Enlightenment aesthetics gives way to the concept of an organising aesthetic (*ibid.*: 231), and so a total system is created, within which objects communicate, and take meaning as parts of a greater whole (*ibid.*: 236). Every object, design choice and built structure is now about connotation (as opposed to being merely useful, or even denoting its usefulness), and the majority of connotations are visual, or built from visual cues. So, on the one hand, the visual design aesthetic takes everything over, but on the other, it is lost to a greater whole within which it is immersed – the fate of all visual objects or phenomena in Baudrillard's theory. Design would become influential in its own right, but the achievement of the Bauhaus, for Baudrillard, is that its totality makes it a marker of what is going on elsewhere, and once it exists, it is as if the entire social world has been designed, as it can be read, sold and consumed for connotation, in ways that had not been accessible to the Arts and Crafts movement or art nouveau. An example of this is the idea of the 'natural', which can now be incorporated as an integral part of a constructed environment (*ibid.*: 234). Once nature has been framed like this, all nature is to be read as framed, as something driven by acculturated structuring of nature.[3] The word 'environment' is a cruelly ironic one, as it signifies the loss of what it claims to be: 'le grand Signifié, le grand Référent Nature est mort, et ce qui le remplace, c'est l'environnement qui désigne, en même temps que sa mort, la restitution de la nature comme modèle de simulation' ['The great Signified, the great Referent, Nature is dead, and what comes to replace it is the environment, which redesigns nature, at the moment of its death, as a simulation model'] (*ibid.*: 254). Ultimately, as simulation spreads, we get 'natural parks', or preserved spaces for 'native populations' (*ibid.*: 255), and this always impacts on the status of the reality of the real object away from the natural park. A later example is Biosphere 2, which aims to reproduce an idealised version of all Earth's habitats, thereby making Earth into Biosphere 1, and the planet becomes something that has always only ever been the first in a sequence of simulations (1992: 126).

Having established the role of an art, design and architecture movement in the advent of simulation, Baudrillard returns to how art reacts to the creeping objectification of the world through design. If all can be placed within a system and understood, then the only way to resist is to disrupt continuity of signification, and this is how surrealism tries to act as an antidote to rationalist modernism. The problem is that even its oddest juxtapositions and cuts in the chain of meanings can be recuperated as communicating systems. This is not just in a general way, but also in the specific case of advertising, as it quickly becomes clear that surrealistic imagery and connections are ideal for commercial use (1970: 247). As Baudrillard will never tire of telling us, modern art is bereft of tools against simulation, and the last vestige of critical perspective in art is in the form of abstract painting (*ibid.*: 243). Baudrillard will go on to cite Marcel Duchamp and Andy Warhol at many points in his œuvre, but as without so within: art becomes a marker of something wider, a convenient shorthand for resistance or collusion with simulation.

Returning to the theme (in 1990) of the aestheticisation of the world and the loss of art as an autonomous category, he writes that '[L'art] a disparu comme pacte symbolique, par où il se distingue de la pure et simple production de valeurs esthétiques, que nous connaissons sous le nom de culture: prolifération des signes à l'infini, recyclage des formes passées et actuelles' ['art has disappeared as symbolic pact, as something thus clearly distinct from that pure and simple production of aesthetic values, that endless proliferation of signs, that recycling of past and present forms, which we call culture'] (1990: 22). This is what he terms the 'transaesthetic', the now complete process of making all aesthetic that the Bauhaus initiated. Now, he argues, the aesthetic flows virally through all other cultural domains, and the same applies to economics in 'transeconomics', sexuality in 'transsexuality'. The success of the Bauhaus vision is now an omnipresent parody, where 'même le plus marginal et le plus banal, même le plus obscène s'esthétise, se culturalise, se muséalise' (*ibid.*: 24) ['no matter how marginal, or banal, or even obscene it may be, everything is subject to aestheticization, culturalization, museumification' (1993: 16)]. Art has fared no better in the intervening years, with contemporary art apparently empty, a vehicle for spectator indifference: we 'fabriquent une profusion d'images *où il n'y a rien à voir*. La plupart des images contemporaines, vidéo, peinture, arts plastiques, audiovisuel, images de synthèse sont littéralement des images où il n'y a rien à voir' (1990: 25) ['we manufacture a profusion of images *in which there is nothing to see*. Most present-day images – be they video images, paintings, products of the plastic arts, or audiovisual or synthesized images – are literally images in which there is nothing to see' (1993: 17)]. While Baudrillard is highly critical of this state of affairs, there is a positive side, which is that the very emptiness first identified by Warhol creates fascination, another fascination 'emerges' (1990: 26). Many would perhaps agree, thinking of blockbuster films heavy on computer-generated imagery (CGI) effects, or the hype around certain contemporary artists, but we should not imagine that fascination replacing aesthetic pleasure is either good or bad for Baudrillard. In this, he is far from Fredric Jameson's concerns, in his book *Postmodernism*, about the 'waning of affect' and attention to surfaces he observes. There is an even more profound difference with the latter: for Baudrillard, contemporary art is not a secondary part of something wider, even of simulation. It is instead a vector, or even agent of the thing it is immersed in, and the emptiness of images that enthral us does not reflect anything any more, it *is* the viral world of simulation.

On many occasions, Baudrillard shows himself to be a thin reader of art, buying into his own theory in a way that pre-empts critical reading, and where in his early books, there are references to several artists and movements, from the 1980s on, and with the exception of Duchamp and Warhol, there is just a blanket condemnation of something he imagines as a homogeneous body of stuff to be dealt with as a category (that has failed) and no more.[4] What better, then, to build a museum that would realise the death of modern art? For this is how Baudrillard conceives of the Pompidou Centre in Paris, on which he writes in the year of its opening, 1977 (Baudrillard 1981: 93–111). He argues that the Pompidou (at that time also labouring under the name 'Beaubourg' in an attempt to suggest continuity with the *quartier* that had been bulldozed to make way for it) is an attempt to resuscitate dying modernity (*ibid.*: 96), but all it does is emphasize the death throes of the modern movement, in showing art that claims to be against art, or that show its ending (such as the crashed cars of sculptor César (*ibid.*: 97)). Those familiar with the building and with more recent contemporary art museums will wonder whether the Pompidou is in fact somehow a harbinger of this 'death of art', and at first it is far from clear, as what Baudrillard argues is that it is the Pompidou's well-meaning sociality that makes it so fatal to art.

The Pompidou was conceived as a new type of museum, a reflection of changed social attitudes and an attempt to make art more accessible, and less isolated from everyday culture. The immense glass building with coloured tubes and vents hardly seems to fit with its surroundings, so we need to look more closely at its structure. When first built, there were no internal divisions, either in the building as a whole or on any floor; the workings of the building – the access, the plumbing, the air conditioning – would all be on show; the plaza would be an integral part of the general 'offre' to help to bring people in, and the museum closer to the city; you could move freely between galleries, café spaces and the large, free, public library. Instead of reading this all as openness,

Baudrillard sees the essential characteristic and purpose as being that of flow: people, air, liquids, art – all can flow and interact (1981: 98). In addition, the building is about itself rather than art, it is standing in for art that now has no place. So it becomes a 'monument de dissuasion culturelle' ['monument of cultural dissuasion/deterrence'] (*ibid.*: 100). The building designed to fascinate the masses will do just that, to the detriment of any residually critical art within.[5] Baudrillard writes that Beaubourg/Pompidou should be left empty (*ibid.*: 98), and then, at some level, it would be continuing the function of critical modern art. But it turns out there will be a new content: the very crowds lured in to the world of high culture. The masses flock to see the spectacle of the failure of art (*ibid.*: 100) and the very success of the building creates a threat to it, as the masses descend, eager to witness the corpse of high culture (*ibid.*: 101). Yes!, shouts Baudrillard, 'Faites plier Beabourg!' ['Make Beaubourg buckle!'] (*ibid.*: 105). Ultimately, Baudrillard's hyperbolic wish becomes true, and the structure of the Pompidou has to be reinforced, the interiors are segregated, the flows much more controlled and subject to payment. Whatever the possibilities for the earlier radicality of the Pompidou, the years since the late twentieth century have seen a retrenchment into ordinariness.

Lastly, Baudrillard compares this museum to hypermarkets (1981: 103); this one has a mass of products and consumers of those cultural products (indeed today museums and the like are part of a 'cultural sector' where we expect public events, plenty of eating facilities, shops, and, as the organising conceit, a collection of art or other objects). The hypermarket is a parallel, totalising universe (*ibid.*: 115), one that sucks the life out of the surrounding towns (*ibid.*: 117), making the town the residue. Hypermarkets are not only the death of towns, but also the death of planning – like the Pompidou, they seek to move planning to a new level, with ultra-practical box warehouses lined with car parks, or malls with 'all your needs under one roof'. This is the plan as implosion, the last gasp of society spiralling inward into enforced sociality (see J. G. Ballard's final novel *Kingdom Come* for an expanded meditation on this idea). The hypermarket is also the premonition of a total immersion visual environment, through CCTV (*ibid.*: 114).[6]

Since the spread of IT software and hardware, and access to the internet, we are accustomed to living in the kind of world Baudrillard mapped out. For the most part, he is critical of this move, but also fascinated, as for him, it is not 'thanks to the media' or thanks to political manoeuvring that we are immersed in simulation. That we are caught up in simulation is an ontological change for Baudrillard, with simulation being something which bits of technology operate within, further removing what last bits of real cling on to the underside of the hyperreal (a world more real than real, where realness is always touted as a supreme value in its own right (*ibid.*: 11–12)).

Something odd happens to the Panopticon (the model for using visibility as a means of control) and we gradually embrace the concept of being ultra-visible. This begins with reality TV, and ends in the 'total screen' we find ourselves no longer in front of, but within. The most literal way this occurs is in the form of being in reality TV, but like the Bauhaus, the deadening of art in the Pompidou, or simulation as a whole, it filters out and affects all behaviours. In *Simulacres et simulation*, Baudrillard writes about the TV series called *An American Family*, filmed in 1971 and broadcast in 1973 (*ibid.*: 48–54). In this piece, Baudrillard sets out the problem for reality TV: in existing, it merges the previously separate worlds of real and representation, thus annulling the 'reality' it purports to show. The cameras have to be ignored by the family (who need to act as if they were not being filmed for display) and the viewer (who is summoned into what claims to be an unmediated environment) (*ibid.*: 49). The rapid profusion of reality TV in the last ten years has led many to question the realness of what is being performed or seen, but, for Baudrillard, this is to dramatically miss the point, which is that reality disappears under the onslaught of reality TV. We are not witnessing a false version of something true, but a change in the structure of 'the real'. We need to see this, he argues, as an example of 'the code', which defines all on the basis of 1/0 (digitality), provides models for everything, then hides itself as model on the interior of the thing made, as DNA does (1976: 89–90). Reality TV will be modelled around norms, or, just as simulatedly, around those outside social norms. Reality TV (of the documentary sort) erases the distinction between being on TV and not: anyone can now be part of reality TV, and may as well be. Initial wariness of CCTV has changed to acceptance, even demands for it, and the absence of an official channel to broadcast the 'slice of life' in your local shopping mall or multi-storey car park has no bearing on how the code of 'reality' combines what used to be seen as real, with what is now shown as 'the real'. Google Street View is the ultimate sign of this, and protestors against it are not defending privacy but the belief that there is a real world to keep hidden from Google's camera vans.

There is much more than the visual at stake here, argues Baudrillard, as reality TV is like a laboratory experiment (1981: 50): what is your life like; what difference does it make having the cameras here; what does it mean to frame the real as real rather than as art. Baudrillard returns to this point in his 2001 text *Télémorphose*, at a point where reality TV has caught up with him, and gradually fills the TV schedules. Recent reality TV has been even more literal, testing participants' capacities to survive within the test environment (*ibid.*: 9ff.). The viewers are also drawn in, through comments, voting and chatshows that comb the details of shows such as *Big Brother*. This system of feedback is part of the test, and part of the continued implosion between what is inside and outside of TV. Writing on *Loft Story*, a French version of *Big Brother*, he muses on what it is we are looking at, and what we are looking for, in looking at reality TV. We are fascinated by the nothingness we see, he writes (*ibid.*: 11). Early versions of these programmes were slower-moving and more 'real' in one way. As far in as series 4 of the British *Big Brother* we could watch one contestant who largely sat on the sofa and read a book, or did nothing. Many viewers also enjoyed the continual coverage of people sleeping through the night. Baudrillard gets beyond the level of journalistic critique in asking whether the nothingness in reality TV is actually quite important, stating that it is not at all about 'voyeurisme et de la stupidité collective' ['voyeurism and collective stupidity'] (*ibid.*: 21); instead it shows that there is never anything to see – all looking reveals a fundamental nothingness in the thing being looked at, and the emptiness of the process – reality TV only seems to be a different species of this, providing us with the 'knowledge' that reality TV isn't really real, not like the real world. This is a point Baudrillard disputes, noting that reality TV is effectively there to make us believe not in its own reality, but in the realness of everything else (*ibid.*: 10).[7]

Baudrillard comments on 'talent' shows in the reality TV format, slightly less interestingly, but he still tries to postulate a counter-intuitive argument. The democracy of talent show TV is an ultimate dream of the masses (he has been praising the radicality of the mass *as mass* since the mid-1970s). It's all about participation, anyone can be a contestant and all can participate through viewing, and voting. This is the ultimate empty democracy (2001: 27). Baudrillard would be very pleased with the problems that have arisen with mass telephone voting, with phone systems crashing, rigged results, unwanted results (like the Finnish metal band Lordi winning the Eurovision in 2005, or the Irish public choosing the puppet turkey Dustin, in 2006, as an entrant for the same competition). Even the rigging of votes is a response to mass viewership: 'we will choose correctly for the masses'. Baudrillard is not praising the idea of content-free democracy (where participation is the end in itself), but what he does like is the exposure of 'real' celebrities as being no more real than the ones that emerge from talent shows. This includes anyone, such as politicians and intellectuals, as well as musicians, etc., who claim to merit their status as a public figure (*ibid.*: 28).

Reality TV ties in to other developments in what might forever be called 'new media'. As noted above, and by Baudrillard, people's attitudes towards being under surveillance have changed. The panoptical world of submitting to control has been replaced by the desire to appear on TV, closed or open circuit. TV is dragged down to its 'degré zéro', as to appear is enough. We might even ask whether anyone seeks Warhol's 'fifteen minutes of fame' – rather they seek visibility through media. Once you link appearing on TV as a goal with social networking sites, web-enabled phones, webcam, Twitter, blogs and so on, Baudrillard's sense of us all living inside a total screen, rather than in front of, or in any way separated from, it (the 'écran total' of the book of the same name that is curiously translated as *Screened Out*) seems feasible. We are living a 'télémorphose intégrale de la société' (*ibid.*: 29) – that is, our complete transformation or metamorphosis into a world of visibility: all images are, at any one time, in existence, and all is imaged. Some of this is not even visual to us, like the tracking that enables Google software, or websites finding suggestions for a consumer – code is the visual culture software inhabits, as shown beautifully in the cascading green code in *The Matrix*.

Baudrillard's argument remains very general on all this, though, targeting the concept of digitally enabled interaction rather than the actual practices, which are far more subtle, and open to manipulation. His view of this screen-based culture is not positive. He argues that computer technology gives us an entirely constructed belief in individuality, and actually humanity has been broken down into constituent parts, a homogeneous mass ('l'indivisibilité de toutes les particules humaines à des dizaines de milliers de kilomètres de distance' ['the indivisibility of all human particles across tens of thousands of kilometres'] (*ibid.*: 31)), spattered on the screen of the world. This mass lives a zombie life, speaking only to other parts of itself (*ibid.*). Regular users of the net, gamers, second lifers, etc. will query this, but the endless proliferation of information via blogs and variants of them is surely not far from Baudrillard's vision. The belief that contact, communication and interaction are good is a product of the 'code' identified by Baudrillard in the 1970s, where models of behaviour supplant behaviour, whether ritual, representational or in some way real. It is the *model* of communication that we live in.

Baudrillard often seems nostalgic for a lost world, but this lost world was no more real than the simulated world we find ourselves in now. In fact it is this one that is most real, and therefore further away from a grounded reality. Ritual-based cultures are the ones which approach this 'lost world' of actual reality most closely – due to what he imagines (in *L'Échange symbolique et la mort*) as a lack of interest in 'the real'. In terms of visual production, he is perpetually drawn to the power of illusion, the last remnant of access to worlds and interactions outside of the real that other societies have or have had. If the simulacrum is the appearance of reality, then it is illusion that prevents us from falling fully into the trap of the flat real. Without illusion, nothing would exist – the perfect world would be like the 1998 film *The Truman Show*, only as real.[8] The removal of illusion begins in an explicit way for Baudrillard, in his 1979 book *De la séduction*, where he charts the distinction between two modes of visual creation: seduction and production.[9] The interest in the potential of illusion to offer something 'other than simulation' continues through *Le Crime parfait* (1995) and *The Vital Illusion* (2000) to *Le Pacte de lucidité* (2004) and strongly informs all his later work and his photography.

As well as the model of a sequence of simulacra defining reality, or a set of different relations to images, Baudrillard also proposes a distinction in the visual realm between seduction and production. The category of 'production' relates to two things: firstly, Baudrillard's schema of the history of simulacra, where the industrial period is paralleled by the growth in representational simulacra, where meaning is to be brought out, probed, discovered, then mastered; secondly, it relates to Foucault's theory of sex as social and scientific production, again in the industrialised West (Foucault 1976). Production is about contained meaning, meaning that is findable, and an overall expectation of resolution. Seduction is about falsity, mystery, and play. It is a 'forme ironique et alternative, qui brise la référence du sexe, espace non de désir, mais de jeu et du défi' ['ironic, alternative form, one that breaks the referentiality of sex and provides a space, not of desire, but of play and challenge'] (Baudrillard 1979: 38). For Baudrillard, production is a masculine form, seduction feminine. At times in the book he reads like a poststructuralist feminist, at others like a simple misogynist, but to summarise, women are more connected to the world of appearances, having been placed there through their social situation. For Baudrillard, this is the place to be, it offers a glimpse of a world not limited to the simulated real.

Seduction is connected to sex acts and the visibility of sex, with pornography the ultimate example of hyperreal sex. In (film) pornography, everything is on show, the demand for realism outpacing the demand for other desires to be sated (*ibid.*: 48). In fact, Baudrillard often makes the comparison the other way round: our heightened demands for news, for high definition, for all of that *now*, is in fact the pornography of the real. Instead, seduction is a way of thinking about appearances that make no claim to be real, that can even be 'plus faux que le faux' ['falser than false'] (*ibid.*). Seduction, like illusion, which Baudrillard uses later to deal with the same questions, is a way of outdoing the system at its own game, and will almost certainly involve what some would imagine to be complicity.

Take Warhol: his images partake of the commercial and pop-cultural worlds, seemingly immersed in simulation, but for Baudrillard, this is so excessive that we are drawn to his works as seductive mysteries. Warhol takes any object, any image, and instead of removing it from its original context and into art, he is actually removing the aesthetic of the object and of the art world (Baudrillard 1995: 111–12). The fascination that is so continually stimulated by simulation is thwarted and turned into an empty, mysterious fascination. According to Baudrillard, this is how Warhol is able to reintroduce illusion to art: 'le règne de l'art est celui d'une gestion conventionnelle de l'illusion, d'une convention qui circonscrit les effets délirants de l'illusion, qui conjure l'illusion comme phénomène extrême' ['the kingdom of art is one where illusion is managed by means of convention, a convention that closes off the limitless disorder of illusion, that conjures away illusion as an extreme phenomenon'] (*ibid.*: 117). Warhol strips away this attempt to master and use illusion, and restores it, perversely, by seeming totally to ignore it. As with the term 'simulation', which does not mean copy of something more real, Baudrillard's use of 'illusion' could mislead at first (appropriately, perhaps). Illusion is not the attempt to pass something off as real, or even to purposely hide something or be enigmatic. Rather it is the attempt to regain a more profound and more philosophically nihilistic illusion, like the *maya*, the world-illusion of Hinduism. This is to be attained by emptying out the lower level illusion of simulation (that is, the imagined real world).[10] This is not just an aesthetic question, it is a question of how rendering the world entirely, in real-time, in high definition and in totality risks destroying the world, the actual, empty world (Google Earth becomes Biosphere 0). This is the 'perfect crime' Baudrillard averts to, at his most Nietzschean, in the book of the same name, and subsequently: 'we are dealing with an attempt to construct an entirely positive world, a perfect world, expurgated of every illusion, of every sort of evil and negativity, exempt from death itself. This pure, absolute reality, this unconditional realization of the world – this is what I call the perfect crime' (Baudrillard 1995: 67).

We are closing in on this perfect crime, the nearer we get to 'virtual reality'. Baudrillard is slightly awkward about this term, and it does not sit too well with a theory of simulation which has already declared 'this' reality to be thoroughly virtual. This is why he writes of 'integral reality', where reality is fully simulated, and no pockets of precious real can subsist. Oddly, we seem to want this, and plunge into reality TV, interactive media, apparently ever-improving media. If you believed there was some sort of agency structuring 'the media' or the world, you might even believe your engagement with Twitter or peer-to-peer (P2P) networks to be somehow liberating, when what is occurring, in Baudrillard's view, is the final visibility of all to all.

As stated above, we, as a global society (we can no longer refer to 'the West' so easily here) are happy or even desperate to become ever more visible. What is so different about this visibility compared to say village life, is the speed, range and detail of it (Baudrillard 1995: 46–7). It's all happening in real time, where 'votre pensée est immédiatement codée par l'ordinateur' ['your thought is instantly coded by computer'] (*ibid.*: 46). Digital technology, itself the product of an epistemic shift to 'the digital' permits us to approach the ironically named 'real time' dream of total communication. Its drive to perfection is also part of this, as machinery strives towards heights of definition never imagined (and for which our eyes did not evolve). Audio and video reach peak after peak, allowing media companies to charge the same amount for newly formatted product as the cost of the old format when it was new. This perfection is the removal of listening and viewing. Sound and vision are replaced by something that has no analogue in the analogue world (1995: 51). The ultimate version (thus far) is CGI, where Baudrillard's vision of the absence of a referent has been made real (Baudrillard 2004: 81).

Baudrillard's reading of how new media technologies interact, and how they are received is very one-dimensional – what is odd about so much CGI in incredibly expensive films (such as the 2008 remake of *The Day the Earth Stood Still*, estimated budget $80 million) is how obviously they are animations, to the point where they have their own mysterious, dreamlike quality. His argument is more effective when we connect media technologies with the drive to visibility, where it is an unquestioned 'good' to be informatically visible. Baudrillard had already noted this relentless positivity in his *La Transparence du Mal*, where he notes how transparency as rhetoric is the way in which goodness is signalled: seeing all somehow equals democratic control. Returning to this fallacy in his last published book of essays, *Le Pacte de lucidité*, he reminds us of the need to resist the sinister charm of positivity and introduce problems, failures, secrets into 'the system' (that is, of simulation). Even supposedly transgressive material falls into the trap of visibility, equating graphic depiction with a clarity of subversion (Baudrillard has been complaining in this vein since the late 1970s). Leaving aside films that have been spiced up by prurient conservatives calling them 'torture porn' (that is, simple horror films with physical violence), we might consider Gunther von Hagens' preserved corpses that travel round 'performing' in *Bodies – The Exhibition.* Here what seem to be flayed bodies are on display, in different poses, maintained through 'plastination' where acetone has replaced body fluids. The show, which on occasion is led by von Hagen's performing of dissections, tickles both the educative part of high-definition reality, and the part that is interested in the uncanny, the threatening. Both sides are annulled in the spectacle of visibility itself.

Reality TV, meanwhile, has showed people dying (internet media have recently been very active here), having operations, inspecting their excrement with an 'expert' – you think of it, it is going on somewhere as reality TV, in a pathetic remake of the Nietzschean view that if nothing is true, everything is possible. The closer we (apparently) get to full reality, the less access we have to illusion, which, for Baudrillard, is the source of creativity. This would suggest a future for art, but Baudrillard has an odd take on this. illusion seems to be so abstract, it cannot be harnessed. Despite this, a surprisingly simple form of resistance is possible: photography.

The category of the image is a special one: in *Simulacres et simulation*, Baudrillard equates all human history as a sequence of thinking and living through different models of what an image is (1981: 17). The image is not just part of our modern simulation, but something specific is happening to it in the contemporary era. Contrary to appearances, it is being destroyed: 'nous tuons les images par le sens' ['we are killing images through meaning'] (2004: 78). The attribution of meaning is removing an almost mystical power from 'the image', and it becomes merely a vehicle for the total visibility of 'integral reality' (*ibid.*: 79). The single image, particularly photographic, is the container of something that escapes meaning, that suggests worlds beyond itself and the one that is the ever flatter 'real world', and this was best done in 'analogique' ['analogue'] (*ibid.*) form. This is because it has a mysterious relation to a referent, rather than being generated by code.

Baudrillard sees the photograph the same way Barthes did in his 1964 essay 'La Rhétorique de l'image' (Barthes 1982: 25–42). The photographic image opens up a narrative and a narrative relation to the viewer (see his *La Chambre claire* on this) in a way that any other narration (for example, in novels, films) precludes. For both writers, the realness of what is shown in the photograph is only a lure, it is the suggestiveness of the photographic image that counts. At the same time, for Baudrillard, it the emptiness of this image that counts, as he believes the mechanical (not electronic) production of an image results in a 'prototype de la littéralité du monde affranchie de la main de l'homme' ['prototype of the literality of a world freed from the hand of man'] (2004: 85). This means the resultant image is part of the 'radical illusion' of the world (*ibid.*), a paradoxical way of getting back to the world. Instead of reproducing the world, what gets reproduced is the absence of reality, the basic illusory quality of the world.

Despite its Nietzschean perversity, this is a very literal view of what photography does, but, despite that, it could be a way of thinking about contemporary photography, by, say Cindy Sherman, Andreas Gursky or countless other art photographers, but Baudrillard seemingly has no interest in anyone else thinking this through, through their photographs. He is interested in himself using photography to summon illusion. This is not just hubris on his part, it is is also a strong, if implicit, claim, that photography is about the practice of it, rather than the art critical reading of it: 'The joy of taking photographs is an objective delight. Whoever has not experienced the objective rapture of the image one morning in town or desert will never in any way understand the pataphysical refinement of the world' (Baudrillard 1999: 129). It would be going too far to see a 'praxis' here, but if it is not exactly theory meeting practice, it is practice mirroring theory. Typically, Baudrillard's photographs are of very banal subjects: empty rooms, small details of objects or interiors, fences, walls, car parks – all in saturated colours and very crisp (see Baudrillard 1999). His photographs leave us with a sense of a super-saturated reality, with simulation outsimulated, made more seductive, made more illusory. This is what to look for when looking for the last traces of visual culture (in Baudrillard's world). Everywhere else it has been swallowed up in the flat totality of simulated reality.

References

Ballard, J.G. (2006) *Kingdom Come*, London: Fourth Estate.
Barthes, R. (1980) *La Chambre claire: Note sur la photographie*, Paris : Gallimard.
—— (1982) *L'Obvie et l'obtus: Essais critiques III*, Paris: Le Seuil.
Baudrillard, J. (1968), *Le Système des objets*, Paris: Gallimard.
—— (1970) *La Société de consommation*, Paris: Denoël.
—— (1972) *Pour une critique de l'économie politique du signe*, Paris: Gallimard.
—— (1973) *Le Miroir de la production*, Paris: Casterman.
—— (1976) *L'Échange symbolique et la mort*, Paris: Gallimard.
—— (1979) *De la séduction*, Paris: Denoël/Gonthier.
—— (1981) *Simulacres et simulation*, Paris: Galilée.
—— (1990) *La Transparence du Mal*, Paris: Galilée.
—— (1992) *L'Illusion de la fin*, Paris: Galilée.
—— (1993) *The Transparency of Evil*, London: Verso.
—— (1995) *Le Crime parfait*, Paris: Galilée.
—— (1997) *Écran total*, Paris: Galilée.
—— (1999) *Sur la photographie*, Paris: Sens & Tonka.
—— (2000) *The Vital Illusion*, New York, Columbia University Press.
—— (2001) *Télémorphose*, Paris: Sens & Tonka.
—— (2004) *Le Pacte de lucidité*, Paris: Galilée.
—— and Nouvel, J. (2000), *Les Objets singuliers: Architecture et philosophie*, Paris: Calmann-Lévy.
Derrida, J. (1967) *De la Grammatologie*, Paris: Minuit.
Foucault, M. (1976) *Histoire de la sexualité vol I: La volonté de savoir*, Paris: Gallimard.
Grace, V. (2000) *Baudrillard's Challenge: A Feminist Reading*, London: Routledge.
Hegarty, P. (2004) *Jean Baudrillard*, London and New York, Continuum.
—— (2008) 'Constructing (in) the "Real" World: Simulation and Architecture in Baudrillard', *French Cultural Studies* 19(3) (Oct.), 317–31.

Jameson, F. (1991) *Postmodernism, or the Cultural Logic of Late Capitalism*, London: Verso.
Merrin, W. (2005) *Baudrillard and the Media: A Critical Introduction*, Cambridge: Polity.
Proto, F. (ed.) (2006) *Mass Identity Architecture: Architectural Writings of Jean Baudrillard*, Chichester: Wiley.

Notes

1 William Merrin engages in a detailed and convincing reading of *The Matrix*, noting connections to Baudrillard that are more interesting than the explicit referencing of the Wachowskis (2005: 116–27).
2 See also Baudrillard 1986 (81–91), on functionality.
3 Baudrillard offers a historicized, technologically driven version of Derrida's reading of Rousseau in *De la Grammatologie* (Derrida 1967: 203–34).
4 'N'importe quel déchet fait fonction d'œuvre d'art' (Baudrillard 1995: 50) ['Any piece of rubbish can act as a work of art']. See also 'Le Complot d'art' (Baudrillard 1997: 205–9). Even where he deals with a specific artist, as he does with Sophie Calle, in 'Suite vénitienne' ['Pursuit in Venice'], the art is a simple window to philosophical speculation about identity, that is, content without form.
5 The years since the mid-1990s have seen an explosion in galleries and museums that outdo their contents and become the aesthetic object being visited (such as the Guggenheim in Bilbao).
6 For more on Baudrillard's views on architecture, see Baudrillard and Nouvel (2000), Proto (2006) and Hegarty (2008).
7 See also his comments on Disneyland providing a similar alibi for the rest of the USA (1981: 26–7).
8 Baudrillard rates this film ahead of *The Matrix* for that very reason (see Hegarty 2004: 140).
9 I will not be dealing in any depth with the sexual politics of this book. For this, see Grace (2000).
10 'Illusion is the general rule of the universe; reality is but an exception' (Baudrillard 2000: 72).

13

Real Time: Bernard Stiegler and the politics of digitalisation

Arthur Bradley

Bernard Stiegler (1952–) is arguably the most original and important French philosopher of technology, media and visual culture to have emerged over the course of the last two decades. He is Director of the Department of Cultural Development at the Centre Georges Pompidou; co-founder of the political group Ars Industrialis and the prolific author of many works such as the multi-volume *De la misère symbolique* [*Of Symbolic Poverty*] and *Mécréance et discredit* [*Non-belief and Discredit*]. It is, however, for his magnum opus *La Technique et le temps* [*Technics and Time*] ([1994] 1998) that Stiegler remains best known in the anglophone world.[1] To put it very simply, Stiegler's entire philosophy is based on a radically new concept of *la technique* (technics) as the originary and fundamental condition of human evolution, culture and philosophy. According to Aristotle's *Physics*, of course, what we call 'technē' [τέχνη] is nothing more than a '*prosthesis*': a tool or instrument that requires an efficient cause [*causa efficiens*] to set it in motion.[2] However, it is precisely this ancient idea of technics – an inert, neutral instrument deployed for the sake of some end external to it – that Stiegler seeks to challenge. For Stiegler, we cannot oppose humanity and technology as if they were entirely separate entities: each only comes into existence through the other. If we tend to define human nature either biologically (as a particular kind of species) or philosophically (as a soul, mind or consciousness), Stiegler argues that humanity is in fact constituted by our relation to technical instruments, systems and structures: we exist by putting more and more of ourselves – skills, memories and consciousness – outside ourselves. In this sense, Stiegler's philosophy of technology might better be described as a new anthropology or even ontology – a science of being in general.

It is not my intention in what follows to offer an account of Stiegler's theory of 'technics' in general – such accounts are now readily available elsewhere – but rather of a specific set of technologies. As we will see, Stiegler is (for all the vast conceptual scope of his philosophy of technology), also an increasingly influential theorist of concrete empirical technologies, and particularly, of visual technologies: writing; photography; cinema; the internet; analogue and digital environments. First, and most obviously, Stiegler's philosophy of 'originary' technicity can be seen as an empirical retooling of Jacques Derrida's famous account of the *arche*-writing, *différance* or supplementation that precedes and underwrites the metaphysical oppositions between nature and culture, the animal and the human. If Derrida articulates a quasi-transcendental *logic* of the supplement – witness, for example, the famous reading of Rousseau in *De la grammatologie* (1967: 203–34) – Stiegler seeks to construct a material *genealogy* of specific, concrete supplements such as tools, alphabetic writing and photography. Perhaps the most significant example of this genealogical approach would be the second volume of *La Technique et le temps – La Désorientation* [*Disorientation*] (1996) – which (in a manner reminiscent of Régis Debray's genealogy of the visual, discussed by Andy Stafford in Chapter 7 in this volume) traces the evolution of mnemo-techniques from the emergence of alphabetic writing via photography all the way up to the digital image. For Stiegler, in fact, the status of the digital image in contemporary society is not simply an aesthetic or even an ontological question but is increasingly one of the most urgent *political* questions we face.

In what follows, I would like to give a conceptual overview of Stiegler's philosophy of technology with particular reference to his phenomenology of the digital image. To begin with, I will briefly recapitulate the central thesis of Stiegler's ongoing project *La technique et le temps*, namely, that there is an essential and constitutive relation between technical prostheses and the human capacity to 'temporalise' (or phenomenologically organise) time. Second, I will focus on Stiegler's increasingly apocalyptic diagnosis of the political implications of this essential relation between technics and time in the contemporary moment. For Stiegler, contemporary capitalism produces what he calls the 'industrialisation' of memory, temporal objects and consciousness: the human capacity to temporalise – itself inherently technical – is now subject to an economic act of appropriation that is without parallel in history. Perhaps the most obvious example of this is the programming of 'live' or 'Real Time' phenomena by the globalised film or television industry which, in his account, collapses the complex human temporalisations of time, as with Baudrillard on Disney, into an endless synthetic present time that can only be consumed passively and uncritically. Finally, and in more detail, I will home in on a specific example of this industrialisation of time: the digital image. On the one hand, Stiegler argues that the digital image represents the paradigmatic site of the techno-capitalist industrialisation of memory. On the other, however, it also creates the conditions for what Stiegler calls a new meta-critical culture that turns passive consumers of the visual image into critical viewers or even into potential image-makers or producers themselves. Such, we will see, are the political stakes of living in Real Time.

1

First, I will describe the broad trajectory of Stiegler's philosophical project as it emerges in his earliest and arguably still best-known work: *La Technique et le temps 1* ([1994] 1998). It is helpful, as a point of entry, to focus on the reason why Stiegler chooses to name this volume *La Faute d'Épiméthée* [*The Fault of Epimetheus*] (Stiegler [1994] 1998: 185–203). To be sure, everyone knows the story of Prometheus – the Titan who steals fire from the Gods – but the role played by his idiotic brother Epimetheus in this narrative has been largely forgotten even though it scarcely makes sense without him. According to Plato's account in the *Protagoras*, the two brothers are ordered by the gods to equip each mortal species with different powers or qualities (*dynameis*) to enable them to survive, but Epimetheus rashly persuades Prometheus to let him do the job himself (Plato 2004: 16–18, 320c–322a). Now, in his haste Epimetheus forgets to allocate any powers at all to human beings – leaving them entirely naked and defenceless – and so Prometheus is forced to steal the gift of skill in the arts (*technai*) from Hephaestus and Athena by way of compensation for this loss. For Stiegler, this mythopoeic account of the origin of man contains a crucial insight into the status of the human that will form the basis of his own philosophy. In Stiegler's account, humanity is constituted by an originary *lack* of defining qualities allegorised by the Epimethean error: this is what he calls our necessary 'default' of origin [*le défaut qu'il faut d'origine*]. What, then, comes to fill this originary lack?

It is actually possible to give a one word answer to this question: *epiphylogenesis*. According to Stiegler, we can distinguish between three different layers of memory: *genetic* memory (which is the biological memory that is programmed into our DNA); *epigenetic* memory (which refers to the experience we acquire during our lifetime and is stored in the central nervous system) and, finally, *epiphylogenetic* memory, which is embodied in technical systems or artefacts like tools, cave paintings, archives and so on. Yet, Stiegler contends that humans are the only living beings who possess this third form of memory: we alone among all life forms have the ability to record, stockpile and transmit our experiences to others in the form of technical artefacts (Stiegler [1994] 1998: 40, 176–7). In Stiegler's eyes, what defines humanity is nothing other than this Promethean process of externalising life onto non-living apparatuses: we are our own outside.[3] If he pursues this argument in many different directions – from Rousseau's mythology of the state of nature, through the palaeontology of André Leroi-Gourhan to the fundamental ontology of Martin Heidegger – Stiegler's most far-reaching thesis is that there is an essential relation between technics and the human experience of time: technical artefacts embody our knowledge of the past and open up the possibility of the future. Perhaps most importantly, however, they also entail the awareness that human time is *finite*. On the one hand, technics embodies the past by enabling us to experience individually what we have never naturally lived: I can, for example, read something (a letter, postcard or book) written by someone long before I was born. On the other, technics opens the possibility of the future by making it possible for us to preserve our own experiences beyond our natural life for generations to come: I can, in the same way, write something (a letter, an email, a book) that is capable of being read long after my own death. For Stiegler, epiphylogenesis represents a quasi-Lamarckian theory of 'artificial selection' where successive genetic and epigenetic experiences are selected, accumulated and transmitted from generation to generation in the form of technical objects. In this sense, Stiegler is able to conclude that technics is '*constitutive*' of temporality (*ibid.*: 17).

For Stiegler, this originary technicity is also the basis for a thoroughgoing rereading or 'deconstruction' of the Western philosophical tradition from Plato to Derrida and beyond. It is Stiegler's contention that the history of Western philosophy is nothing other than the history of the Epimethean 'forgetting' of its technical origins: 'Epimetheus is not simply the forgetful one ... he is also the one who is forgotten. The forgotten of metaphysics' (*ibid.*: 186). According to the first volume of *La Technique et le temps*, Western thought consistently transforms the technical constitution *of* human temporalisation into a series of metaphysical oppositions *between* technics and time that relegates the latter to a purely incidental or supplemental position. To put it crudely, Stiegler argues that the philosophy of time has always sought to oppose two ideas of time: a pure, primary and technics-free time versus a secondary, corrupt, technological time. First, of course, Plato sets Western metaphysics in motion by opposing the divine recollection of the immortal soul [*anamnēsis*] to artificial memory [*hypomnēsis*] in the *Meno*. However, this gesture can be traced all the way up to the epoch of the supposed closure of metaphysics, Stiegler argues. Just as Plato opposes *anamnēsis* to *hypomnēsis*, so Marx, for instance, opposes the qualitative time of labour to the empty quantitative time of capital; Bergson opposes clock-time to *la durée*; Husserl opposes the primary retention of the temporal object to the secondary memory of it, Heidegger opposes ontological time to vulgar countable time and, last but not least, Benjamin, Levinas, the later Derrida and now Giorgio Agamben oppose an incalculable messianic time to homogenous historical or chronological time. If, however, Stiegler is right to say that technical recording systems are the basis for the human experience of temporalisation as such – no retention of the past and no anticipation of the future without technics – then such attempts to pit two concepts of time against one another are revealed to be nothing more than the most dogmatic Platonism. Such, at least, is the remarkable wager on which *La Technique et le temps* stakes everything: all time – whether anamnesic or hypomnesic, qualitative or quantitative, calculable or incalculable, messianic or historical – is technical all the way down.

What provisional remarks can we make about Stiegler's philosophy of technology before we go any further? It is well known that his corpus has received a somewhat mixed reception in both the francophone and the anglophone philosophical community over the last decade or so which accuse it of everything from a phenomenological or linguistic idealism to a reductive Marxian materialism or determinism. As I have already hinted, the vast majority of this criticism surrounds what is, in my view at least, the single most original, if fraught, aspect of Stiegler's work: its reworking of the empirico-transcendental opposition between technics and time. On the one hand, the Derrida scholar Geoffrey Bennington charges Stiegler with offering a reductive, technologically determinist and scientifically positivist account of Husserl, Heidegger, Derrida and the (post-)phenomenological tradition more widely: he confuses a 'valid and necessary claim about originary technicity' derived from Derrida's account of *arche*-writing with 'a positivistic claim about techno-science' (Bennington 1996: 175–216). On the other hand, the embodiment theorist Mark B. N. Hansen has accused Stiegler of not going far enough in his materialist critique of Derrida, Heidegger and the phenomenological tradition: he remains complicit in the idealist disembodiment of 'a richly and multiply embodied experience' (2004: 584–626). Either Stiegler is guilty of illicitly reducing a quasi-transcendental logic to a state of matter, it would seem, or of falsely elevating a state of matter into a transcendental logic. To be sure, Stiegler's philosophy is not unproblematic (as we will see in the remainder of this discussion) but in his defence, we might reply that such empirico-transcendental doubling is less an unwitting *confusion* than an (exhaustively worked-out) argument that, regardless of its ultimate merits, at least deserves to be taken seriously. Perhaps Stiegler's almost contradictory philosophical reception – where he is simultaneously criticised for being excessively transcendentalist *and* empiricist or not empiricist or transcendentalist *enough* – might be a symptom of what is really going on in his thought: a reorganisation of the empirico-transcendental opposition in terms of the technicity of temporalisation. Such a complex field of force cannot be reduced to one side of the empirico-transcendental opposition because, as we have seen, what it describes is a dynamic, recursive and mutually constitutive relation between man and matter where neither holds the secret to the other: 'the human inventing the technical, the technical inventing the human' (Stiegler [1994] 1998: 137).[4] If *La Technique et le temps* is capable of generating such a diametrically opposed set of readings, in other words, it may be because all his critics are (at least half-) right: what Stiegler calls the constitutive technicity of time demands *both* a quasi-transcendental logic of technicity *and* a quasi-empirical history of technical supplements at one and the same time. In my own view, Stiegler's twin-track approach in *La Technique et le temps* – oscillating back and forth between transcendental critique (metaphysics, phenomenology, deconstruction) and empirical history (evolutionary biology, palaeontology, techno-science) without ever coming to rest in one or the other – might most profitably be seen as a kind of (post-) Derridaean double reading: what is taking place throughout is an attempt to articulate an aporia of origin – *le défaut qu'il faut d'origine* – which is neither inside philosophy nor outside it (Bradley 2011).

2

Second, and with the broad outline of Stiegler's project in place, I would now like to turn in more detail to the contemporary political implications of the technical constitution of temporalisation. It is generally agreed that the second volume of *La Technique et le temps* is written in a different register from the first: we move from a set of fairly abstract philosophical discussions to a series of pointed empirical and sociological analyses of specific technologies. As Stiegler himself rehearses it, the question of *why* technics and time are co-related has already been answered, so we must now turn to the matter of *how* that co-relation plays itself out across, and as, history ([1994] 1998: 15). Yet, once again, it would be a little reductive to see this empirical turn as simply the post hoc application of a pre-existing transcendental logic – in the same way that, say, Hegel's *Logic* paves the way for his *History* and *Nature* – for it would never have been possible to articulate the 'why' of originary technicity in the first place without the 'how' of empirical technics. For Stiegler, then, it is quite simply essential to trace the evolution of empirical technics from the emergence of alphabetic writing through the printing press, photography and phonography all the way up to the epoch of digitalisation in order to bear out his overarching thesis. On the one hand, he argues that the process of technogenesis is defined by what he calls an ever-increasing 'orthography' [*orthographie*] of inscription: each new mnemo-technique affords a greater exactitude of preservation of the past and anticipation of the future. On the other, however, he also insists that the evolution of ever more exact forms of technics also produces a massive and globalised disorientation [*désorientation*]: each new form of technology increasingly and violently collapses the difference between past and future into a technically produced and determined 'now'. In Stiegler's thought, as we will see, this process of disorientation is embodied in the evolution of so-called 'Real Time' ['temps réel'] media.

It is important to fill in a little of the phenomenological background to Stiegler's critique of 'Real Time' technologies if we are to appreciate its political force. According to Edmund Husserl's *Lectures on the Phenomenology of Internal Time Consciousness* (1905), what we call the 'now' of perception is in fact a synthesis of the retention of what has just passed (the no longer now) and the protention of what is about to arrive (the not yet now) (Husserl 1964: 50–1). To exemplify this argument, Husserl gives a phenomenological account of what happens when we listen to a melody: he says that we are simultaneously remembering the note just passed and anticipating the note to come when we listen to any individual note of the tune. Just as we do not hear one note at a time when we listen to a piece of music, Husserl argues, so we do not perceive time as an endless series of discrete present moments or 'nows'. If Husserl's classic analysis of the human process of temporalisation recognises that what we call the 'present' of perception is always a synthesis of past and future, Jacques Derrida argues that the phenomenologist does not fully capitalise upon his own insight: Husserl still stresses the originary 'present' impression at the expense of the retentions and protentions that also comprise the process of perception. For Derrida, Husserl's phenomenology of time depends upon a problematic and ultimately unsustainable opposition between what he calls 'primary retention' – the recollection of the note 'just-passed' that, as we have seen, is included in the 'now' of listening to a melody – and 'secondary retention': this is the longer memory we may have of listening to the same melody yesterday, a memory I can hear again in my imagination today, but which (on Husserl's account at least) plays no role in the theatre of perception. In Derrida's view, Husserl's decision to include the 'just-passed' in the process of temporalisation inevitably opens the door for the entry of secondary memory and imagination as well and, with them, the deconstruction of the residual metaphysics of his phenomenology of time: what still seems to be the experience of a living, immediate, if distributed, present in Husserl turns out to be shot through with the absence that is the absolute historical past (Derrida 1973).

For Stiegler, Derrida's critique of Husserl's opposition between primary and secondary retention is axiomatic but, as he argues in *La Désorientation*, it is lacking in one crucial respect: what neither Husserl nor Derrida appreciate is that there is a *third* form of retention at play in the phenomenology of time. To put it in a word, this third or 'tertiary' memory is what we have earlier called our 'epiphylogenetic' memory. Neither the primary retention of what has just passed nor the secondary retention of what happened yesterday or last week, tertiary memory is the technical retention of experiences *we have not personally lived through* but which nonetheless can be actualised by us in our conscious lives. Why, then, does tertiary memory perform such a constitutive role in our experience of time? First, Stiegler insists that – contra Husserl – what we call primary retention is *always* contaminated by secondary memory. If I listen to the same melody two, three or four times in a row,

I will hear something slightly different each time: this is why I can say that a good piece of music 'grows' on me with repeated hearings. What is happening here is that the *secondary* memory of the first hearing is influencing the *primary* retention of the second hearing: the secondary memory forms what Stiegler calls the 'criteria' or 'horizon of expectation' from *out of which* the primary retention is able to select what to retain in every new hearing. Now, Stiegler wishes to take this argument one step further by arguing that this secondary memory is itself contaminated by what Husserl calls 'image consciousness' or *tertiary* memory. Given what Heidegger calls our finitude – the fact that we are thrown into a world that is not of our making – consciousness cannot simply be constitutive *of* its objects but must be constituted *by* them: I am the product not simply of my own life experiences but of experiences that were not lived by me – tradition, culture, habitus – but that I have retained and reactivated through mnemo-technical systems. Such tertiary memories form my horizon of expectation: they are the criteria that I use to select what to retain in every new perception (Stiegler 1996: 258). Perhaps the best example of this in the current context is that the entire phenomenological architecture of internal time consciousness could not have been constructed before the epoch of phonographic recording: it is only because we have the power to listen to *the exact same melody many times in succession* that we can begin to articulate the interplay of primary, secondary and tertiary memories (*ibid.*: 257). The differences we perceive between repeated hearings of the same melody when a live performer sings one song several times in a row, for instance, can always be attributed to the minute but ineradicable variations in the performance itself. This possible explanation can be ruled out when we listen repeatedly to a phonographic recording of the same song, however, because we know that any perceptible differences cannot reside on the side of the object. Why else, in other words, can what we know to be *an identical temporal object* be temporalised so differently every time we hear it – if not that the primary retention of each new hearing is actively selecting from a secondary and tertiary horizon of expectation? Just as primary retention is conditioned by secondary retention, then, so this condition *is itself conditioned* by the possibility of exact repetition afforded by tertiary forms of retention. In this way, Stiegler is able to conclude that tertiary memory forms the ground for the human temporalisation of time: 'This is true in general, but the tertiary recollection that is the phonogram makes it obvious' (Stiegler 2007: 33).

In his later work, however, Stiegler begins to stress the *political* stakes of tertiary memory in increasingly dire, even apocalyptic, terms: we are in the midst of nothing less than a war of, and for, memory. It is Stiegler's contention, remember, that the unique strength of the human race is its ability to exteriorise itself: we put more and more of our memory, knowledge and capacity into external technical apparatuses. At the same time, though, this exteriority is also humanity's greatest vulnerability, because *whoever controls such tertiary memory systems necessarily also controls the human experience of time* (*ibid.*: 17). To Stiegler's eyes, the contemporary epoch is thus characterised by what he calls the 'industrialization' of time, memory and desire (Stiegler 1996: 119–216). During the eighteenth- and nineteenth-century Industrial Revolution, it was only labour power that was the subject of technological subsumption but in the twentieth- and twenty-first century it is nothing less than consciousness itself. On the one hand, we can see this revolution in the global commodification of tertiary memory systems like films, radio and television programmes: Hollywood, in particular, and America in general, effectively monopolises the criteria by which the world temporalises time. On the other, we can also witness it at work in what Foucault and later Giorgio Agamben call bio-politics: the politicisation of life itself by the technoscientific control of biological or cognitive processes. However, the single most pervasive index of the techno-capitalist industrialisation of memory for Stiegler is the proliferation of what are called 'live' [*en directe*] or 'Real Time' technologies.[5] From live television or radio programmes, through digital streaming of images on the internet, all the way up to locative media accessible through wireless networks and handheld interfaces, Real Time claims to offer something quite without parallel in the history of media: the absolute simultaneity of recording and transmission. Why, though, do 'live' media pose such an existential threat to the human temporalisation of time? For Stiegler, everything seems to hinge on the fact that Real Time is not *really time*: what we perceive to be happening 'live' or immediately when we watch television is, of course, actually the product of a technological synthesis operating so quickly that it is below the minimal threshold of phenomenological time consciousness (Stiegler 1996: 78). Just as we cannot register the discrete twenty-four frames that comprise a single second of cinematic time, in other words, so the infinitesimal differences between recording and transmission that comprise the time of, say, a live radio or television programme are not accessible to our perceptual ratios. Perhaps more importantly, however, Stiegler argues that Real Time thereby collapses the critical gap between primary retention and secondary/tertiary memory and, with it, the possibility of selecting what to retain and what not to retain in perception. If I listen to a melody yesterday, I will have a horizon of expectation from which to select when I hear it again today, but when I watch or listen to a programme in Real Time there is no 'yesterday', no possibility of stopping, or slowing down, or reflecting upon, what I have seen and heard – just a permanent, continuous, live 'now' that has always already selected my primary retentions for me (*ibid.*: 148–9, 277). Such is the position of the consumer in the age of industrial reproducibility: what we represent today is nothing less than a new proletariat condemned to consume time mechanically, indiscriminately and destructively (Stiegler 2004).[6]

What, if we may pause briefly once more, are we to make of Stiegler's politics of technology? It might seem difficult, at face value, to square the apparent technophilia of Stiegler's ontology – which consistently stresses that there is *nothing* outside technics (Stiegler [1994] 1998: 14) least of all humanity – with the seeming technophobia of his politics. As Jean-Michel Salanskis argues in one of the most rich and insightful francophone reviews of *La Technique et le temps*, Stiegler's thesis that time is, at bottom, technical seems to be forgotten among an almost classically Heideggerian or even Marxian critique of contemporary technology from the vantage point of some more primordial 'human' time (Salanskis 2000: 235–78). Nowhere is this (Epimethean?) forgetting more problematic than in the critique of Real Time, which seems to fly in the face of everything Stiegler has told us thus far about time. To put it bluntly, why – if *all* temporalisation is conducted through tertiary memory – is Real Time any less 'real' than, say, the time afforded by analogue recording, alphabetic writing or even the first flint tool? First, then, I wish to flag up a concern that will reappear in the final section of this chapter: Stiegler may well leave himself open to the very charge he levels against the history of metaphysics by appearing to valorise one simple, homogeneous and a-historical time of consciousness over and against technicised time. Such a valorisation is, as we will see, particularly manifest in his consistent stress on *temporisation*, on delaying or slowing down the speed of the technical synthesis of Real Time, until it coincides with the perceptual synthesis that makes criticism possible. However, it is important to be clear about what Stiegler is – and is not – saying about the industrialisation of time before we attempt to question, or criticise, it. For me, Stiegler's real target in his critique of Real Time technology cannot simply be the de-temporalising power of the technology itself – such de-temporalisation itself represents a new, and entirely unprecedented, mode of temporalisation – so much as its *hegemony over temporalisation* (Stiegler 1996: 165): Real Time monopolises both the production and consumption of tertiary memory today and, with it, the human experience of time.[7] Just as Heidegger's much-misunderstood critique of *das Gestell* [enframing] is really inspired by its stranglehold over the process of *alētheia* [unconcealment] – rather than some romantic nostalgia or technophobia – so Stiegler's critique of Real Time concerns its monopolisation over the processes of temporalisation: Real Time leaves us with no other way of temporalising time (Heidegger 1977: 27).[8] Perhaps the real difference between Stiegler and Heidegger, although this is the subject of another essay, would concern the *technicity* of temporalisation itself: Stiegler would insist that what Heidegger calls the essence [*Wesen*] of technology – the process of presencing by which it comes into unconcealment and which is deemed to absolutely precede ontic technology – is *itself given technically* (Stiegler, 1996: 205). Finally, though, Stiegler's constant emphasis upon the irreducibly technical constitution of time also raises the crucial question of what – if anything – can be done about the temporal crisis generated by Real Time technologies. If Heidegger's belief that ontological time is simply more originary than technical time means that he can take for granted the possibility of obtaining a free relationship to *das Gestell* – even if it is one that currently remains obscure to the questioner – Stiegler is compelled to find a solution to the problem of Real Time from within the possibilities afforded by technical time itself. In other words, Stiegler can only resist the contemporary hegemony of Real Time technologies by appealing, not to some allegedly pre-technical Heideggerian 'piety of thinking', but to the evolution of new forms of technicisation that, in turn, make possible new forms of temporalisation.

3

Finally, then, I wish to offer a brief assessment of Stiegler's attempt to construct what he calls a new 'politics of memory' [*politique de la mémoire*] which is capable of resisting the industrialisation of memory embodied by Real Time media. It is important to begin, though, by recalling once again his abiding thesis that there is a constitutive relation between technics and temporalisation and, thus, whatever political import his thought possesses must necessarily flow from this premise.

As we have just seen, Stiegler argues that any critical response to technics must arise from *within* the absolutely specific technological condition it seeks to address rather than through an appeal to some ontological ground apparently uncontaminated by technics such as Heideggerian Being. For Stiegler, what defines our own technological epoch is digitalisation and, consequently, a great deal of his philosophy is concerned with articulating the positive, critical and creative possibilities afforded by the emergence of new digital environments. Just as every revolution in technology carries with it a concomitant revolution in temporalisation – from the fabrication of the first flint axe to the taking of the first photograph – so, too, he argues, the digital revolution makes possible new ways of synthesising time. In Stiegler's account then (what we might call a digital *pharamakon* following Derrida, combining both poison and remedy) it is to the very media that generated the crisis of Real Time in the first place – by arrogating all power over temporalisation to technology – that we must look in order to reassert a measure of human agency over the way we experience time. So, how does Stiegler substantiate such a claim?

It is possible to find one – albeit very speculative and provisional – answer to this question in Stiegler's filmed interviews with his mentor Derrida which were published in abridged form as *Echographies de la télévision* [*Echographies of Television*] (Derrida and Stiegler 2002). As this fascinating set of exchanges makes clear, Derrida and Stiegler are agreed upon the fundamental threat posed by digitalisation: what Real Time technologies preside over is the de-temporalisation of the complex tissue of protentions and retentions that comprise the phenomenology of time (Derrida and Stiegler 2002: 129). Yet, as Richard Beardsworth notes, where the two philosophers appear to differ is upon the question of how this de-temporalisation can be *re-temporalised* – how we can invent new ways of temporalising time that break the stranglehold of Real Time – and this critical difference also helps to clarify Stiegler's own politics (Beardsworth 1998). To be sure, Derrida himself always acknowledges that a politics of technology cannot simply be a 'spectatorial critique, a theoretical vigilance' (Derrida and Stiegler 2002: 63) – which presumes that it can somehow stand outside of what it criticising – but, nonetheless, he frequently depicts the critique of Real Time as principally a *philosophical* task in which technics does not meaningfully participate: 'Any such demonstration already appeals, in and of itself, to philosophy' (*ibid.*: 5). If Derrida calls upon philosophy alone to solve the problem of Real Time, it may be because – for all his critiques of

Heideggerian ontology – there is still an element within deconstruction that sees empirical technology as a second-order manifestation of an a priori philosophical logic or condition, namely, *différance*: 'The real time effect is itself a particular effect of "différance"' (*ibid.*: 129). For Stiegler, though, Derrida's deconstruction of technology would risk falling into the same trap as Heidegger's questioning after technology: both create a philosophical *deus ex machina* which somehow stands above technology – whether it be ontological time or the quasi-transcendental condition of possibility of time called *différance* – and to which we can appeal in order to pass judgement upon technology's vicissitudes. In the later Derrida's appeals to a 'messianism without messianism' – the advent of an incalculable ethical alterity that is simply *inimical to* technological calculability – this philosophical piety arguably reaches its logical conclusion (Bradley 2006).

Such a (quasi-)transcendental solution is, of course, out of the question in Stiegler's philosophy: the essence of technology is nothing but technological. It is this message that comes through very strongly in his own contribution to *Echographies of Television* which is an essay entitled 'The Discrete Image' ['*L'image discrète*'] (Derrida and Stiegler 2002: 145–63). At the core of this essay, we find the argument that the widespread dissemination of new media, publicly available technological archives, together with advanced techniques of editing, manipulation and consumption create the space for a new 'critical culture' of the image capable of 'discretising' or breaking down the apparent continuity of Real Time syntheses into its component parts. First, and most crucially, Stiegler argues that the very possibility of the digital image carries with it a radical phenomenological uncertainty concerning the existence of its *noemata*. If Roland Barthes ([1980] 1981) argued that all photography (regardless of its actual authenticity) conjures up a spontaneous belief in the 'reality' of its referent – because an analogue photograph is literally the imprint of the photons emanating from its 'noeme' – Stiegler insists that this belief has been thrown into crisis by the emergence of the digital image. However, such a crisis (*krisis*) is also the space in which a new critical culture of the image (*krinein*, to judge or discern) can emerge, one capable of challenging the industrialisation of temporality. For Stiegler, the digital image – where photons are pixelated and then converted into a binary code which is permanently open to manipulation – paves the way for a new critical phenomenology of the reality claims of all imagery: '*A more knowing belief, and by the same token, a less insipid and credulous one: this is what the things we fear about the analogico-digital photo would also make possible*' (Derrida and Stiegler 2002: 152, Stiegler's emphasis). Now, the most important aspect of this 'knowing belief' that digitalisation makes possible is its capacity to interrupt the 'reality effect' (*effet de réel*) generated by Real Time recording and transmission and, thus, to restore a measure of spectatorial agency over our consumption. By giving us the power to 'discretise' the pseudo-continuous flow of Real Time imagery – whether by freezing it, rewinding it or replaying it several times in a row in order to watch it differently – new media technologies recuperate the secondary and tertiary horizon of expectation that Real Time media conflate into an all-consuming primary retention: we thus regain the critical power actively to select and organise our perceptions that the industrialisation of temporality had arrogated for itself. Perhaps most importantly, however, new media do not simply enable us to consume Real Time technologies less naively – which is to say more analytically – but even to become technological *producers* ourselves: witness, for instance, the crisis in the music industry over the last decade generated by the illegal sampling, downloading and remixing of music in the form of mash-ups (see, for example, Lévy 1998).

In summary, then, Stiegler's politics of memory would claim to be neither a Heideggerian recuperation of a forgotten Being nor the Derridean affirmation of an incalculable future but a present state in the ongoing co-invention of the human and the technical. It is, however, possible to admire the materialist force of Stiegler's logic here while still being able to detect what I earlier called a certain idealist tendency to revalorise the opposition between human and technical forms of temporalisation. According to a theorist of embodiment like Hansen, for example, Stiegler's affirmation of human temporality is actually something to be celebrated: the politics of memory enable 'personal lived consciousness' to regain enough agency to 'live time' according to 'its own rhythms' (Hansen 2006: 304). To my eyes, Stiegler's philosophy is not quite so anthropocentric as this suggests: it consistently stresses that what Hansen calls 'personal lived consciousness' is structurally constituted by what it has never personally lived and that whatever 'rhythms' it possesses are thus never purely and simply its 'own'. By the same token, we must bear in mind that whatever agency the subject possesses over its processes of temporalisation has always been given *through* technical mediation and nowhere is this more true than in the case of digitalisation: 'the grammatical operator is, above all, technology itself' (Derrida and Stiegler 2002: 161). Yet, all this being said, I do still think there is a sense in which Stiegler risks reifying the dynamic relation between the human and the technical – which co-constitute each other – into a hard and fast opposition between two discrete, mutually exclusive, entities. On the one hand, the 'who' of human time consciousness is occasionally depicted as if it were a technics-free zone existing independently of the technical synthesis: Stiegler speaks of the need to 'give time time' [*donner du temps au temps*] (*ibid.*: 86) in his discussions with Derrida as if 'time' could somehow take place outside of its technical embodiments. On the other hand, the 'what' of the technical synthesis is just as reductively depicted as an essentially inhuman operator evolving quite autonomously of human time consciousness: Stiegler somewhat tendentiously contends that Real Time technology has accelerated to the point where it no longer has any relation whatsoever to our perceptual ratios (Stiegler 1996: 160–1).[9] For me, though, Stiegler's residual idealism can perhaps best be witnessed in the constant stress he places on *temporising* the Real Time flow: giving time time (Derrida and Stiegler 2002: 86); checking or putting on the brakes [*freiner*] (*ibid.*: 77), slowing down (if it wishes to) the technical hare until the (as it were) perceptual tortoise has time to catch up. If the evolution of the technical synthesis has always implied the evolution of the spectatorial synthesis (*ibid.*: 161) – because transformations in technology always bring about transformations in perception, consciousness, memory – it is to say the least curious that the political response to Real Time should seem to be couched in terms of what we can only call *devolution*. Perhaps – although this is a question for another discussion – we can also witness something of this in Stiegler's more recent focus on taking care [*prendre soin*], paying attention to, and assuming responsibility for, the long-term transmission of knowledge as opposed to remaining caught in short-term drive-oriented consumption (Stiegler 2008). To what extent must the politics of memory necessarily be a question of *reducing* the speed of the digital synthesis of time to that of some pre-digital spectatorial synthesis or, as Derrida briefly suggests elsewhere in *Echographies*, could they not just as easily be conceived as a matter of digitally *accelerating* the spectatorial synthesis itself (Derrida and Stiegler 2002: 77)?

So, what, to draw this discussion to a close, can we conclude about Stiegler's attempt to construct a new digital politics of memory capable of interrupting the unending flow of sound and light called Real Time? To do him justice, Stiegler himself seems to make no grand claims for his own politics: '*Il ne s'agit pas de "sortir de la crise", mais d'entrer dans la critique*' ['it's not a matter of "getting out of a crisis", but of entering into a critique'] (Stiegler 1996: 171). It would be reductive – for all his critique of the globalised malaise [*mal-être*] induced by global industrialised consumption – to see Stiegler as merely a latter day member of the Frankfurt School bemoaning a new culture industry. As Hansen again argues (2006: 305), Stiegler does not succumb to the 'utopian hope (or delusion) that new media would somehow displace and succeed mass media' but simply that it makes possible *a more critical reception* of mass media. Yet, with the benefit of more than a decade's hindsight, it could be argued that even this modest faith in the possibility of a new metacritical culture of the image risks looking a little utopian. For Stiegler, speaking and writing in the early 1990s, it is intriguing that the main responsibility for creating this culture falls, not to the individual or collective consumer/producer of media, but to the state: he approvingly cites the so-called French 'cultural exception' [*l'exception culturelle*] (where francophone media were subsidised and protected under the terms of the 1993 international GATT agreement) as an instance of political resistance to the global hegemony of American culture (Derrida and Stiegler 2002: 73–99ff.). If we put to one side the question of whether the philosopher is right about the cultural exception – it could just as easily be argued that it has produced a synthetic francophone monoculture that is the mirror image of its Hollywood rival – we might still feel that Stiegler's 'top-down' statism here sits awkwardly alongside the 'bottom-up' technological individuation he champions elsewhere. Given the increasing prevalence of the new media environments Stiegler is talking about, the cultural exception has, if anything, been rendered increasingly *redundant* as a mode of critique: any francophone internet user can, of course, access anglophone culture anytime and anywhere, wirelessly. Perhaps most depressing of all, however, is the fact that the very infrastructure of Stiegler's politics of memory – the digital technologies that ostensibly enable us to question the industrialisation of time – have quickly become an instrumental part of the capitalist order he seeks to resist: what the philosopher depicts as new and revolutionary forms of media in the mid-1990s have now been at last partially absorbed into mass media in the form of, say, Google, YouTube and Apple's iTunes; social-networking sites such as MySpace, Facebook or Twitter, view-on-demand digital television and such user-generated content as blogs, podcasts and mobile-phone photography. In what we might almost see as the capitalist gesture par excellence, the critique of the industrialisation of time is *itself becoming industrialised* under the pretext of offering greater individuation of consumption and production. Such, it seems, is one depressing fate of Stiegler's politics of digitalisation: the greater personal agency it promised over the machinic flow of the image is now being sold to the spectator by the culture industry *itself* as ever-increasing freedom of consumer choice, here, now and in Real Time.

References

Aristotle (1999), *Physics*, trans. R. Waterfield, intro. and notes by D. Bostock, Oxford: Oxford World's Classics.

Barthes, R. ([1980] 1981]) *Camera Lucida: Reflections on Photography*, trans. R. Howard, New York: Hill & Wang.

Beardsworth, R. (1998) 'Towards a Critical Culture of the Image: J. Derrida and B. Stiegler's *Echographies de la télévision*', *Tekhnema: Journal of Philosophy and Technology* 4 (http.tekhnema.free.fr/ 4Beardsworth.html).

Bennington, G. (1996) 'Emergencies', *Oxford Literary Review* 18 (1996), 175–216.

Bradley, A. (2006) 'Derrida's God: A Genealogy of the Theological Turn', *Paragraph* 29(3) (Nov.), 21–42.

—— (2011) *Originary Technicity: The Theory of Technology from Marx to Derrida*, London: Palgrave Macmillan.

Derrida, J. (1967) 'Ce dangereux supplément', in *De la grammatologie*, Paris: Éditions de Minuit, 203–34.

—— (1973) *Speech and Phenomena and Other Essays on Husserl's Theory of Signs*, ed. and trans. D. Allison, Evanston, IL: Northwestern University Press.

—— and Stiegler, B. (2002) *Echographies of Television: Filmed Interviews*, trans. J. Bajorek, Cambridge: Polity.

Dillon, M. and Fletcher, P. (2008) 'Real Time: The Instant of My Death', *Journal for Cultural Research* 12(4), 389–402.

Hansen, M. B. N. (2004) 'The Time of Affect, or Bearing Witness to Life', *Critical Inquiry* 30(3) (spring), 584–626.

—— (2006) 'Media Theory', *Theory, Culture & Society* 23(2–3), 297–306.

Heidegger, M. (1977) 'The Question Concerning Technology', in *The Question Concerning Technology and Other Essays*, trans. W. Lovitt, New York: Harper & Row, 3–35.

—— (1988) 'Martin Heidegger *im Gespräch mit* Richard Wisser', in

Antwort: Martin Heidegger im Gespräch, ed. G. Neske and E. Kettering, Pfullingen: Verlag Günter Neske.

Husserl, E. (1964) *The Phenomenology of Internal Time Consciousness*, trans. J. Churchill, Bloomington, IN: Indiana University Press.

Leroi-Gourhan, A. (1993) *Gesture and Speech*, trans. A. Bostock Berger, Cambridge, MA: MIT Press.

Lévy, P. (1998) *Becoming Virtual: Reality in the Digital Age*, trans. R. Bononno, New York: Plenum.

Plato (2004) *'Protagoras' and 'Meno'*, trans. by R. C. Bartlett, Ithaca, NY: Cornell University Press.

Salanskis, J.-M. (2000) 'Ecce Faber', *Les Temps Modernes* 55(608), 235–78.

Stiegler, B. (1996) *La Technique et le temps 2: La Désorientation*, Paris: Galilée.

—— ([1994] 1998) *Technics and Time 1: The Fault of Epimetheus*, trans. R. Beardsworth and G. Collins, Stanford, CA: Stanford University Press.

—— (2001) *La Technique et le temps 3: Le Temps du cinéma et la question de mal-être*, Paris: Galilée.

—— (2002) 'Derrida and Technology: Fidelity at the Limits of Deconstruction and the Prosthesis of Faith', trans. R. Beardsworth, in T. Conley (ed.), *Jacques Derrida and the Future of the Humanities*, Cambridge: Cambridge University Press, 238–70.

—— (2004) *De la misère symbolique 1: L'époque hyperindustrielle*, Paris: Galilée.

—— (2007) '*Anamnēsis* and *Hypomnēsis*: The Memories of Desire', trans. A. Bradley and F.-X. Gleyzon, in A. Bradley and L. Armand (ed.), *Technicity*, Prague: Charles University Press, 15–41.

—— (2008) *Prendre soin: De la jeunesse et des générations*, Paris: Flammarion.

Notes

1 Bernard Stiegler ([1994] 1998, 2001)). In the 'Avertissement' to the third volume, Stiegler mentions a fourth and possibly even a fifth volume which, at the time of writing, have yet to appear: *Symboles et diaboles ou les guerres des spirites* (which treats Plato and Derrida) and *Le défaut qu'il faut*. All further references to these works will be given in the text. Unless otherwise indicated, all translations from the French and the German are my own.

2 Aristotle, *Physics* (1999: 33–6, 192b–193b). In Book 2, Aristotle writes: 'Of

things that exist, some exist by nature, some from other causes. "By nature" the animals and their parts exist, and the plants and the simple bodies (earth, fire, air, water) – for we say that these and the like exist "by nature". All the things mentioned present a feature in which they differ from things which are not constituted by nature. Each of them has within itself a principle of motion and of stationariness (in respect of place, or of growth and decrease, or by way of alteration). On the other hand, a bed and a coat and anything else of that sort, *qua* receiving these designations i.e. in so far as they are products of art – have no innate impulse to change.'

3 It is worth noting that an important precursor for Stiegler's thought here is the palaeo-anthropology of André Leroi-Gourhan. In Leroi-Gourhan's account, the history of humanity is the history of its exteriorisation onto technical tools and support systems: 'The whole of our evolution has been oriented towards placing outside ourselves what in the rest of the animal world is achieved inside by species adaptation' (1993: 42).

4 As Stiegler himself consistently observes, the relation between the 'who' of humanity and the 'what' of technics is 'transductive' in Gilbert Simondon's sense of a relation whose constitutive terms do not pre-exist the relation (1998: 152; 1996: 14–15). Perhaps another precursor for originary technicity might be Francisco Valera's concept of a structural coupling of organism and environment. In Valera's later theories of biological autopoiesis, he moves beyond the emphasis on autonomy that marked his classic work with Maturana to argue that bio-systems operate through a complex feedback loop of input and output whereby each new input from the environment introduces minor deviations into the system: this idea is also alluded to by Stiegler as a way of conceptualising the co-evolution of the human and the technical (Stiegler 1998: 158; 1996: 204).

5 See Michael Dillon and Paul Fletcher (2008), for an incisive genealogy and critique of Real Time media.

6 One can see clear parallels between Stiegler's critique of the reality effect generated by Real Time technologies such as television and that of other key French theorists of the visual image such as Jean Baudrillard, Régis Debray and Paul Virilio.

7 To be sure, Stiegler is frequently ambiguous on this crucial point: 'Ce que nous appelons le "temps réel" n'est pas donc le temps; c'est peut-être même la détemporalisation du temps, ou l'occultation du temps; et c'est encore, cependant, le temps, industriellement "gagné", c'est-à-dire aussi perdu' ['What we call "real time" is thus not time; it is perhaps even the de-temporalisation of time, or the occultation of time; and yet it is, nonetheless, time, "gained" industrially, which is also to say lost'] (Stiegler 1996: 62).

8 For Heidegger, it is clear that his critique of *das Gestell* as the dominant mode of unconcealment is in no way a romantic, pastoral or otherwise anti-technological gesture: 'To start with, it must be said that I am not *against* technology. I have never spoken *against* technology, nor against the so-

called demon of technology' (1988: 25).

9 In Salanskis's review essay, he accuses Stiegler of conflating two quite different Real Time technologies with two quite difference purposes. On the one hand, there are 'real time' digital computing systems that operate quite independently of, and far more quickly than, human time consciousness. On the other hand, there are 'real time' media that, while operating at a speed beyond the threshold of perception, are still explicitly designed to produce a phenomenon – the 'live event' – which is accessible to perceptual consciousness (2000: 274).

Part VI
Afterword

14

Interview with Bernard Vouilloux

Nigel Saint and Andy Stafford

NS & AS: What do you think of our choice of thinkers in this book and of the way in which we discuss them?

BV: What I could say about every chapter would confirm my general view, which is that your English-speaking readers are very fortunate, since there is no equivalent volume in French. However, I'd also like to add a couple of points. To reinforce what you say in your introduction about your decision to include Merleau-Ponty and Metz, I'd first underline how any selection of thinkers that is organised thematically, in which the way the thinkers are discussed reflects the organisation of the volume into five themed parts, emphasises certain aspects of their thought: reading Damisch via the question of dreams justifies his inclusion in the group devoted to new genealogies in art history (Part II), whereas a reading that focused on *Théorie du nuage* (1972) and its semiological considerations of painting would have led to his inclusion in Part III of your book. Nuancing your mapping of visual theory in fact does it the most justice, since after all you avoid sowing the illusion of encyclopaedic coverage and are offering a series of readings that privilege plurality and current perspectives; indeed, the work of most of the thinkers under discussion are still 'in progress'. Besides, there is also the issue of the English-language context: certain authors are already well known to your audience – for example Sartre, Lacan, Lévi-Strauss, Barthes, Lyotard, Deleuze, Foucault, Derrida whose contribution to the study of the visual and of the image has been fundamental (hence your

A first version of this text was based on the interview recorded in Paris on 27 November 2009. It was transcribed and edited by Nigel Saint. Additional questions were sent by both editors by email and answered in writing. An agreed version was then translated by Saint.

inclusion of some of them in your introduction), but for the purposes of your volume I can see that it wasn't necessary to place them alongside the thinkers your collection aims to bring into the limelight, even if one can still regret the absence of certain figures.

Thus I'd like to mention, for the record as it were, Yve-Alain Bois, who is well known to readers of English, since he has taught in the US for many years and curated, with Rosalind Krauss, the 1996 Centre Pompidou exhibition *L'Informe*, which Didi-Huberman's exhibition a year later, *L'Empreinte*, responded to: Bois, like Damisch and Marin, was linked to an art theory review called *Macula* which was very influential, even if it was fairly short-lived (six issues between 1976 and 1979). The name of this review gives me the opportunity of mentioning Jean Clay, its founder, who shortly afterwards created the publishing house of the same name; indeed, Clay isn't just a fine publisher, he's also produced some great texts himself. We should also note the work of Jean-Claude Lebensztejn, who has written on contemporary art (Stella, Morley) as well as topics as diverse as Pontormo's *Diary*, the notion of *sprezzatura*, Seurat's paintings, Fauvism and Expressionism, etc. Bois, Clay and Lebensztejn were part of a group of theorists who shook things up in French art history. With stronger links to philosophy, Marie-José Mondzain has developed her work on icons and theology into an enquiry into the status of the visual and images in contemporary society. Another interesting development is the work of Jacques Rancière, who, originating in political philosophy, began writing on the cinema quite early on and who, since *Le Partage du sensible* (2000), has been evolving ideas that have reached a considerable public, both abroad and in France. Finally, we ought also to mention all those working today at the research centre created by Damisch and Marin at the École des Hautes Études en Sciences Sociales (EHESS), namely the Centre d'Histoire et Théorie des Arts (CEHTA), for example Giovanni Careri and Éric Michaud, as well as the rapid expansion that has occurred in photography studies since the classic studies by Barthes, Krauss and Jean-Marie Schaeffer: Andre Rouillé's revisiting of the indexical paradigm, Michel Poivert's rereading of modernism, and the links with literature in text/image studies explored by Philippe Ortel, Jérôme Thélot and Daniel Grojnowski.

The second point I'd like to make concerns something that the monograph-style approach doesn't always allow one to see, even if your contributors have supplied contexts for the thinkers they are studying: I'm referring to the networks and effects of influence that provide the framework for a period of thought. For example, Nancy's work implies that of Derrida and of Lacoue-Labarthe (whose writings on art were collected in one volume in 2009), two authors he was very close to in every respect while at the same time producing his own distinctive work. Similarly one cannot read Stiegler without many references to Derrida, and to understand Buci-Glucksmann requires an acquaintance with Deleuze. One also needs to stress that phenomenology developed after Merleau-Ponty with Mikel Dufrenne, Henri Maldiney, and many others. By the way, it was through Maldiney that Deleuze, when he came to write *Logique de la sensation* (1981), found the distinction introduced early in the twentieth century by Riegl between optic and haptic vision. Riegl was read comparatively late in France: most French art historians were unaware of him and it needed all of Maldiney's enthusiasm for German thought to resurrect these categories (Maldiney was also one of Ludwig Binswanger's great interpreters). When it comes to Baudrillard, one should also mention Paul Virilio, whose research also focuses on the changes affecting images in the information age and who explores the question of technology more directly than Baudrillard, just as Stiegler pays a lot of attention to technology too. Still on the question of Baudrillard, we need to recall the particularly French episode of the 'contemporary art polemic' which broke out at the end of the 1980s and which led to some very trenchant position-taking (with Jean-Philippe Domecq, Marc Fumaroli, Jean Clair and Jean Molino on one side and Didi-Huberman and Philippe Dagen on the other), as well as certain analytical studies of the debate (by Yves Michaud and Nathalie Heinich).

NS & AS: As you've mentioned, our book is divided into Parts I–V: phenomenology, new histories of art, semiology, the body and the digital. At the same time, it is noticeable that in your book *L'Œuvre en souffrance* (2004) you point out that when trying to combine different theoretical approaches one should not skate over the details, for example in relation to phenomenology and semiology. How may we best arrive at an overview of visual theory and a sound strategy for combining different theories?

BV: By opting to work on French theories of the visual, or, to put it another way, theories of the image, you have of course chosen a complex topic. A survey of art history in France would naturally have been simpler. This is because we know what a painting or a sculpture is, and we understand what we mean by an architectural project. These objects not only have a history, but they are also basically material objects. Even if they've evolved and changed, you can frame them and establish the relevant disciplinary parameters. Heinich's sociological approach to the category of 'art' deals precisely with both this establishment of parameters and the current questioning of them. She has studied the interplay of representations and values that underpins the three principal systems of legitimation in the art world: the artisanal corporations; the liberal academies of art; and the purely vocational artists.

With the image, things get more complicated because there are at least four dimensions involved. First, there's the perceptual image – whether visual or sound: the image as unit of perception. Second, there's the physical image, the image as an object: a painting, an engraving, a drawing, a photograph, a film, they are all images. Third, there's the mental image, studied by traditional psychology or cognitive science: we use it when we represent things, for our 'ways of worldmaking', as in Goodman's title (1978). Fourth, and lastly, there is what we call, but only since the beginning of the nineteenth century, the verbal image, which nevertheless comprises the whole rhetorical tradition concerning comparison, metaphor and metonymy. The image therefore opens up an extremely complex set of problems. And one needs to add that while the image can be analysed in terms of representation, it can also be discussed in terms of investment, within an economy that can be psychical (or 'libidinal', as Lyotard put it), or determined by the media, or influenced by the market.

Thus one sees how the questions provoked by the study of images are linked to various aspects of key debates in the fields of philosophy and the human sciences. This book therefore faces the considerable difficulty of dealing with an object of study prone to dispersion. In this respect the intellectual trajectory of certain of your thinkers is revealing. We have Régis Debray, for example, who started out writing about politics and literature, and only came to 'mediology' quite late on. Alongside him there are others who from the outset put images, and in particular the images of art, at the centre of their work: I'm thinking of course of Metz, Schefer, Buci-Glucksmann, Thierry de Duve, Damisch, Marin, Arasse and Didi-Huberman. Finally there are others for whom the turn to the image represents an inflection, more or less late on in their work, of their thinking developed in other fields, as was the case for Merleau-Ponty and Baudrillard, and is the case today for Nancy and Stiegler. They all deploy conceptual tools that lead us to rethink a certain number of transdisciplinary concepts, such as memory, corporeality, duration, space, etc., which explains the audience they've reached beyond the confined circles of specialists. By the same token, if philosophy is well placed to put the different research questions originating in the human sciences into perspective, then you haven't taken the easier option of offering a survey of the philosophy of art or of aesthetics in France.

The art historian – I am caricaturing the matter somewhat – who is mainly concerned with attributions and dating, doesn't run the same risk of being spread too thinly or of encountering endless pluralities of meaning, but nor is there the same opportunity to expand his or her readership. An enterprise such as yours therefore has to be able to deal with the challenge of objects that are prone to dispersion and diffraction. Nowadays the study of the image overlaps with many other fields of enquiry.

NS & AS: Is it helpful to think about the potential difference between the image and the visual? In our volume we offer, almost, an 'anti-definition' of the image, resisting any attempt to define the image, preferring to speak of the visual so as not to limit the image. Is that different from your four-part categorisation of the image?

BV: It's true that my wish to clarify the concept of the image could seem to be opposed in some way to the theories we're discussing in relation to your book. However, I'd like to digress a little, if I may, by mentioning part of my own intellectual development: I read Lyotard, Deleuze and Derrida pretty early on, followed by Damisch and Marin, and then I encountered analytical philosophy via Goodman (even if he isn't the most representative example). He's quite a marginal and unusual figure within Anglo-Saxon philosophy – in some respects he's close to Wittgenstein (in the way he discusses symptoms) and there's also a pragmatist dimension (the attention to contexts and the notion of apprenticeship). At the time I felt the need to organise and tidy up my conceptual tools very carefully, in the manner of Wittgenstein, so the influence of Goodman helped me to think more clearly. Nevertheless I don't think there's a fundamental difference between the conception of the image that I was developing and the visual theories discussed in your book.

Crafted images, in my view, involve both representation and resemblance. They are representative in so far as representation is based on a relation where 'x stands for y': that is to say that representation is underwritten by the beliefs and convictions that are central to the unity of a cultural community. Therefore I understand the term differently from its use in art history, where it is used either for any sort of figurative art or for the paradigmatic system of figurative painting established in the Quattrocento and theorised by Alberti. Resemblance, on the other hand, is based on a 'being like' relation: the perception of similarities (of form, colour, texture, etc.) is enabled by a skill that human beings share with a certain number of animal species. Of course these two aspects of the image are separate from one another: twins look like each other, but one doesn't represent the other.

Following the critique of 'representation' (as commonly understood) by the different arts during modernity – a reinterpretation that in fact constitutes the key to that period – there has been a tendency to reject resemblance a little too hastily, despite its great richness in anthropological terms. For example, if we consider the Roman *imago*, the term refers to a Roman funerary mask that is cast directly from the face of the deceased. These masks didn't just represent (stand for) the spirits of the ancestors, they resembled the ancestors, since otherwise the family tie would not have been *recognised*, in both senses of the word. Looking at the processes involved in making the *imagines* we uncover the cultural 'thickness' of the practice, involving recognition, acknowledgement, family ties, funeral rites, etc. That's why the notion of resemblance seems to me to be crucial when discussing iconicity. However, we do need to bear in mind a third term when it comes to physical, material and crafted images made by human hands: the figurative system in which a representation that resembles is produced. If we neglect this third term, if we think simply of the image as a representation that resembles then we turn it into an absolute category and end up having to confront the paradoxes and *aporiae* of 'true' resemblances.

Let me explain. To understand the role of this third term, what I'm calling the figurative system, in the mediation of the relationship between representation and resemblance, we might compare our situation with that of seventeenth-century private collectors. Masks from countries outside Europe, for example, ended up in cabinets of curiosities among the *naturalia*: a cultivated gentleman would not have thought of placing them alongside his collection busts or portraits, because for him they didn't belong in such company. This is because representation that resembles was then considered according to a single category that was defined by the ideology of perspective which I've already alluded to and endorsed by the Vasarian grand narrative of art history, in which the history of modern representation could only be understood as a story of increasing progress in the portrayal of appearances. Nowadays our approach is completely different, since the global circulation of images, reproduced with endless variations, has made us used to the move from one figurative system to another: whatever the image, whether Japanese print, Mongolian painting or African mask, even if we've only seen a few examples, rather than judging them according to a single standard, we try to relate to them on their own terms and to place them in their context, with due consideration of their origins and objectives.

To sum up, resemblance is a term affecting both subject and object, as they say in analytical philosophy: when we say that an object 'resembles', it means or it should mean that it 'resembles for' (somebody). I'm entitled to say that for a Picasso his portrait of Kahnweiler resembles the subject, whereas a contemporary of Arnauld and Nicole would have stated simply that there was no resemblance, because at the time an absolute model of resemblance was taken for granted. Hence we realise how the question of resemblance leads us into the anthropology of perceived resemblances and of taxonomies, classifications and recognised families of objects that we assemble, all of which of course appeals to those working on the interpretation of images. A further extension of this topic can be pursued though comparisons with the animal kingdom, looking at decoration and ornamentation, including animal ornamentation, in the field of aesthetics. This could be a direction for further research, without necessarily subscribing to a naturalist approach to culture.

NS & AS: Perhaps there remains the problem of working with the term representation for those who are concerned about the word 'presence' at its heart. And yet hasn't the proper theorisation of representation always refuted any straightforward path to true presence, so that you are not really envisaging its displacement by resemblance?

BV: First, we have to set out the historical development of what we commonly understand by 'representation', indicating its epistemic turning points. We can begin our account in Greece or with the establishment of the system of perspective during the Quattrocento; it's equally possible to argue for the importance of the conceptualisation that occurs between Descartes and Port-Royal, etc. Meanwhile, representation is also a logical concept used to describe the fact, for example, that we associate certain utterances that we produce or perceive with representations. Then in his *De anima*, Aristotle refers to *phantasiai*, a term that has less to do with representation and more to do with appearance, from the Greek *phainein*, 'to show' or, in the passive, 'to be seen'. You can see that there's a continual need to clarify the terms and concepts involved.

What is more, it's not because a concept has been critiqued or even deconstructed that we have to cast it aside and avoid it. Avoidance isn't the best way to resolve a problem. We have to be guided by the fact that people did once believe in images, for example in the image as a double, an aspect demonstrated very clearly by the work of Jean-Pierre Vernant, David Freedberg and Jack Goody. Beliefs and convictions attach themselves to representations and we need to think through the implications of this fact. The etymology of 'representation' can be traced back to the phrase *rem praesentem facere*, 'make the thing present'. The thing that is present, according to Benveniste, is not a thing that may be in front of us, but a thing that is yet to come, that is ahead of us in time, as it were, imminent and about to arrive. Iconic representation functions through a dynamic of suspense that we associate with the fetish: something is blocked that may yet be released. Just as in the case of resemblance, there is still much to discover about representation: we need to continue to study it, not just as a historical concept with various manifestations and theoretical developments (even a doctrine, in the form of *mimesis*), but also in its anthropological dimension, by looking at the production of representations in societies without writing or far away from the European context – a topic explored by Philippe Descola's exhibition at the Quai Branly Museum, *La Fabrique des images* (2010–11).

I'd like to return to the issue of the differences between the image and a painting or sculpture, etc. I think it's a crucial and fertile question, even if it may lead us in a different direction from the perspectives chosen by your volume. We could put it this way: while Arasse works on painting, Didi-Huberman works on the image. What occupies Arasse's attention is the pictorial object, a painting:

there is a very specific field of study involved, focusing on the pigments of colours applied to a canvas. We only have to recall the way Arasse discusses the left side of Fragonard's *The Lock* at the end of his book *The Detail* (1992). As for Didi-Huberman, if we think of his use of Benjamin's concept of the dialectical image or his work on Warburg, especially on the *Atlas Mnemosyne* (1929), then we see that he is a thinker who deals with images. He is therefore concerned with images in their plurality. The image is composed of many things: perception, the psyche (including cognition, memory, dreams and fantasy) and the verbal are all interwoven in the artefact. The same point applies to Debray's mediology: the image is part of a network or grouping, with each image referring to another through counterpoint, echo and resonance; Debray's 'videosphere' is what Yves Michaud would call the 'gaseous image', dispersing in all directions.

By contrast, someone concentrating on painting is affected by the almost dazzling uniqueness of the object, which the notion of aura helps us think about. However, if we look a little more closely the situation becomes more complicated: while in my view Damisch is indeed primarily a theorist of painting, his structural methodology and studies via series (found in the work of his teacher Pierre Francastel), as well as his interest in phenomenology and psychoanalysis, tend to pluralise and dematerialise a painting, resulting in a focus on painting as thought (as he likes to say, 'painting thinks'); and in the case of Marin, who was first a theorist of the image, as seen in his foundational work on Pascal and Port-Royal, the studies he made of representation's semiotic mechanisms also led him to examine in great detail these functions as they impacted on the construction of individual paintings. Despite these nuances, however, I believe we can extend this polarity between painting and image and deploy it in quite a different field from visual theory. It can be used to observe differences between writers like Stendhal and Pierre Michon, who write about painting, and Flaubert and Pascal Quignard, who write about the image.

NS & AS: Several chapters in this volume analyse the style of writing of the selected thinker. May we ask you to say more about the links between theory and writing? The critic Paul Ardenne has stated that there is no such thing as specifically 'French' contemporary art, but are we able to say that there is a certain French way of writing about visual theory, perhaps one that is essayistic?

BV: In order to appreciate the importance of language in the way an image is thought, you need to begin with our relationship with the visual object. This may lead to the experience of a kind of strangeness, involving the feeling of otherness: visual experience, however small the object in question, unsettles and disrupts our usual ways of thinking. It's no accident that writers are adept at detecting the way visual images disturb us – I'm thinking of course of well-known texts by Mallarmé, Proust and Beckett, but also particular passages in the works of Melville, Tanizaki, Nabokov and Calvino. When the visual is engaged within a text in some way, the process will inevitably have a self-reflexive element, once a text isn't just saying something about an object or work, but also commenting on the relation between subject and object. Such a reflexive aspect can be found in the majority of authors in your volume, even if we don't need to go so far as to pinpoint a *linguistic turn* as such. One of Nancy's first books, after all, was an anthology of German Romantic poetic theory that he edited with Lacoue-Labarthe. For his part, Marin also explored this dimension with some fervour in *De l'entretien*, which was published posthumously in 1997, and there are examples in the work of Damisch, although his attitude to writing has certainly been a complex one; we could also refer to the unclassifiable and fascinating *Zigzag*, published by Lebensztejn in 1981 in the 'Philosophie en effet' collection created by Derrida, Lacoue-Labarthe, Nancy and Kofman. This matter of the relation to language and writing is absolutely vital. However, to be clear, we need to emphasise that it's not an aesthetic relation, since the authors concerned are not appealing to some academic ideal of 'good writing', which is based on the notion of a norm, nor are they trying to evoke 'the sensations of art', as famously practised by Roberto Longhi in his *Officina ferrarese* where he describes a vision of Cosmè Tura by multiplying alliteration, assonance and metaphors in a sort of hyperliterary exercise that seeks to emulate the visual effects. Our authors don't write like that: ever since Merleau-Ponty's essay 'Le Doute de Cézanne' (1945), the attention to language has been a sign of the reflexivity of a text that engages with the otherness of the visual object.

From the moment when art history, following the German model of the discipline, sought to acquire scientific methods and objectives, it quickly came to consider as aesthetic affectation any emphasis placed on the kind of artistic or literary writing found in the work of Longhi or indeed of Henri Focillon. What was encouraged at the time was a sort of textual neutrality or transparency, resulting in

France in a simple prose style endorsed by the universities. If the question of the writing of art history hasn't been addressed much in France, it's also because this country came to the theory of the discipline comparatively late: the epistemology of art history and of literary studies is a very recent concern. We have the works of Germain Bazin (albeit pretty unsound), Édouard Pommier and, quite recently, Roland Recht on the history of art history, as well as Lynne Therrien's study of the foundations of the discipline at the end of the nineteenth century, but on the whole such studies aren't numerous and are pretty recent when one compares them to efforts from elsewhere, especially Germanic and Anglo-Saxon countries. As early as 1953 Panofsky contributed such an essay to a collective volume on the contribution of immigrants to intellectual life in the USA, with chapters devoted to the individual disciplines. The turn to epistemology or disciplinary critique took place abroad but not in France. It's as if the question of writing was deemed to have been sorted out so that all that remained to be done was to focus on the appreciation of the style of writing, judged according to the criterion of taste: so and so writes well, while another does not.

Some of the authors under discussion have been criticised for writing in a 'mannered', 'precious' or 'over-complicated' style, since their style is noticeable. There is in effect at times a kind of violence which can take a variety of forms, or at any rate a degree of distortion that draws attention to the medium of writing. How could it be otherwise? If you're engaged in thinking seriously about the complexity and opacity of the image, then you are necessarily aware of the opacity, blind spots and ignorance pervading language. Here we may mention Schefer, who's never had any link with academia, like Jean-Christophe Bailly (close to Lacoue-Labarthe and Nancy), who is an equally interesting case: both produce texts that are 'essays' in the strictest sense of the term, by which I mean a certain French tradition including Paulhan, Bataille, Sartre, Blanchot, Caillois, etc. At first Schefer wrote extremely theoretical works, like *Scénographie d'un tableau* (1969), still the best example we have of the impossibility of applying semiology to painting, at least in the way semiology was conceived in the 1970s. Then we saw a different Schefer, whose books were published by POL, a notable literary publisher. Schefer is not of course the first experimental writer on the visual outside academia: a well-known case is Georges Duthuit, who was one of the rare figures in the inter-war years to value the work of Riegl: it's no accident that the person who's set out to save Duthuit from oblivion is a major poet, namely Yves Bonnefoy.

NS & AS: At the same time would you say that there is a risk in any theorising about the image of slipping into mere analogy – between text and image, photography and painting, indeed 'ekphrasis' and essayism?

BV: Well, we shouldn't be too hard on analogy. It's definitely useful in a heuristic way, when deployed to link the less well known to the better known, drawing our attention to what is prominent in a field. Nevertheless, if you restrict your understanding of analogy to this view you have essayism (which I'd distinguish from the essay) or what we might still call impressionism. In France there used to be impressionistic criticism, Émile Faguet's for example, which set itself in opposition to Lanson's positivist criticism. I'd situate in this context the invention around 1880 of the notion of literary impressionism, promoted by Ferdinand Brunetière and Paul Bourget. This is clearly a good example of analogy, with the process working in the following way: some of the characteristic traits of so-called 'impressionist' writers (the Goncourt brothers, Huysmans, Daudet, Loti), such as the substantivation of the adjective (e.g. 'the black of the caps'), function in a text as touches of colour do in a painting, with the thing as it is perceived occurring before it is named, as Proust noted. There is a whole system of overlooked parallels, which posit the existence of a level of pure sensation, freed from conceptualisation, which the painter can access if he or she looks at things with a child's 'innocent eye' (as in Ruskin); in the same way in literature the impressionist sentence, preferring adjectives to nouns, could be described as phenomenalist. When considering the analogies found in essayism, as for example in the key case of literary impressionism, two lines of enquiry are conceivable, quite apart from the simple imitation of this tradition, as practised by some critics.

The first position, the one I adopted when I worked on this question, consists in unpacking the system of analogies by detailing its presuppositions and by demonstrating its reliance on certain epistemological foundations: as unconvincing as it may seem today (the theory of linguistics and of perception have rendered it obsolete), it was needed at a certain moment.

The second position would try to look beyond the superficial aspects of analogy in order to uncover the links between language and the visual when considered in historical terms. If we accept that the limitations on the viability of switching from one medium to another (word to image, word to sound, image to music, etc.), we still have to consider whether such links are due to historical circumstances or not. If the answer is yes, then these links could take place in a number of ways: through the modelling of one work on another (we often use the term 'influence' here); or via the actualisation of conceptual schemata, in the manner of the 'symbolic forms' of Cassirer; or due to historical determinism, as in the Hegelian view of the Zeitgeist, in which certain cultural forces gain ascendancy (an idea taken up by Spengler); or, lastly, as a result of the epistemic thinking of a particular period (I'm thinking here of Foucault).

I should qualify this prospect of a many-layered research project by stressing that such attempts to study analogy have so far only met with limited success, since the argument that certain words or phrases are more significant than others leads to exaggeration, even if the study of language inevitably involves a degree of abstraction. We should not confuse the way linguistic signs work (by using letters and sounds to refer to things) with the subsequent representations that words may lead us to imagine. In my own work I sought to overcome all these difficulties by reprising the notion of the dispositive, which was first used in the 1970s.

It's a bit different in the case of the links between photography and painting, where an art form that already existed allowed an emerging form to find its models. This modelling occurred both in practice (the early photographers had all been trained as painters) and in the discourse of the new medium. In fact photography only became a separate art form once it was practised and described in an autonomous manner, once the dead ends of pictorialism had been overcome. At the same time it's interesting to note that photography speeded up the process, which had been under way since the Renaissance, by which painting was becoming autonomous. Here we have the well-known view, reiterated in particular by Valéry, that photography had taken away the ancillary task of 'imitation' from painting.

NS & AS: In the context of essayism, what part would 'orality' play in the relationship between text and image?

BV: More than the voice, orality could indeed lie at the heart of what concerns us here. While writing in fact depends on the denial of orality, nevertheless writing is haunted by it as if by the ghost of the community which writing addresses (as hard as this is to specify). In this way writing draws on a long tradition of speech, attaining authority as it does so: this was how Benjamin saw the storyteller (the *Erzähler*, the one who recounts and who counts). Writing is 'silent speech': behind written signs there is an open mouth but no sound. Without this shadow cast by speech, written signs would be like the unreadable forms of a painting, which Simonides's aphorism likened to silent poetry, since to know how to read is to know how to pronounce. We can see therefore that orality has a paradoxical relationship with language and this is also the case with the gaze. In French we talk of 'devouring someone with one's gaze'. Every gaze is motivated by desire, the drive to devour, to absorb and ingest: the gaze gets hungry.

Two paradigmatic scenes sum this situation up for me. The first one means a lot to me personally because I took great delight in talking to Louis Marin about it a few months before he died. It comes from the *Mémoires de Saint-Simon* (1739–49): it concerns the stratagem thought up by the young Saint-Simon to get around the very devout Abbé de Rancé's objections to having his portrait painted (1696–97). He arranged for the painter Hyacinthe Rigaud, whom he commissioned to do the portrait, to pretend to be a total idiot when he met Rancé. Rigaud therefore gazed at him from every possible angle, devouring and lapping up every detail, pausing from time to time to slip away into an adjacent room to sketch out the aspects he'd captured in this way. The second concerns Francis Ponge, who recounted the episode in one of his texts on Braque. At the end of the war, Ponge went to see the artist after Jean Paulhan had shown Braque (and other artists) Ponge's *Parti pris des choses* (1942). Coming down from the studio, Ponge spotted from the stairs a painting by Braque hanging in the dining room which depicted a platter of fish. We often talk about how fish have their mouths and eyes wide open – in French we say 'to be as dumb as a carp' or 'to look at someone (idiotically) with eyes like fried whiting'. Ponge states that he felt an 'aesthetic choke': his throat tightened, his tongue became stiff. In other words he experiences a brief episode of aphasia which is linked to the enormous trouble he felt with language at the end of his adolescence. He overcame this initial difficulty by inventing a rhetorical style based on a real exchange, taking the side of things, but also taking words into account. The scene at Braque's house occurs at a moment when he's going to move on to a second phase, leading a few years later to *Tentative orale* (1947) and *La Rage de l'expression*

(1952). In these works the aim is to show the different stages of a text's writing as it tries to represent the object, whether soap, field, fig or table. This exemplary scene ought to remind us that when it comes to the image, to the visual, we have lots to learn from writers and poets, which brings us back to what we were saying about the links between *theory* (which deals with vision, but through ideas) and *writing*.

NS & AS: May we move on to address the question of institutions (academies, art schools, research institutes, universities, secondary schools) in more detail? Have institutions greatly influenced the way our thinkers have written about the visual, or have our thinkers attempted to offer individual, even rebellious, takes on the images they discuss?

BV: France is divided into two great tropisms or tendencies: the conservatism of an old peasant nation, for whom nothing must be wasted and everything must be carefully conserved; and the frequent desire for radical innovation, starting from a tabula rasa, and revolution. When the two attitudes are combined, you have a very complex set of structures. The place where we're holding this interview is very significant in this respect. We're at the INHA, the Institut National d'Histoire de l'Art, sitting in fact in the office of Michel Laclotte, who was Director of the Louvre from 1987 to 1995. INHA is a meta-institution, consisting of institutions that existed already: the CNRS (Centre National de la Recherche Scientifique), the EHESS, which we've already mentioned, the EPHE (École Pratique des Hautes Études) and a certain number of Parisian universities who are listed in the entrance hall and on the banners hanging in the Arcade [see Plate 13]. Entering this building, a foreign academic must feel quite bewildered at the complexity of the structure of French institutions.

To return to our main topic, let's call it art, the visual and images, one needs to be aware that art history is taught in universities in ad hoc departments of art history and, outside the university sector, at the École du Louvre. Art history, aesthetics and the kind of visual theory we're discussing is also taught in fine art departments, mainly by philosophy specialists. We also need to add to this picture those philosophers who work on aesthetics in philosophy departments, as well as the teachers in art schools such as the École Nationale Supérieure des Beaux-Arts de Paris (ENSBA). What may seem very puzzling to outsiders is the division that can indeed exist between art history departments, who are a bit like the official guardians of the discipline, and the other departments or institutions. We could account for this division in the following way: art history thinks of itself primarily as history. To put it bluntly, the history of art is practised like the history of anything else: the aim is to place the selected objects in their historical context, looking at questions of patronage and the commissioning of artworks, collectors, the diffusion of works, the networks of workshops, etc. Meanwhile in fine art departments, the emphasis is placed instead on the image, the visual, in other words on the iconic object. This approach examines what sort of history is involved in the study of such an object, thus getting closer to the particular historicity of the image.

Among the group of thinkers studied in this volume, Arasse is the most respected by art historians. He began work with André Chastel, France's most famous art historian, who held sway over the discipline's institutions until the 1980s. Arasse related how coming across *The Art of Memory* (1966) by Frances Yates, which he translated, led him to reflect on the mobilisation of strands of memory in front of a painting, so that an image is a surface where we project our ideas and which requires us to finish it. This work meant that he encountered a whole range of issues that he would probably not have encountered had he remained in the strictly academic confines of art history. Even so, he arrived at EHESS fairly late in his career, joining Damisch and Marin there. Beforehand he'd directed the French Institute in Florence and then taught at the University of Paris I for several years. In fact Arasse's success has been largely posthumous, since what made him known to the non-specialist public was the series of elegant interviews he gave to France Culture a few months before his death and which were published in book form as *Histoires de peintures* (2004, with accompanying CD). Since then, most of Arasse's texts have been collected or republished, but this recognition has happened belatedly.

If we're saying that the 'centre' is defined by the academic institution of art history as it is taught at university, then we have to acknowledge the fact that all our thinkers belong to peripheral or marginal institutions. If they teach at universities, they don't teach in art history departments. This doesn't mean that they find it difficult to reach a wider audience, quite the opposite: there's a surprising mismatch between their institutional position and their readership, which includes students of art history (this may explain some of the heated reactions they provoke). The question of institutions is therefore far from being insignificant. It reveals something of the way in which theories are inscribed within force fields of ideas, with tensions and divisions that are reflected in institutional affiliations.

NS & AS: Could we also consider the francophone question, since there seem to be very few 'francophone' and/or 'post-colonial' theorists of the visual. Apart from a few names here and there, such as Khatibi and Bidima, what are the possible reasons for the absence from this volume of figures from beyond France?

BV: This is a general problem found in many other areas of thought and which may be explained by the difficult relationship that exists between France and its former colonies or former spheres of influence. The secular republican and Jacobin model of integration or assimilation, which dominated for so long, has been found to have limitations, notably that of cultural homogenisation. If France showed itself incapable of benefiting from the intellectual riches of the countries it used to rule, so those who might have contributed something in these countries either chose not to do so in a form that they didn't consider theirs or turned instead towards artistic or literary production. At the same time, where there are figures who've maintained an interest in theory, some of them have restricted themselves to polemics and score-settling. It's striking that certain prominent intellectuals have entrenched themselves in somewhat old-fashioned positions, for example the views expressed by Edward Said in *Orientalism* (1978). This was definitely a necessary book and it was very timely, but thirty years after its publication we cannot just go on repeating it: there are many other directions for research now, linked especially to globalisation. We need to consider, for example, how our approach to visual objects may have been formed by the fact of colonialism. This work has yet to be carried out in France: the research questions addressed by post-colonial studies are only mentioned very tentatively in this country. First, because for a long time France's colonial past remained – indeed still is – a politically sensitive subject: it wasn't until 1999 that the French state officially recognised that there had been an Algerian War (we used just to talk about 'events'). So once again we see how paradoxical French society is, vacillating between conservative reaction and the desire to disrupt everything, so that we're looking at a country that experiences a particularly pronounced form of the 'afterwardsness' phenomenon, or *Nachträglichkeit*, as described by Freud: it took the French state as long to acknowledge its colonialist policies as it did to recognise its official involvement, under the Vichy regime, in the organisation of the destruction of European Jews (let me stress that I'm not making any parallel between the two phenomena).

In the particular case of the Maghreb, of which I have personal experience having lived there, we have to remember that the image doesn't have the same status in these societies as it does in ours. The interdiction on representation in the Islamic, as in the Jewish, religion has certain exceptions but is generally sufficiently strong to have led either to a very stylised figurative tradition, primarily featuring animals or plants, or to the development of decorative and ornamental art. What is at stake is not (or not simply) the fact that artworks housed in the great European museums are difficult to see, since that problem can be alleviated by the dissemination of books, images on the internet and, in the case of the United Arab Emirates, the planned building of 'Louvre 2' in Abu Dhabi; it's also a matter of the problem of the image. We should acknowledge our debt to the work of Abdelkébir Khatibi, who showed us how to work on this topic, employing the customary tools of his time, mainly those of semiology.

Turning to artisanal and artistic traditions in black Africa, we may note that intercultural traditions only really surface in the work of artists. There are few intellectuals from former French-ruled countries who have engaged with these issues. Yet it would be interesting to see what an art historian or visual culture specialist in one of these countries would make, for example, of the Western academic discourse that has attached itself to Picasso's 'borrowings' from African art. The debate was initiated at the large *Primitivism* exhibition organised by William Rubin at New York's Museum of Modern Art in 1984, then pursued with the *Magiciens de la Terre* exhibition at the Centre Pompidou in Paris in 1989, which featured artists from countries without any recognisable artistic institutions, and recently explored further at *African Remix* in 2005 (also at the Pompidou), which again asked the question: what does it mean to be a painter or artist today in Abidjan or Dakar?. However, we still don't have any reflections, from the perspective of these other places, on the ideas and concepts that concern us in this volume. It seems that political concerns hide cultural or intellectual questions. In any event, there won't be any debate until the intercultural tensions have been resolved. In order to consider non-Western approaches, we have to refer to the work of American academics such as Clifford Geertz,

Thomas McEvilley, James Clifford or Sally Price, since they belong to a society where minorities are important and they have developed the conceptual tools needed to discuss these issues.

NS & AS: Finally, with regard to your own work, you have already mentioned aspects of your intellectual development and you've spoken very valuably and generously about the classification of images, representation and writing, as well as other topics. Would you say a little more about your methodological principles as a researcher and theorist?

BV: I'd like to mention three aspects of my work. My first principle would be to give sufficient attention to verbal language. That is where my work began, investigating the aporiae troubling certain semiological approaches to the visual arts. I was not concerned with establishing whether the image is structured like a language, to use Lacan's famous formula about the unconscious, but looked instead at how language causes certain things to happen to the image – what it does to an image and what it makes an image do – and I then looked in turn at what the image does to discourse and makes it do. Of course my aim was not to show that an image could be reduced to how discourse accounted for it. My starting point was rather that we can only show what an image is and what it does by highlighting the role of the medium of language, which we tend to consider as a transparent or neutral intermediary. In other words, to adopt Ponge's title *Le Parti pris des choses*, it is only possible to 'speak for' the image by 'taking proper account' of language, which as Peirce taught us is our major interpretative tool, as Benveniste showed us is the only medium capable of taking on board the other semiotic systems and as Goodman argued is endowed with a 'formative force'.

The second methodological principle to mention concerns intellectual wariness about the untested assumptions of common sense that underwrite many analogies between media and which become hardened into dogmatic views about history and aesthetics: for example, in debates surrounding *ekphrasis* and *Ut pictura poesis*, which you mention in your introduction, and literary impressionism, which I've already talked about in this interview. I'm perfectly willing to categorise this aspect of my work as 'metatheoretical'. I should emphasise that the aim is not to establish a super-theory but to reflect on theoretical objects in order to dismantle the presuppositions and to bring to light the weaknesses and to try to think more clearly. Just as my first principle didn't aim at a sort of 'pantextuality' and didn't rely on logocentric positions, my work on theories of the visual and textual doesn't adopt a 'meta' position that seeks to promote a theory of all theories. The 'meta' here doesn't imply an overview, but a lateral view, a step to the side, a degree of displacement; it comes from a general sense of disquiet that consists in questioning the limits of an officially recognised disciplinary field backed up by academic institutions, by linking research questions that do not usually come into contact.

My third methodological principle is the logical corollary of these first two. Whether I'm working on discursive formations or theoretical objects, and especially if they belong to different disciplinary traditions (literary studies, art history, aesthetics), it's a matter of expanding the corpus of works and of replacing them in a longer time frame. I'm not sure if this is really a methodological principle or rather an intellectual necessity that I felt early on in my career: the need, when I work on an author, to reconstitute the chains of reasoning, to draw out the internal coherence or the inner theory, even if the author is not especially theoretical; the need to work on heterogeneous historical corpora – in my case, mainly from the second half of the seventeenth century through to the contemporary period; the need to refer to other periods and topics, for example the rhetorical treatises of antiquity or the notion of manner in fifteenth- to eighteenth-century Italian literature devoted to the arts. In short, the need to try to grasp everything involved in, and all the consequences of, particular historical sequences or theoretical problems, but not to master them. Such a programme can of course only be carried out by one individual with the tools at his or her disposal, adopting Lévi-Strauss's 'bricolage' technique or Michel de Certeau's 'poaching' method. If I had to use one word to sum myself up, I wouldn't say a ferryman (*passeur*), since that evokes a founding figure who transmits knowledge and therefore sounds pretentious, but instead I'd compare myself to a transporter bridge (*pont transbordeur*)![1]

Note

1 A *pont transbordeur* features at the beginning of Jacques Demy's film *Les Demoiselles de Rochefort* (1967).

Index

Note: numbers in **bold** refer to images on that page.